OBSTETRIC INTENSIVE CARE MANUAL

Notice

OBSTETRIC INTENSIVE CARE MANUAL

Second Edition

Editor
Michael R. Foley, MD
Medical Director, Phoenix Perinatal Associates
an affiliate of Obstetrix Medical Group of Phoenix, PC
Phoenix, Arizona
Director, Obstetric Intensive Care Unit
Banner Good Samaritan Regional Medical Center
Phoenix, Arizona
Clinical Professor of Obstetrics and Gynecology
Department of Obstetrics and Gynecology
University of Arizona School of Medicine
at the Arizona Health Sciences Center, Tucson, Arizona

Assistant Editors
Thomas H. Strong, Jr., MD
Associate Director, Maternal Fetal Medicine
Phoenix Perinatal Associates
an affiliate of Obstetrix Medical Group of Phoenix, PC
Phoenix, Arizona
Associate Clinical Professor of Obstetrics and Gynecology
Department of Obstetrics and Gynecology
University of Arizona School of Medicine
at the Arizona Health Sciences Center, Tucson, Arizona
Assistant Clinical Professor of Obstetrics and Gynecology
Department of Obstetrics and Gynecology
University of California, San Francisco, Fresno, California

Thomas J. Garite, MD
Professor and Chairman
Obstetrics and Gynecology
University of California, Irvine
Irvine, California

McGRAW-HILL
Medical Publishing Division

New York Chicago San Francisco Lisbon London Madrid Mexico City
Milan New Delhi San Juan Seoul Singapore Sydney Toronto

The McGraw-Hill Companies

Obstetric Intensive Care Manual, Second Edition

1 2 3 4 5 6 7 8 9 0 DOC/DOC 0 9 8 7 6 5 4

ISBN 0-07-144483-1

This book was set in Times Roman by International Typesetting and Composition.
The editors were Andrea Seils and Michelle Watt.
The production supervisor was Phil Galea.
Project management was provided by International Typesetting and Composition.
RR Donnelley was printer and binder.

This book was printed on acid-free paper.

Library of Congress Cataloging-in-Publication Data

Obstetric intensive care manual / edited by Michael R. Foley,
Thomas H. Strong Jr., Thomas J. Garite.—2nd ed.
p. ; cm.
Includes bibliographical references and index.
ISBN 0-07-141055-4
1. Obstetrical emergencies—Handbooks, manuals, etc. 2. Obstetrics—Handbooks, manuals, etc. I. Foley, Michael R. II. Strong, Thomas H. III. Garite, Thomas J.
[DNLM: 1. Intensive Care—Pregnancy. 2. Pregnancy Complications. 3. Emergencies—Pregnancy. WQ 240 O134 2004]
RG571.O266 2004
618.2′025—dc22 2003061415

To Lisa, Bonnie, Molly, and Michael for their unending loving support.
To Bette and Ray for giving me this opportunity.

Michael R. Foley

To Cstephani, Rebekah and my parents for the patience and gentle lessons that sustain me every day.

Thomas H. Strong, Jr.

To Cathy, thank you for your never ending support.

Thomas J. Garite

Contents

Contributors

Tamerou Asrat, MD
Clinical Associate Professor in Obstetrics and Gynecology
Department of Obstetrics and Gynecology
University of California
Irvine, California

Robert D. Auerbach, MD
Associate Clinical Professor of Obstetrics and Gynecology
Yale University School of Medicine
Yale-New Haven Hospital
New Haven, Connecticut

Thomas M. Bajo, MD
Associate Professor of Critical Care
Good Samaritan Regional Medical Center
Phoenix, Arizona

Michael A. Belfort, MD, PhD
Director
Maternal-Fetal Medicine
Utah Valley Regional Medical Center
Provo, Utah

Linda R. Chambliss, MD
Associate Director
Maternal-Fetal Medicine
Maricopa Integrated Health Systems
Phoenix, Arizona
Clinical Professor of Obstetrics and Gynecology and Family and Community Medicine
University of Arizona Health Sciences Center

Steven L. Clark, MD
Professor of Obstetrics and Gynecology
University of Utah School of Medicine
Salt Lake City, Utah

William H. Clewell, MD
Director, Fetal Medicine and Surgery
Phoenix Perinatal Associates
an affiliate of Obstetrix Medical Group of Phoenix, PC
Phoenix, Arizona
Clinical Professor of Obstetrics and Gynecology
University of Arizona College of Medicine
Tucson, Arizona

Kristin H. Coppage, MD
Maternal-Fetal Medicine Fellow
Department of Obstetrics and Gynecology
University of Cincinnati
Cincinnati, Ohio

Steven C. Curry, MD
Department of Medical Toxicology
Banner Good Samaritan Medical Center
Associate Professor of Clinical Medicine
University of Arizona College of Medicine
Phoenix, Arizona

Lisa A. Dado, MD
Valley Anesthesiology Consultant
Phoenix Children's Hospital
Phoenix, Arizona

Gary A. Dildy III, MD
Professor
Section of Maternal-Fetal Medicine
Department of Obstetrics and Gynecology
Loaisiana State University Health Science Center
School of Medicine in New Orleans
New Orleans, Louisiana

John P. Elliott, MD
Director, Division of Maternal Fetal Medicine
Banner Good Samaritan Medical Center
Associate Director, Maternal Fetal Medicine
Phoenix Perinatal Associates
an affiliate of Obstetrix Medical Group of Phoenix, PC
Phoenix, Arizona

Michael R. Foley, MD
Medical Director, Phoenix Perinatal Associates
an affiliate of Obstetrix Medical Group of Phoenix, PC
Phoenix, Arizona
Director, Obstetric Intensive Care Unit
Banner Good Samaritan Regional Medical Center
Phoenix, Arizona
Clinical Professor of Obstetrics and Gynecology
Department of Obstetrics and Gynecology
University of Arizona School of Medicine
at the Arizona Health Sciences Center,
Tucson, Arizona

Karrie E. Francois, MD
Associate Director, Maternal Fetal Medicine
Phoenix Perinatal Associates
an affiliate of Obstetrix Medical Group of Phoenix, PC
Phoenix, Arizona

Thomas J. Garite, MD
Professor and Chairman
Obstetrics and Gynecology
University of California
Irvine, California

Alfredo F. Gei, MD
Assistant Professor
University of Texas Medical Branch
Galveston, Texas

Cornelia R. Graves, MD
Director, Obstetrical Critical Care
Associate Professor of Obstetrics and Gynecology and Medical Administration
Vanderbilt University
Nashville, Tennessee

Afshan B. Hameed, MD
Clinical Instructor, Department of Obstetrics and Gynecology
Division of Maternal Fetal Medicine, UCI
Clinical Assistant Professor
Department of Medicine
Keck School of Medicine
University of Southern California
Los Angles, California

Cathleen M. Harris, MD, MPH
Associate Director, Maternal Fetal Medicine
Phoenix Perinatal Associates
an affiliate of Obstetrix Medical Group of Phoenix, PC
Phoenix, Arizona

Charles J. Lockwood, MD
Professor and Chairman
Department of Obstetrics and Gynecology
Yale University School of Medicine
New Haven, Connecticut

William C. Mabie, MD
Clinical Professor
Department of Obstetrics and Gynecology
University of South Carolina
Greenville, South Carolina

Stephanie R. Martin, DO
Associate Director, Maternal Fetal Medicine
Phoenix Perinatal Associates
an affiliate of Obstetrix Medical Group of Phoenix, PC
Phoenix, Arizona

Jennifer McNulty, MD
Staff Perinatologist
Women's Hospital
Long Beach Memorial Medical Center
Assistant Professor
Division of Maternal Fetal Medicine
Department of Obstetrics and Gynecology
University of California, Irvine
Irvine, California

Keith S. Meredith, MD
Medical Director, Phoenix Neonatal Operations
Phoenix Children's Hospital
Medical Director, Phoenix Perinatal Associates—Neonatal Division
an affiliate of Pediatrix Medical Group
Phoenix, Arizona

Robert A. Myers, MD
Director, HIV In-Patient Service
Maricopa Medical Center
Phoenix, Arizona
Instructor Mayo Medical School
Rochester, Minnesota

Michael P. Nageotte, MD
Executive Careline Director
Long Beach Memorial Hospital
Professor, Department Obstetrics and Gynecology
University of California, Irvine
Irvine, California

Jordan H. Perlow, MD
Associate Director, Maternal Fetal Medicine
Banner Good Samaritan Regional Medical Center
Associate Director, Maternal Fetal Medicine
Phoenix Perinatal Associates
an affiliate of Obstetrix Medical Group of Phoenix, PC
Phoenix, Arizona

Robert Raschke, MD
Assistant Professor of Clinical Medicine
Good Samaritan Regional Medicine Center
Phoenix, Arizona

George R. Saade, MD
Professor
Department of Obstetrics and Gynecology
Divisions of Maternal-Fetal Medicine and Reproductive Sciences
The University of Texas Medical Branch
Galveston, Texas

Philip Samuels, MD
Associate Professor of Obstetrics and Gynecology
The Ohio State University College of Medicine and Public Health
Residency Program Director
The Ohio State University/Mt. Carmel Health Program in Obstetrics and Gynecology
Columbus, Ohio

Baha M. Sibai, MD
Professor and Chair
Department of Obstetrics and Gynecology
University of Cincinnati College of Medicine
Cincinnati, Ohio

Bob Silver, MD
Associate Professor, Chief
Maternal-Fetal Medicine
University of Utah Health Sciences Center
Salt Lake City, Utah

Thomas H. Strong, Jr., MD
Associate Director, Maternal Fetal Medicine
Phoenix Perinatal Associates
an affiliate of Obstetrix Medical Group of Phoenix, PC
Phoenix, Arizona
Associate Clinical Professor of Obstetrics and Gynecology
Department of Obstetrics and Gynecology
University of Arizona School of Medicine
at the Arizona Health Sciences Center
Tucson, Arizona
Assistant Clinical Professor of Obstetrics and Gynecology
Department of Obstetrics and Gynecology
University of California, San Francisco
Fresno, California

Victor R. Suarez, MD
Fellow, Maternal Fetal Medicine
Department of Obstetrics and Gynecology
University of Texas Medical Branch
Galveston, Texas

David J. Watts, MD
Department of Medical Toxicology
Good Samaritan Regional Medical Center
Phoenix, Arizona

Foreword

The *Obstetric Intensive Care Manual*, developed by Drs. Michael Foley and Thomas Strong, Jr. six years ago, was a best seller. McGraw-Hill is now publishing this new edition.

The second edition has many new features and enlists an additional Senior Editor, Dr. Thomas Garite, a recognized expert in maternal-fetal medicine and the Editor-in-Chief of the *American Journal of Obstetrics and Gynecology*. A number of distinguished clinicians and academicians also have been asked to contribute chapters in their specific areas of expertise, bringing an expanded knowledge base to this second edition: George Saade (Galveston, Texas), Michael Belfort (Provo, Utah), Karrie Francois (Phoenix, Arizona), Stephanie Martin (Phoenix, Arizona), Charles Lockwood (New Haven, Connecticut), Baha Sibai (Cincinnati, Ohio), Alfredo Gei (Galveston, Texas), Mike Nageotte (Long Beach, California), Jennifer McNulty (Long Beach, California), Cathleen Harris (Phoenix, Arizona), Keith Meredith (Phoenix, Arizona), Connie Graves (Nashville, Tennessee), and Bob Silver (Salt Lake City, Utah).

Before these new authors came on board, the first manual was thoroughly evaluated by being "field tested" by fellows, residents, and practicing physicians. This field-testing led to additional topics and revisions for this new edition. The principle questions for such a revision are: What is needed in a manual that can be stuck in a pocket and is most useful in deciding on the care of the critically ill patient? Will you take care of the patient or refer the patient to another care center?

The anxiety of caring for the critically ill patient is tremendous. Some of this is predicated on escalating malpractice costs. No matter what you do for these patients the end results may leave something to be desired. Sometimes there is no place to send critically ill patients and the burden of responsibility is on your shoulders, and this manual will not only provide you with scholarly information but will help you be a "hands on" physician. You can begin working with the patient now and make a referral or get further help later.

It is hoped that this handbook will be in the hands of all obstetric caregivers. If you care for obstetric patients, you cannot predict emergencies, but this manual will better prepare you for the emergencies and the complexities that arise in obstetric intensive care.

This new manual contains 27 different chapters about the pregnant patient who encounters an emergency or an urgent problem with her pregnancy. This book will help the practitioner make proper choices for care of the patient. "Hands on" is the basis of medicine and where it all starts; you can go from there with your mental algorithm on what to do. This manual will assist you in your thinking.

Good luck on your learning on this complicated topic of intensive care and enjoy your education.

Frederick P. Zuspan, MD
Professor and Chairman Emeritus
Department of Obstetrics and Gynecology
The Ohio State University College of Medicine
Columbus, Ohio
Editor-In-Chief Emeritus
American Journal of Obstetrics and Gynecology

Preface

Most, if not all, practitioners in the field of obstetrics will undoubtedly, at some point in their career, willingly or otherwise, find themselves caring for a critically ill parturient. Unfortunately, but quite predictably due to the nature of our business, we are often unprepared to deal with these rare, emergent complexities at a moment's notice. We are not afforded the luxury of having the time to page through a comprehensive textbook in order to review the problem at hand. What is needed, when we find ourselves "up to our eyebrows in alligators," is a handy, brief, pragmatic source that provides a short review of pathophysiology and diagnostic methods while placing a primary focus on "what to do and how often" type management.

The second edition of *Obstetric Intensive Care Manual* has evolved from "in the trenches" type testing. What worked well was expanded, what was missing was added, and what did not work well was remodeled. I am extremely indebted to Drs. Strong and Garite for their fabulous editorial assistance during the preparation of this second edition. As always, I am grateful to my mentors Dr. Frederick P. Zuspan and Dr. Steven G. Gabbe, and my colleagues at Phoenix Perinatal Associates–Obstetrix Medical Group of Phoenix for their guidance and friendship over the years in preparation for "real life" practical obstetric care delivery. Thank you to all the outstanding contributing authors, past and present, for making this book a valuable asset to obstetric care providers worldwide.

> "To know what you do not know is the best.
> To pretend to know when you do not know is disease."
> *Lao Tzu*

As educators and caregivers, we should strive to capably manage and understand the true essence of "disease."

Michael R. Foley, MD
Phoenix, Arizona
March 2004

Acknowledgment

Drs. Foley, Strong, and Garite are extremely indebted to Susan Weisman for her outstanding editorial assistance during the preparation of this book. We all appreciate her good humor, wit, and graciousness.

OBSTETRIC INTENSIVE CARE MANUAL

1 Basic Hemodynamic Monitoring for the Obstetric Care Provider

William C. Mabie

INTRODUCTION

The cardiovascular system can be monitored in a variety of ways as shown in Table 1-1. Transthoracic or transesophageal echocardiography has advantages. It can be used to assess ventricular dimensions, mass, and function, as well as valvular morphology and function. Echocardiography aids in the differential diagnosis of shock due to hypovolemic shock (poorly filled hyperdynamic left ventricle), cardiogenic shock (focal wall motion abnormality), septic shock (global decrease in contractility), and pulmonary embolism (right ventricular dilatation). Echocardiography has its disadvantages: (1) it is operator dependent with a long learning curve; (2) it gives only a single snapshot in time; and (3) it is expensive compared to other modalities. Thoracic electrical bioimpedance is inaccurate. Transesophageal Doppler and pulse contour analysis are emerging technologies that require more studies to document accuracy. This chapter will concentrate on Swan-Ganz pulmonary artery catheter (PAC) monitoring.

Clinicians are painfully aware of how difficult it is to accurately assess perfusion status in critically ill patients. Pioneering studies of critical illness were primarily descriptive—a series of bedside observations of vital signs, urine output, and orthostatic change in blood pressure. Researchers had little in the way of invasive monitoring and developed their insights based primarily on physical examination. The PAC had been used in the cardiac catheterization lab since the 1940s. In 1970, a flow-directed, balloon-tipped pulmonary artery catheter was introduced by Dr. H.J.C. Swan and Dr. William Ganz. Over the past 30 years, many of our clinical concepts of the pathophysiology of myocardial infarction, cardiogenic shock, septic shock, acute respiratory distress syndrome, cardiovascular surgery, and trauma resuscitation and surgery have developed through use of the Swan-Ganz catheter. In pregnancy, the hemodynamics of normal pregnancy and the effects of anesthesia were studied, as well as the hemodynamics of severe preeclampsia, eclampsia, pulmonary edema, refractory hypertension, mitral stenosis, and peripartum cardiomyopathy. The hypothesized benefit of PAC monitoring was that, by understanding the disease process, one could tailor therapy to the individual patient. In addition, one could transfer the knowledge gained to other patients and manage them without necessarily using a Swan-Ganz catheter.

Currently about 1.5 million Swan-Ganz catheters are used in North America annually. Thirty percent are used in cardiac surgery, 30 percent in cardiac catheterization laboratories and coronary care units, 25 percent in high-risk surgery and trauma, and 15 percent in medical intensive care units. About one-third of sick patients in medical and surgical ICUs undergo PAC monitoring. The PAC has been refined so that, in addition to pressures and intermittent cardiac output, one can obtain nearly continuous cardiac output, right

TABLE 1-1 Methods of Hemodynamic Monitoring

Noninvasive	Invasive
Auscultation	Arterial catheter
Vital signs	Arterial blood gases
Urine output	Central venous pressure catheter
Electrocardiogram	Swan-Ganz catheter
Pulse oximeter	Transesophageal echocardiography
Transthoracic echocardiogram	Transesophageal Doppler
Thoracic electrical bioimpedance	Pulse contour analysis

ventricular end diastolic volume index, and continuous mixed venous oxygen saturation.

But, like fetal heart rate monitoring, the Swan-Ganz catheter was introduced into practice without supportive clinical outcome data. Now there is great controversy about its use because of complications, cost, and lack of evidence of patient benefit. A discussion of three recent developments will summarize the current state of opinion on the Swan-Ganz catheter.

In 1996, Connors et al. published a large, prospective cohort study which showed increased mortality, length of stay, and cost with use of pulmonary artery catheters in a mixed medical and surgical population. Although they attempted to control for selection bias by using a *propensity score*, the lack of randomization raises the possibility of unknown sources of bias. In particular, the study did not account for the practice style of many intensivists which was to initiate empiric therapy and then utilize invasive monitoring in those patients who did not respond to treatment. Thus, use of the catheter may have been a marker for greater severity of illness. This study generated intense interest in the lay press and resulted in calls for a moratorium on its use.

In 1997, the National Institute of Health sponsored a consensus conference to scrutinize the efficacy and safety of the PAC. The participants noted several problems. Clinical trials were too few and were not randomized. The trials were not designed with enough equipoise for physicians to allow their patients to be randomized to management without a PAC. There was too much crossing over from standard care in the control group to use of the PAC. The catheter is only a monitoring device. The therapy chosen may be ineffective or harmful. There is little agreement on best treatment for the hemodynamic abnormalities. In future trials, treatment must be protocolized and factorialized. The major problem may be the user, not the device. A knowledge deficit disorder still persists. Several studies have shown that physicians and nurses make errors in obtaining and interpreting hemodynamic data. Since the conference, a randomized trial of 1000 patients with acute lung injury/ARDS has begun. Patients will be randomized to receive either a central venous catheter or a PAC. A second randomization will be performed in which the patient will receive a liberal or a conservative fluid management strategy. A treatment algorithm will manage vasopressor therapy and diuretic use. Finally, a broad-ranging, standardized educational program for physicians, nurses, and other health care professionals who use the PAC is being developed.

In 2003, Sandham et al. published a prospective trial of 1994 elderly, high-risk surgical patients randomized to goal-directed therapy guided by a PAC or to standard care without the use of a PAC. The primary outcome was in-hospital mortality. There was no benefit of therapy directed by PAC (mortality 7.7 vs. 7.8 percent), and there was a higher rate of pulmonary embolism in the catheter group (8 vs. 0).

INDICATIONS FOR INVASIVE HEMODYNAMIC MONITORING

With improved understanding of pathophysiology, the Swan-Ganz catheter is used less frequently now than in the 1980s and 90s. Nevertheless, indications for considering pulmonary artery catheterization in obstetric patients are listed below.

- Refractory or unexplained pulmonary edema
- Refractory or unexplained oliguria
- Massive hemorrhage
- Septic shock
- Acute respiratory distress syndrome
- New York Heart Association Class 3 and 4 cardiac disease
- Intraoperative or intrapartum cardiovascular decompensation
- Respiratory distress of unknown cause

The Swan-Ganz catheter is useful in differentiating cardiogenic from noncardiogenic forms of pulmonary edema. It may also be used to guide diuretic therapy and manipulations of cardiac output such as preload and afterload reduction or inotropic therapy.

Definitons of hemodynamic terms are given below.

Wedge Pressure Also known as the pulmonary artery occlusion pressure (PAOP), wedge pressure is a measure of left ventricular preload. The pulmonary artery wedge pressure is obtained with a balloon-tipped catheter advanced into a branch of the pulmonary artery until the vessel is occluded, forming a free communication through the pulmonary capillaries and veins to the left atrium. A true wedge position is in a lung zone where both pulmonary artery and pulmonary venous pressures exceed alveolar pressure (West Zone 3).

Preload Initial stretch of the myocardial fiber at end diastole. Clinically, the preload to the right and left ventricles (end-diastolic pressures) is assessed by the central venous pressure and wedge pressure, respectively.

Afterload Reflected by both the wall tension of the ventricle during ejection and the resistance to forward flow in the form of vascular resistance (vasoconstriction). The pulmonary vascular resistance (PVR) and the systemic vascular resistance (SVR) are the primary afterloads for the right and left ventricles, respectively, in a normal heart.

Contractility The inherent force and velocity of myocardial contraction when preload and afterload are held constant.

In patients with oliguria, the catheter may be used to assess volume status. In preeclampsia it has been shown that central venous pressure is not adequate for assessing volume status. The change in wedge pressure and cardiac output in response to a fluid challenge is the most important guide to intravascular volume. While invasive hemodynamic monitoring is not necessary for acute resuscitation from hemorrhagic shock, it is useful in the subsequent 24 to 72 hours to guide fluid therapy in complex cases in which it is not clear if internal bleeding is continuing or if oliguria, pulmonary edema, liver dysfunction, or severe coagulopathy are present. In septic shock, invasive monitoring allows manipulation of cardiovascular parameters with fluid and inotropic therapy as well as assessment of response to therapy through such parameters as oxygen delivery and consumption. In the acute respiratory distress syndrome, the catheter is used to exclude cardiogenic pulmonary edema and to guide supportive therapy with mechanical ventilation, positive end-expiratory pressure, intravenous fluids, diuretics, and inotropic agents. New York Heart Association Class 3 and 4 cardiac patients may require invasive monitoring to guide fluid and drug therapy, as well as for anesthesia management during labor and delivery. The cause of sudden intraoperative or intrapartum cardiovascular decompensation may be clarified by obtaining wedge pressure and cardiac output. The final indication includes patients in whom the contribution of cardiac or pulmonary disease to respiratory distress is unclear by clinical examination. The pulmonary artery catheter can help differentiate heart failure from pneumonia, pulmonary thromboembolism, amniotic fluid embolism, acute respiratory distress syndrome, or chronic pulmonary disorders.

INSERTING THE SWAN-GANZ CATHETER

The Swan-Ganz catheter is most commonly inserted through the internal jugular vein or the subclavian vein. It may also be inserted through the basilic vein in the arm or the femoral vein. Several commercial trays containing the necessary equipment are available for central venous cannulation using the Seldinger technique (i.e., over a guidewire). The procedure is performed under continuous electrocardiographic monitoring. The equipment needed for inserting the Swan-Ganz catheter is shown in Fig. 1-1. The technique for venous cannulation and passing the catheter through the heart will not be described here. Unless the obstetrician is performing at least 12 of these

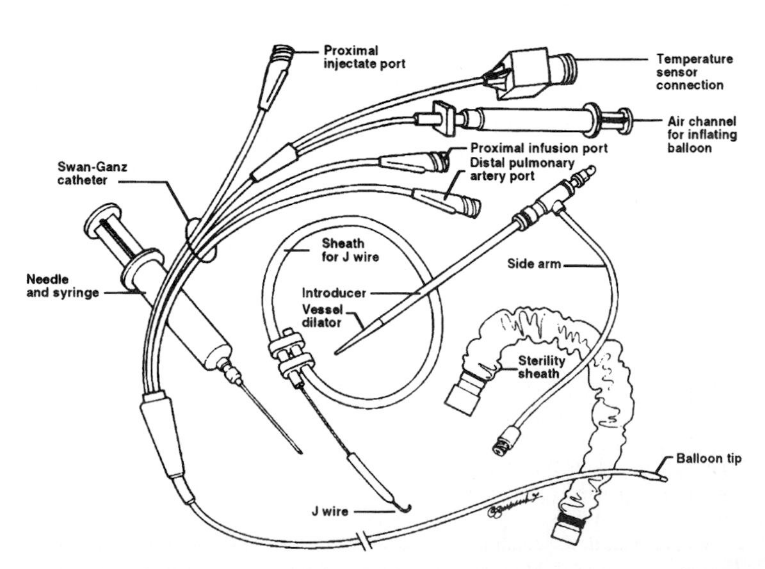

FIG. 1-1 Equipment needed for inserting the Swan-Ganz catheter. (*Source: From Mabie WC: Critical care obstetrics. In: Gabbe SG, Niebyl JR, Simpson JL (eds), Obstetrics: Normal and Problem Pregnancies, 3rd edn., New York: Churchill Livingston, 1996; Chapter 18, pp. 533–559.*)

procedures per year, it may be safer for the patient to have this done by an anesthesiologist, internist, or cardiologist, who has more experience. Even though someone else inserts the catheter, the obstetrician is frequently called upon to troubleshoot or to manipulate the catheter if it is not wedging, the waveform is damped, or the nurses do not trust the numbers. I will therefore discuss the waveforms seen as the catheter passes through the heart.

HEMODYNAMIC WAVEFORMS

The right atrial pressure tracing (Fig. 1-2A) consists of three distinct waves *a*, *c*, and *v*. The *a* wave is a small wave due to atrial systole. The declining pressure that immediately follows the *a* wave is called the *X* descent. The *c* wave may or may not appear as a distinct wave. It reflects the increase in right atrial pressure produced by closure of the tricuspid valve. The negative wave following the *c* wave is called the *X′* descent. The *v* wave is caused by right atrial filling and concomitant right ventricular systole, which causes the leaflets of the closed tricuspid valve to bulge back into the right atrium. The *Y* descent immediately follows the *v* wave. The pressure changes produced by the *a*, *c*, and *v* waves are usually within 3 to 4 mmHg of each other so that the mean pressure is taken. The normal resting mean right atrial pressure is 1 to 7 mmHg. Elevated right atrial pressures may occur in the following conditions: right ventricular failure, tricuspid stenosis and regurgitation, cardiac tamponade, constrictive pericarditis, pulmonary hypertension, chronic left ventricular failure, and volume overload.

The phases of systole and diastole in the right ventricular pressure tracing can be divided into seven events (Fig. 1-2B). Systolic events include (1) isovolumetric contraction, (2) rapid ejection, and (3) reduced ejection. Diastolic events

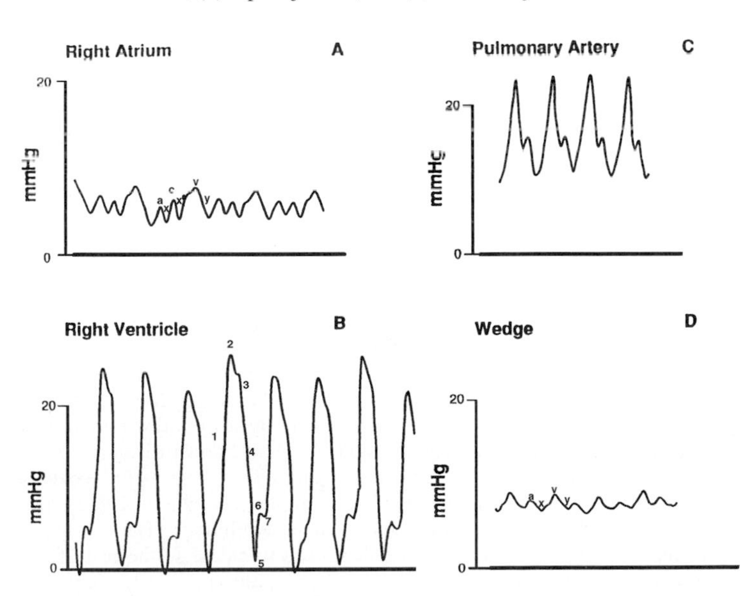

FIG. 1-2 (A-D) Pulmonary artery catheter placement. Waveforms and normal pressures. (*Source: Daily EK, Schroeder JP: Hemodynamic Waveforms: Exercises in Identification and Analysis. St. Louis: CV Mosby, 1983.*)

include (4) isovolumetric relaxation, (5) early diastole, (6) atrial systole, and (7) end diastole.

The pulmonary artery pressure tracing is seen in Fig. 1-2C. There is a sharp rise in pressure followed by a decline in pressure as the volume decreases. When the right ventricular pressure falls below the level of the pulmonary artery pressure, the pulmonary valve snaps shut. This sudden closure of the valve leaflets causes the dicrotic notch in the pulmonary artery pressure tracing. Normal pulmonary artery systolic pressure is 20 to 30 mmHg. Normal end-diastolic pressure is 8 to 12 mmHg. Elevated pulmonary artery pressures are seen in pulmonary disease, primary pulmonary hypertension, mitral stenosis or regurgitation, left ventricular failure, and intracardiac left-to-right shunts. Hypoxia increases pulmonary vascular resistance and pulmonary artery pressure.

When a small branch of the pulmonary artery is occluded by inflation of the balloon on the Swan-Ganz catheter, the pressure tracing reflects left atrial pressure. The waveform looks similar to the right atrial pressure tracing described above (Fig. 1-2A). The *a* wave of the wedge pressure is produced by left atrial contraction followed by the *X* descent (Fig. 1-2D). The *c* wave is produced by closure of the mitral valve, but is usually not seen. The *v* wave is produced by filling of the left atrium and bulging back of the mitral valve during ventricular systole. The decline following the *v* wave is called the *Y* descent. The normal resting mean wedge pressure is 6 to 12 mmHg. Elevated wedge pressure is seen in left ventricular failure, mitral stenosis or regurgitation, cardiac tamponade, constrictive pericarditis, and volume overload.

DETERMINING THE HEMODYNAMIC PROFILE

Thermodilution cardiac output is determined using the Fick principle in which a known quantity and concentration of a detectable marker travels a known distance, to a point where its concentration is measured. From this information the quantity of blood passing the reference point can be calculated. With thermodilution cardiac output, temperature is the marker; and it is given as a bolus of saline through the proximal central venous port of the Swan-Ganz catheter. The change in temperature is measured approximately 30 cm downstream at a thermistor near the tip. Cardiac output is measured using five (10 cc) injections of iced or room temperature saline. Highest and lowest values are discarded with the mean of the three remaining values recorded. The value for the first injection is usually high because of heat gained by the injectate in cooling the catheter. In general, the greater the difference in temperature between the saline bolus and the blood, the more accurate the cardiac output determination. Instead of requiring a bolus of saline, the continuous cardiac output Swan-Ganz catheter has a copper coil proximal to the thermistor which heats the blood passing by it by a few hundredths of a degree centigrade. The heated blood travels a known distance to the thermistor where the change in temperature is measured. This technique does not result in a continuous cardiac output measurement, but it is repeated every 10 seconds so that for practical purposes it is continuous. The following measured hemodynamic variables are then used to calculate the rest of the hemodynamic profile: heart rate, blood pressure, pulmonary artery pressure, pulmonary artery wedge pressure, central venous pressure, cardiac output, and patient's height and weight. The derived variables include cardiac index, stroke volume and index, systemic vascular resistance and index, pulmonary

TABLE 1-2 Derived Hemodynamic Parameters

Parameter	Abbreviation	Formula	Units
Pulse pressure	PP	BP syst – BP diast	mmHg
Mean arterial pressure	MAP	BP diast + 1/3PP	mmHg
Cardiac index	CI	$\frac{CO}{BSA}$	L/min/m^2
Stroke volume	SV	$\frac{CO \times 1000}{HR}$	mL
Stroke index	SI	$\frac{SV}{BSA}$	mL/beat/m^2
Systemic vascular resistance	SVR	$\frac{MAP - CVP}{CO} \times 80$	dyn/s/cm^{-5}
Systemic vascular resistance index	SVRI	SVR × BSA	dyn/s/cm^{-5}/m^2
Pulmonary vascular resistance	PVR	$\frac{\overline{PAP} - PCWP}{CO} \times 80$	dyn/s/cm^{-5}
Pulmonary vascular resistance index	PVRI	PVR × BSA	dyn/s/cm^{-5}/m^2
Left ventricular stroke work	LVSW	SV × MAP × 0.136	g/m
Left ventricular stroke work index	LVSWI	$\frac{LVSW}{BSA}$	g/m/m^2
Right ventricular stroke work	RVSW	SV × $\overline{PAP}$ × 0.136	g/m
Right ventricular stroke work index	RVSWI	$\frac{RVSW}{BSA}$	g/m/m^2

Key: BP syst, systolic blood pressure, BP dias, diastolic blood pressure; CO, cardiac output, HR, heart rate, BSA, body surface area; $\overline{PAP}$, mean pulmonary artery pressure; PCWP, pulmonary capillary wedge pressure.

vascular resistance and index, and left and right ventricular stroke work and indices (Table 1-2 provides formulas).

OXYGEN TRANSPORT

Arterial oxygen content (CaO_2) is the sum of the oxygen bound to hemoglobin and that dissolved in plasma as described by the equation:

$$CaO_2 = (Hgb \times 1.36 \times SaO_2) + (PaO_2 \times 0.003)$$

where 1.36 is the amount (in milliliters) of oxygen bound to 1 g of hemoglobin (Hgb); SaO_2 is the arterial oxygen saturation; and 0.003 is the solubility coefficient of oxygen in human plasma. If SaO_2 is 1.0 or 100 percent saturated, Hgb is 15 g/dL, and PaO_2 is 100 mmHg, then

$$\begin{aligned} CaO_2 &= (15 \times 1.36 \times 1.0) + (100 \times 0.003) \\ &= 20 + 0.3 \\ &= 20 \text{ mL/dL} \end{aligned}$$

The amount of oxygen dissolved in the plasma usually does not make a significant contribution to CaO_2.

Mixed venous blood gives an estimate of the balance between oxygen supply and demand. For example, in low cardiac output states with a high rate of peripheral oxygen extraction, mixed venous oxygen tension (PvO_2) is low. Normal PvO_2 ranges from 35 to 45 mmHg and mixed venous oxygen saturation (SvO_2) ranges from 0.68 to 0.76. Clinical concern for tissue hypoxia arises when the PvO_2 falls below 30 mmHg and/or the SvO_2 falls by 5 to 10 percent over 3 to 5 minutes or to a value below 0.60. Mixed venous oxygen content is measured on blood drawn from the pulmonary artery rather than from the superior vena cava, inferior vena cava, or the right atrium. This is necessary because oxygen saturation in the inferior vena cava is higher than in the superior vena cava. Drainage of coronary sinus blood into the right atrium contaminates that chamber with markedly desaturated blood, owing to the high myocardial oxygen extraction rate. After blood from the three sources passes through the right ventricle into the pulmonary artery it is thoroughly mixed resulting in a true "mixed venous" sample.

Mixed venous oxygen content is calculated as follows:

$$CvO_2 = (Hgb \times 1.36 \times SvO_2) + (PvO_2 \times 0.003)$$

If Hgb = 15 g, $SvO_2 = 0.75$, and $PvO_2 = 40$ mmHg, then

$$\begin{aligned} CvO_2 &= (15 \times 1.36 \times 0.75) + (40 \times 0.003) \\ &= 15 + 0.12 \\ &= 15 \text{ mL/dL} \end{aligned}$$

The arterial-venous oxygen content difference is described by the equation:

$$A\text{-}VO_2 = CaO_2 - CvO_2$$

Substituting the above calculations,

$$A\text{-}VO_2 = 20 - 15 = 5 \text{ mL } O_2/\text{dL}$$

The normal range of the arterial-venous oxygen content difference is 3.5 to 5.0 mL/dL. Oxygen delivery (DO_2) is the product of arterial oxygen content (CaO_2) and cardiac output (CO) as expressed by the equation

$$DO_2 = CO \times CaO_2 \times 10$$

If cardiac output equals 5 L/min, then

$$DO_2 = 5 \times 20 \times 10 = 1000 \text{ mL/min}$$

Oxygen delivery is normally about 1000 mL/min. Oxygen consumption is the amount of oxygen that diffuses into the tissues and is expressed by the equation:

$$\begin{aligned} VO_2 &= CO \times (CaO_2 - CvO_2) \times 10 \\ &= 5 \times 5 \times 10 = 250 \text{ mL/min} \end{aligned}$$

Oxygen consumption is normally about 250 mL/min.

Oxygen delivery and consumption can also be indexed to body surface area. Normal values for the oxygen delivery index are 400 to 550 mL/min/m^2 and for the oxygen consumption index are 110 to 150 mL/min/m^2.

Low SvO_2 and PvO_2 may indicate the presence of shock; however, in two settings these parameters may be artificially elevated. Patients with cirrhosis have arteriovenous shunting throughout the body, so that the oxygen carried in the blood is unavailable for metabolism in the tissues at the capillary level. In the case of septic shock, there may be arteriovenous shunting as in cirrhosis or there may be a metabolic defect such that the oxygen and substrate are there, but the cells do not pick it up.

A second concern pertaining to studies of the relationship between oxygen delivery and consumption relates to the concept of mathematical coupling. The same variables are used in calculating both oxygen delivery and consumption causing movement in the same direction. This concern has been substantiated by studies using different techniques for measuring oxygen delivery and consumption.

Shoemaker et al. popularized the concept of supranormal oxygen delivery in resuscitation from shock using aggressive volume expansion with crystalloid, colloid, and blood and inotropic support with dobutamine. The therapeutic goals were a cardiac index above 4.5 L/min/m^2, oxygen delivery index above 600 mL/min/m^2, and oxygen consumption index above 170 mL/min/m^2. Other studies have shown that it is difficult to achieve such physiologic goals, and that such therapy is associated with no benefit or with increased morbidity and mortality. Although Shoemaker et al. were treating high-risk general surgical patients and many of the negative studies treated a more heterogeneous population, the inconsistent results indicate that there is a little role for maximizing oxygen delivery.

OXYHEMOGLOBIN DISSOCIATION CURVE

Some familiarity with the oxyhemoglobin dissociation curve is necessary to understand oxygen transport and the influence of shifts in the curve. Acidosis, increased red cell 2,3-diphosphoglycerate (DPG), and fever shift the curve to the right, thus reducing the hemoglobin affinity for oxygen and increasing oxygen unloading in the tissues. Alkalosis, reduced red cell 2,3-DPG, and hypothermia cause the curve to shift to the left with the opposite effects on tissue oxygenation. As seen in Fig. 1-3, hemoglobin is 50 percent saturated (P_{50}) at a PaO_2 of 27 mmHg. A PaO_2 of 60 mmHg correlates with an oxygen saturation of about 90 percent. Therefore, little is gained in oxygen saturation by increasing PaO_2 much higher than 60 mmHg. On the other hand, below PaO_2 of 60 mmHg, small changes in PaO_2 result in large changes in oxygen saturation. A PaO_2 less than 20 mmHg is incompatible with life.

HEMODYNAMIC SUPPORT

Cardiac output is determined by four factors: preload, afterload, heart rate, and contractility. Hemodynamic therapy directed at each of these factors is summarized in Table 1-3. According to the Frank-Starling principle, the force of striated muscle contraction varies directly with the initial muscle length. The relationship between myocardial fiber length and fiber shortening can be graphically described by the curve in Fig. 1-4. Fiber length can best be equated with preload or filling volume of the ventricle. To allow clinical estimation of preload the pressure correlate of the filling volume is used, i.e., right or left ventricular end-diastolic pressure. Varying compliance will alter the pressure-volume relationship. For example, a poorly compliant left ventricle resulting from myocardial hypertrophy or ischemia requires higher intracavitary pressure to achieve a specific end-diastolic volume or fiber stretch.

Afterload is defined as the wall tension of the ventricle during ejection. This is best reflected by the systolic blood pressure. In the absence of aortic or pulmonary stenosis, vascular resistance in the appropriate bed—systemic

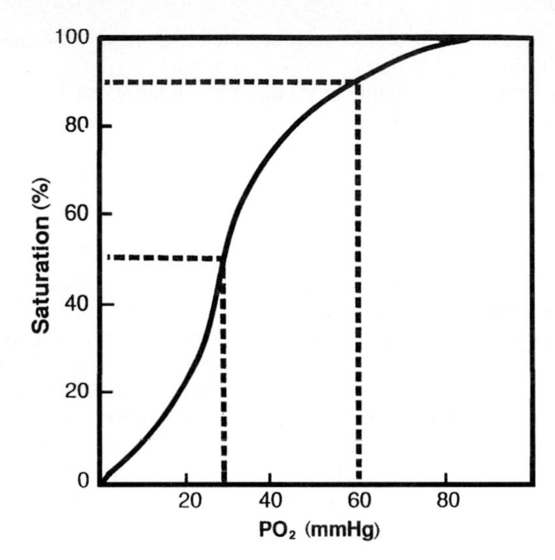

FIG. 1-3 The oxyhemoglobin dissociation curve of normal blood. Hemoglobin is 50 percent saturated at a PaO_2 of 27 mmHg. A PaO_2 of 60 mmHg correlates with an oxygen saturation of about 90 percent. (*Source: From Mabie WC: Critical care obstetrics. In: Gabbe SG, Niebyl JR, Simpson JL (eds), Obstetrics: Normal and Problem Pregnancies, 3rd edn., New York: Churchill Livingston, 1996; Chapter 18, pp. 533–559.*)

or pulmonary—will determine the afterload for that side of the heart. The effect of afterload on ventricular output is shown in Fig. 1-5.

Heart rate has a marked effect on cardiac output (i.e., cardiac output = heart rate × stroke volume). Increases in heart rate are accomplished at the expense of diastolic filling time, systolic emptying time being rate independent.

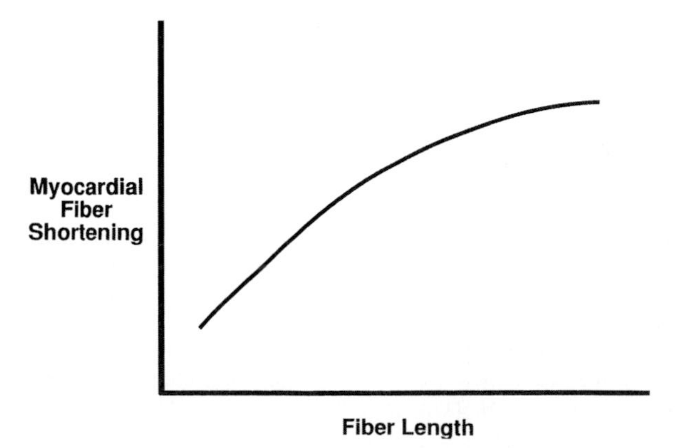

FIG. 1-4 Starling curve relating myocardial fiber length to fiber shortening. (*Source: Rosenthal MH: Intrapartum intensive care management of the cardiac patient. Clin Obstet Gynecol 1981;24:789–807.*)

TABLE 1-3 Hemodynamic Therapy

Decreased preload	Decreased afterload	Heart rate	Contractility	Increased preload	Increased afterload
Crystalloid	Volume	Usually not	Dopamine	Diuretics	Arterial dilators
Colloid	Vasopressors	treated unless	Dobutamine	Furosemide	Hydralazine
Blood	Phenylephrine	complete heart	Epinephrine	Ethacrynic acid	Nifedipine
	Inotropic vasopressors	block treated	Digoxin	Bumetanide	Nicardipine
	Norepinephrine	with pacemaker	Intraaortic	Venodilators	Mixed A-V dilator
	Epinephrine		balloon pump	Furosemide	Nitroprusside
	Vasopressin		Biventricular	Morphine	Venous dilator
			assist device	Nirtroglycerin	Nitroglycerin
					Alpha-beta blocker
					Labetalolol

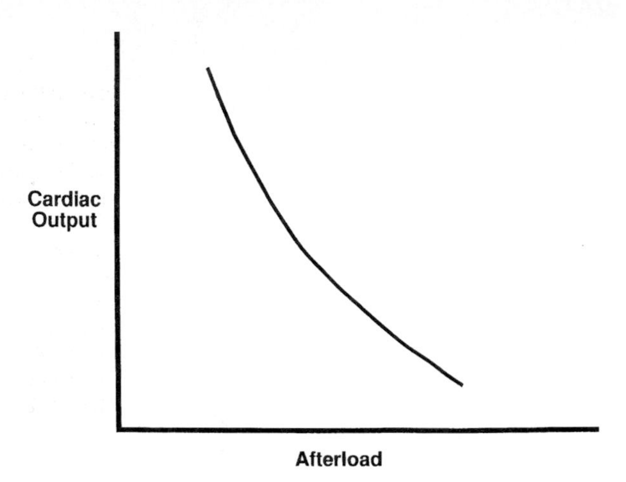

FIG. 1-5 Relationship of afterload to cardiac output at a constant preload. (*Source: Rosenthal MH: Intrapartum intensive care management of the cardiac patient. Clin Obstet Gynecol 1981;24:789–807.*)

Marked increases in heart rate may lead to circulatory depression when they cause myocardial ischemia or when reduced diastolic filling or loss of atrial "kick" prevent adequate ventricular preload. As a general rule, a heart rate that exceeds the difference of 220 and the patient's age in years reduces cardiac output and myocardial perfusion.

Contractility is defined as the force of ventricular contraction when preload and afterload are held constant. An increase in contractility is associated with an increase in stroke volume despite no change in preload. Factors that affect contractility include sympathetic impulses, catecholamines, acid-base and electrolyte disturbances, ischemia, loss of myocardium, hypoxia, and drugs or toxins. A third heart sound, distant heart sounds, and a narrow pulse pressure suggest impaired contractility. Radionuclide ventriculograms and two-dimensional (2D) echocardiography allow determination of ventricular size and contractile state. Effects of altered myocardial contractility on cardiac output at a given preload are shown in Fig. 1-6.

Figure 1-7 uses the Starling curves to summarize the effects of increases and decreases of preload, afterload, and contractility on ventricular function. The therapeutic rationale for supporting the cardiovascular system based on the Frank-Starling relationship is illustrated in Fig. 1-8.

The primary adjustment to improve low cardiac output is to optimize preload using volume administration. Because of the lack of correlation between measurements on the right and left sides of the heart in patients with significant cardiopulmonary disease, pulmonary capillary wedge pressure (PCWP) is monitored to optimize left ventricular preload and to avoid pulmonary edema. If blood pressure and cardiac output do not respond to fluids (e.g., PCWP of approximately 15 mmHg), then a positive inotropic agent may be needed to increase myocardial contractility. Dopamine is the drug of choice in most situations. It is utilized because its activity is modified at different doses. At 2 to 3 μg/kg/min, renal and splanchnic vasodilatation occur. Positive inotropy occurs up to 10 μg/kg/min. Vasoconstriction predominates over

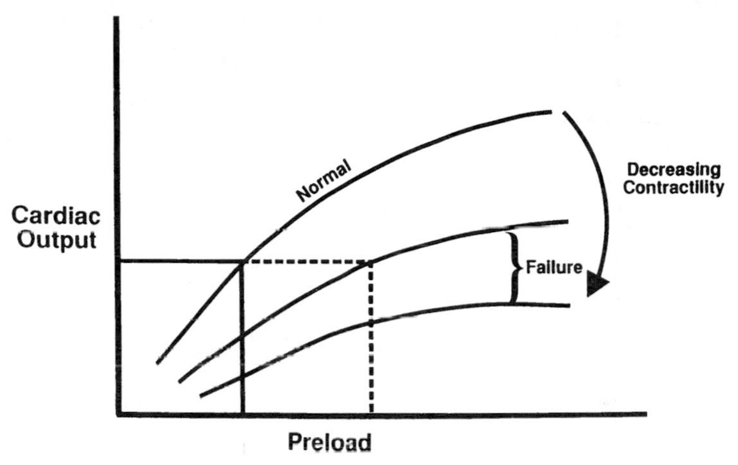

FIG. 1-6 Cardiac function curves demonstrating downward displacement secondary to decreased contractility and failure. Dotted line represents increased preload demands in failure. (*Source: Rosenthal MH: Intrapartum intensive care management of the cardiac patient. Clin Obstet Gynecol 1981;24:789–807.*)

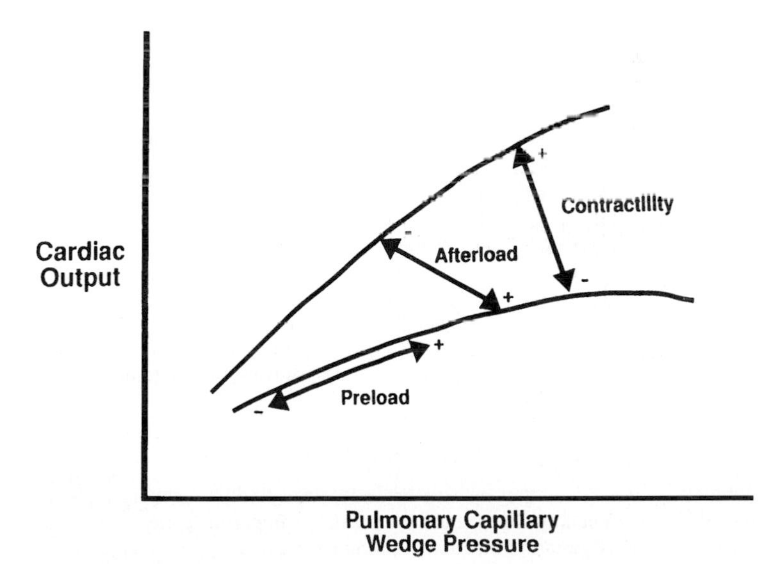

FIG. 1-7 Alteration in Starling curve of ventricular function caused by increases and decreases in preload, afterload, and contractility. (*Source: Rosenthal MH: Intrapartum intensive care management of the cardiac patient. Clin Obstet Gynecol 1981;24:789–807.*)

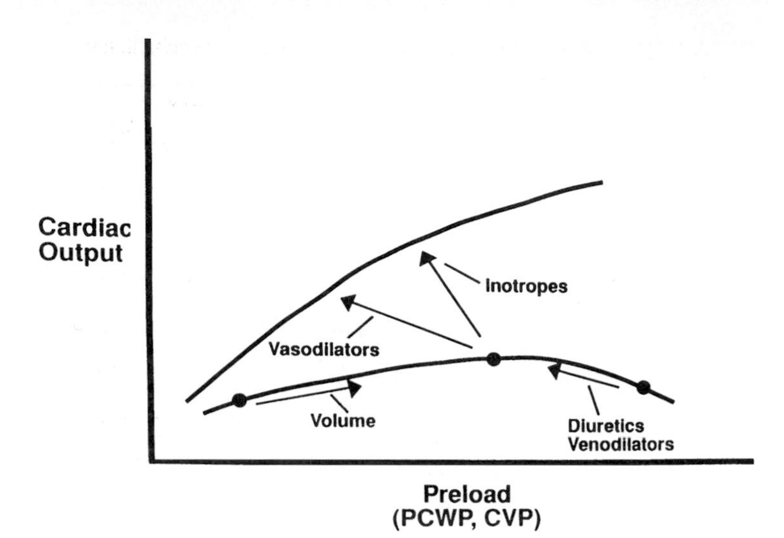

FIG. 1-8 Treatment approaches for altered hemodynamic states based on Starling's law of the heart. PCWP, pulmonary capillary wedge pressure; CVP, central venous pressure. (*Source: Rosenthal MH: Intrapartum intensive care management of the cardiac patient. Clin Obstet Gynecol 1981;24:789–807.*)

10 μg/kg/min. These dose ranges reflect a predominance of action only. There is a great deal of overlap and individuality of response. The usual therapeutic range for dopamine in clinical practice is 3 to 20 μg/kg/min. When the requirement exceeds this, a more potent inotropic vasopressor such as norepinephrine is substituted at a dose of 1 to 30 μg/min. If the systolic blood pressure is quite low (less than 70 mmHg) after fluid resuscitation, norepinephrine is the drug of first choice.

Afterload may be manipulated with vasodilators in cardiac failure or in low cardiac output states secondary to severe hypertension. Vasodilators have varying effects on arterial and venous resistances. Nitroglycerin, predominantly a venodilator, may cause a greater reduction in preload than in afterload. Nitroprusside, an equal arterial and venular vasodilator, may be preferred; however, marked decreases in systemic vascular resistance result in hypotension, poor perfusion, and myocardial ischemia. The use of a vasodilator requires careful observation of the adequacy of intravascular volume and the net effect on cardiac output.

HEMODYNAMICS OF NORMAL PREGNANCY

Table 1-4 summarizes the invasive hemodynamic findings in normal pregnancy as determined by Clark et al. Ten normal primiparous patients between 36 and 38 weeks gestation underwent pulmonary artery catheterization, arterial line placement, and central hemodynamic assessment in the left lateral recumbent position. Studies were repeated in the same patients between 11 and 13 weeks postpartum. Mean arterial pressure, central venous pressure, and pulmonary artery wedge pressure remained unchanged during pregnancy. Cardiac output increased about 40 percent due to an increase in both heart rate and stroke volume. Systemic and pulmonary vascular resistances fell.

TABLE 1-4 Hemodynamic Values in Healthy Nonpregnant, Pregnant, and Postpartum Subjects

Parameters	Units	Nonpregnant	36–38 weeks gestation	Postpartum
Heart rate	beats/min	60–100	83 ± 10	71 ± 10
Mean arterial pressure	mmHg	90–110	90.3 ± 5.8	86.4 ± 7.5
Central venous pressure	mmHg	1–7	3.6 ± 2.5	3.7 ± 2.6
Pulmonary artery wedge pressure	mmHg	6–12	7.5 ± 1.8	6.3 ± 2.1
Cardiac output	L/min	4.3–6.0	6.2 ± 1.0	4.3 ± 0.9
Stroke volume	mL/beat	57–71	74.7	60.6
Systemic vascular resistance	dyn/s/cm^{-5}	900–1400	1210 ± 266	1530 ± 520
Pulmonary vascular resistance	dyn/s/cm^{-5}	<250	78 ± 22	119 ± 47

Data from Clark et al.: *Am J Obstet Gynecol* 1989;161:1439–1442.

SUGGESTED READING

Bernard GR, Sopko G, Cerra F, et al.: Pulmonary artery catheterization and clinical outcome. National Heart, Lung, and Blood Institute and Food and Drug Administration Workshop Report. *JAMA* 2000;283:2568–2572.

Clark SL, Cotton DB, Lee W, et al.: Central hemodynamic assessment of normal term pregnancy. *Am J Obstet Gynecol* 1989;161:1439–1442.

Connors AF Jr, Speroff T, Dawson NV, et al.: The effectiveness of right heart catheterization in the initial care of critically ill patients. *JAMA* 1996;276:889–897.

Daily EK, Schroeder JP: *Hemodynamic Waveforms: Exercises in Identification and Analysis*. St. Louis: CV Mosby, 1983.

Hayes MA, Timmins AC, Yau EHS, et al.: Elevation of systemic oxygen delivery in the treatment of critically ill patients. *N Engl J Med* 1994;330:1717–1722.

Mabie WC: Critical care obstetrics. In: Gabbe SG, Niebyl JR, Simpson JL (eds), *Obstetrics: Normal and Problem Pregnancies*, 3rd edn., New York: Churchill Livingston, 1996; chapter 18, pp. 533–559.

Mabie WC, Sibai BM: Treatment in an obstetric intensive care unit. *Am J Obstet Gynecol* 1990;162:1–4.

Rosenthal MH: Intrapartum intensive care management of the cardiac patient. *Clin Obstet Gynecol* 1981;24:789–807.

Sandham JD, Hull RD, Brant RF, et al.: A randomized controlled trial of the use of pulmonary-artery catheters in high-risk surgical patients. *N Engl J Med* 2003;348:5–14.

Shoemaker WC, Appel PL, Kram HB, et al.: Prospective trial of supranormal values of survivors as therapeutic goals in high-risk surgical patients. *Chest* 1988; 94:1176–1186.

Snyder JV: Oxygen transport: The model and reality. In: Snyder JV, Pinsky MR (eds), *Oxygen Transport in the Critically Ill*. Chicago: Year Book Medical Publishers, 1987; pp. 3–15.

2

Transfusion of Blood Components and Derivatives in the Obstetric Intensive Care Patient

Stephanie R. Martin   Thomas H. Strong, Jr.

INTRODUCTION

Obstetric hemorrhage remains one of the leading causes of maternal death in the United States, often necessitating the transfusion of blood products as a life saving measure. More commonly, the practitioner encounters less acute situations and must decide which blood products, if any, are most appropriate for the patient. In this chapter, we will address the blood products currently available for transfusion, the indications for their use and potential risks. We will also discuss alternatives and techniques to avoid transfusion, including available colloid solutions, use of the "autologous transfusion device" and acute normovolemic hemodilution (ANH).

In modern obstetric practice, transfusion of whole blood is uncommon. Whole blood which has not been separated into its various components contains clotting factors, platelets, and red blood cells. However, one unit of whole blood also contains roughly 500 mL of fluid and poses a significant risk of circulatory overload when many units are used. The major limitation to the use of whole blood is the inability to store the product beyond 24 hours. After 24 hours of extra-vascular storage, platelets and granulocytes are completely lost and 2,3-diphosphoglycerate is depleted. Without this important compound, the oxygen carrying capacity of the red blood cell is significantly compromised. After one week of storage, the labile clotting factors (factors V and VIII) are also lost. Other changes which occur include an increase in the plasma level of potassium and ammonia.

In contemporary medical practice, whole blood is separated into its components (red blood cells, platelets, fibrinogen and other clotting factors) and stored. Blood component therapy allows the physician to treat specific derangements in the patient's blood. The decision to transfuse a blood product must be individualized to the clinical scenario. The potential benefits of improved oxygen carrying capacity and improved clotting must be weighed against the potential risks, particularly infectious complications.

RISKS OF TRANSFUSION

Infections

The most common causes of transfusion-associated infections are the human hepatitis viruses. Hepatitis B is most commonly diagnosed, occurring in 1 of 137,000 units of blood. Since 1999, improved donor screening techniques have decreased the incidence of hepatitis C.

As is widely known, the HIV virus is uniformly fatal. The risk of acquiring this virus ranges from 1 in 40,000 to 1 in 1,000,000 units of transfused blood products depending upon where in the country one resides. While a screening test is available for HIV antibodies, it can take six months or more for a patient to convert following infection. Blood donated by an HIV-infected person during this window would give a false negative antibody screen.

Clinically significant cytomegalovirus (CMV) infections usually occur in immunocompromised patients. However, a small but significant portion of persons in the population has never been exposed to CMV and has no natural immunity to it. While CMV infection in the adult is usually a benign, subclinical process, primary infection in the fetus can have devastating effects. Therefore, only CMV seronegative blood products should be administered to the seronegative patient.

On rare occasions, bacterial and endotoxin contamination can occur in donated blood products. Bacterially infected blood could potentially lead to septicemia in the patient who receives it. Other diseases which are less frequently transmitted through transfusion include malaria, parvovirus, Epstein-Barr virus, Babesia and T-cell viruses.

Immunologic

Antigens on red and white blood cells typically trigger transfusion reactions. There are two types of transfusion reactions: hemolytic and nonhemolytic. The hemolytic variety occurs in 1 out of every 6000 transfusions and is fatal in 1 out of every 100,000 units of blood transfused. The ABO-system antigens are usually responsible for hemolytic reactions. The nonhemolytic transfusion reaction is much more common (1 per 100). Usually characterized by febrile or urticarial reactions, the incidence of nonhemolytic reactions can be reduced by using leukocyte-poor blood products. Alloimmunization can result in platelet antibodies which may prevent therapeutic response in the thrombocytopenic patient who receives platelet transfusion. Rarely, graft-versus-host disease can occur following transfusion of some blood components (platelets, white blood cells, etc.) into an immunocompromised individual.

Those blood products that are most commonly used in pregnancy are generally subdivided into cellular or plasma components (Table 2-1).

Cellular Components

Red Blood Cells

- Most patients requiring replacement of red blood cells should receive packed red blood cells (RBC).
- One unit of packed RBCs contains roughly 250 mL of RBCs, 50 mL of plasma and has a hematocrit of approximately 80 percent. The decreased plasma volume of packed cells minimizes the risk of fluid overload.
- Transfusion of one unit of packed RBCs into a 70 kg person will usually increase the hemoglobin level by 1 g/dL.
- Like whole blood, packed RBCs have a shelf life of approximately six weeks when stored at 1 to 6°C.
- Frozen RBCs can be stored at –70°C for years, but the freezing process destroys white blood cells (WBC) which may be present in the unit of blood.

TABLE 2-1 Blood Components

Component	Contents	Indications	Volume (mL)	Shelf life	Expected effect
Packed RBCs	Red cells, some plasma, few WBCs	Correct anemia	300	42 days	Increase Hct 3% per unit, Hgb 1 g/unit
Leukocyte-poor blood	RBCs, some plasma, few WBCs	Correct anemia, reduce febrile reactions	250	21–24 days	Increase Hct 3% per unit, Hgb 1 g/unit
Platelets	Platelets, some plasma, RBCs, few WBCs	Bleeding due to thrombocytopenia	50	Up to 5 days	Increase total platelet count 7500/mm^3 per unit
Fresh frozen plasma	Fibrinogen, plasma, clotting factors V, XI, XII	Treatment of coagulation disorders	250	2 h thawed, 12 months frozen	Increase total fibrinogen 10–15 mg/dL per unit
Cryoprecipitate	Fibrinogen, factors V, VIII, XIII, von Willebrand factor	Hemophilia A, von Willebrand's disease, fibrinogen deficiency	40	4–6 h thawed	Increase total fibrinogen 10–15 mg/dL per unit

- When WBCs have been removed from a unit of blood, the blood is considered to be "leukocyte-poor" and possesses a decreased risk of febrile transfusion reactions.
- Gravidas who exhibit cardiovascular instability, hemoglobin levels below 8 to 9 g or evidence of fetal compromise should be considered as candidates for RBC transfusion.

Autologous Blood

Autologous transfusion is the collection and reinfusion of the patient's own RBCs. Therefore, donor and recipient are identical. Exclusive or supplemental use of autologous blood can reduce or eliminate many transfusion-related complications. Until recently, pregnant women were not allowed to donate blood because the effects of maternal intravascular volume changes upon the fetus were unknown. However, a growing database suggests that it is safe for certain pregnant women to donate blood in the third trimester.

It is not unreasonable to encourage pregnant patients at increased risk for blood transfusion (e.g., placenta previa) to consider autologous blood donation. However, the obstetric care provider should not deny the option of autologous donation to low-risk patients. The guidelines for autologous blood donation during pregnancy are as follows:

- A minimum predonation hemoglobin of 11 g/dL.
- Because RBCs may be refrigerated in liquid form for only six weeks, initiation of autologous blood donation generally occurs no earlier than six weeks before their anticipated use. The last donation should be planned at least two weeks before the estimated date of delivery.
- One week should elapse between donations.
- Autologous blood should be used selectively. The unnecessary transfusion of autologous blood increases the risk of circulatory overload.
- Due to the special logistics of autologous blood, autologous donor candidates should be aware that this technique is more costly than homologous transfusions.
- Patients should be aware that autologous blood donation does not completely eliminate the possibility of homologous transfusion.

Platelet Concentrates

Platelets are separated from whole blood and suspended in small amounts of plasma. They can be collected from a single donor or from multiple donors. Platelet concentrates are indicated for the treatment of hemorrhage due to thrombocytopenia or platelet dysfunction (thrombocytopathia). The cause of thrombocytopenia or thrombocytopathia must be determined. For example, in the presence of immune thrombocytopenic purpura (ITP), where platelets are destroyed via an antibody-mediated process, corticosteroids rather than platelets probably represent the best therapy. Additionally, patients taking aspirin preparations can experience potentially serious bleeding despite normal platelet counts. When ordering a platelet transfusion, the following should be considered:

- In the pregnant patient, thrombocytopenia is considered to be present when the platelet count falls below 100,000/mm^3. Bleeding following major surgery or trauma rarely occurs when the platelet count is 50,000/mm^3 or greater, assuming normal platelet function. When the platelet count ranges from 20,000 to 50,000/mm^3, bleeding with major surgery or trauma can occasionally occur. Platelet transfusion may be performed prophylactically in nonbleeding patients with platelet counts of 20,000 platelets/mm^3 or less. When the platelet count falls to 10,000/mm^3, bleeding with trauma or surgery is likely. Spontaneous bleeding can occur once the platelet count drops below 10,000/mm^3.

- Among patients receiving massive transfusions within a short period of time, dilutional thrombocytopenia can occur. Following replacement of one blood volume, 35 to 40 percent of a patient's platelets usually remain. Most patients who receive rapid replacement of 1 to 2 blood volumes do not develop bleeding problems, however. Platelets should not be given in the setting of massive transfusion unless significant thrombocytopenia or clinically abnormal bleeding occurs.
- One unit of platelets is equivalent to the number of platelets typically found in one unit of whole blood and will typically increase the platelet count in a 70-kg patient by approximately 7500 platelets/mm^3. Typically, the platelet count will equilibrate within 10 minutes of transfusion. As a result, the platelet count can be assessed immediately following completion of the transfusion.
- Platelet concentrates contain sufficient numbers of serum-bound RBCs to cause alloimmunization to red cell antigens. Therefore, the possibility of Rh immunization by red cells should be considered in Rh-negative female recipients.
- Platelet transfusion is contraindicated in thrombotic thrombocytopenic purpura (TTP).

Plasma Components

Fresh-Frozen Plasma (FFP)

FFP is plasma extracted from whole blood within six hours of collection and frozen. A typical unit of FFP contains 250 mL of fluid and 700 mg of fibrinogen. FFP is indicated to correct deficiencies of multiple clotting factors in bleeding patients. Clotting factor deficiencies can arise from liver disease, vitamin K deficiency or disseminated intravascular coagulation. FFP may also be used for specific factor deficiencies (factors II, V, VII, IX, X, and XI) when specific component therapy is not available. FFP is also indicated when rapid reversal of warfarin is indicated. Warfarin causes a deficiency of the vitamin K dependent factors (II, VII, IX, and X). While vitamin K will eventually reverse this deficiency, FFP can affect a more rapid recovery.

- One unit of FFP will typically increase the fibrinogen level by approximately 10 to15 mg/dL. When FFP is indicated, 15 mL/kg is a reasonable guideline for the initiation of FFP therapy (target serum fibrinogen level is ~100 mg/dL).
- It should be kept in mind that 30 minutes are required to thaw FFP in the blood bank.
- When only Factor VIII, von Willebrand's factor or fibrinogen is needed, cryoprecipitate is a more appropriate therapeutic choice. Inappropriate uses of FFP include use of this blood component for volume expansion or as a nutritional supplement.

Cryoprecipitate

Cryoprecipitate is extracted from whole blood which has been frozen and then allowed to thaw at refrigerator temperatures. The product is a cold insoluble fraction of FFP which precipitates under these conditions. Cryoprecipitate is rich in factor VIII (80 to 120 units), fibrinogen (200 mg) and also contains von Willebrand's factor and factor XIII. One unit of cryoprecipitate will raise the fibrinogen level by the same amount as one unit of FFP (10 to 15 mg/dL). However, as one unit of cryoprecipitate consists of only 40 mL of fluid, it more efficiently raises the fibrinogen level than does a 250 mL unit of FFP. Indications for the use of cryoprecipitate include the treatment of von Willebrand's disease, factor VIII deficiency and fibrinogen deficiency. Since cryoprecipitate is a single donor product, it has a lower risk of hepatitis and HIV transmission than pooled clotting factor concentrates.

Colloid Solutions

Intravenous fluids containing particles that will not pass through a semipermeable membrane and are larger than 10,000 daltons are known as colloids. Compared to crystalloid solutions, colloids are more expensive, less readily available and may be associated with anaphylactoid reactions. Colloids tend to produce greater elevations in colloid oncotic pressure than crystalloids. They also produce greater increases in plasma volume and deplete extracellular fluid. Patients receiving a colloid solution must be adequately prehydrated with crystalloids (see Table 2-2).

Effective management of hypovolemic shock is more dependent upon successful fluid resuscitation than the fluid actually used. Which solution is used is a function of medical philosophy and risk-versus-benefit analysis.

Albumin

Albumin solutions may rapidly restore intravascular volume, especially if serum albumin levels are less than 2 g/dL. Use should be limited to patients with decreased plasma volume and adequate extracellular volume. Albumin is available in concentrations of 5 percent or 25 percent. When 25 g of albumin are infused, intravascular volume will increase by roughly 450 mL over 60 minutes as a result of the considerable oncotic activity of albumin. However, the benefits are only transient and may result in complications such as pulmonary edema if administered excessively because supplemental albumin is rapidly redistributed throughout the extracellular space, disappearing from the circulation at a rate of up to 8 percent per hour. In the setting of shock or sepsis, the rate can approach 30 percent per hour. Other potential benefits provided

TABLE 2-2 Colloid Infusions

Colloid	Dose (mL)	Crystalloid volume expansion equivalent	Estimated duration of effect (h)
Albumin			
5% solution	500–700	Similar to crystalloid	24
25% solution	100–200	3.5 times crystalloid	24
Hetastarch	500–1000	Similar to crystalloid	24–36
Dextran (70)	500	1050 mL over 2 h	24

by supplemental albumin include (1) limitation of lipid peroxidation by scavenging free radicals, (2) binding of free fatty acids and lysozymes, (3) inhibition of pathologic platelet activation, and (4) inhibition of factor Xa by antithrombin III.

Dextran

Dextran is a large, glucose polymer solution available with polymers having mean molecular weights of 40,000 (dextran 40) or 70,000 (dextran 70). A 6 percent dextran 70 solution is most commonly used for similar indications as 5 percent albumin. Dextran 40 is rarely used for volume expansion. A 500 mL infusion of dextran produces intravascular volume expansion of 1050 mL over two hours and improves capillary blood flow by reducing viscosity and red cell aggregation. As with albumin, the effects of dextran are temporary and may be associated with pulmonary edema if used too aggressively.

In doses exceeding 20 mL/kg/24 h, dextran may also foster hemorrhage by reducing platelet and clotting factor activation and by binding with fibrin to produce less stable clots. It should be used cautiously in patients with hypovolemia, who due to hemorrhage, may already have a coagulopathy. Rarely can dextran induce potentially fatal anaphylactoid reactions in patients who have received dextran previously. Dextran may also interfere with laboratory cross-matching of blood by reducing red blood cell aggregation. Therefore, blood typing and cross-matching should be performed prior to administering dextran.

Hetastarch

Hydroxymethyl starch is a synthetic molecule available as a 6 percent solution in normal saline (Hespan). Like albumin and dextran, it possesses considerable oncotic activity and can induce intravascular fluid expansion. However, hetastarch increases colloid oncotic pressure more effectively than albumin and lasts 24 to 36 hours. The dose should not exceed 20 mL/kg/24 h. Hetastarch may also prolong prothrombin and partial thromboplastin times, decrease platelet counts and reduce clot tensile strength. Therefore, it should be used cautiously in patients who may have a coagulopathy. Hetastarch may also artifactually increase serum amylase levels.

Red Blood Cell-Saving Devices

The salvage of shed blood has been a topic of research since early in the nineteenth century. The first reported case of autologous transfusion occurred over 100 years ago. Since that time, transfusion of blood lost during surgery or following trauma has become an accepted treatment modality. Autologous blood, collected preoperatively or intraoperatively, offers a variety of advantages over homologous blood. As a perfectly compatible source, autologous blood eliminates the risk of infectious disease transmission or isoimmunization.

Because of the theoretic risk of inducing amniotic fluid embolism by transfusing blood contaminated with amniotic fluid, the use of autologous transfusion devices during obstetric procedures has been limited. However, over 400 cases of successful transfusions using autologous transfusion devices have been reported in published literature. This safety record has prompted The American College of Obstetricians and Gynecologists to recommend consideration of this technology for patients at risk for intraoperative hemorrhage.

Once the operating field is cleared of amniotic fluid, the suction device is changed and the blood is collected into the Cell Saver. The Cell Saver can provide a unit of blood with a hematocrit of 50 percent in approximately three minutes. In patients where blood loss is anticipated to be excessive, more than one Cell Saver may be employed.

Acute Normovolemic Hemodilution

Patients at risk for significant intraoperative hemorrhage may be candidates for acute normovolemic hemodilution (ANH). Immediately preoperatively, blood is collected from the patient into special storage bags containing an anticoagulant obtained from the blood bank. At the same time, the patient is given large amounts of crystalloid in a 3:1 ratio resulting in a dilutional effect and a decrease in the maternal hematocrit. Blood lost intraoperatively is therefore more dilute. After blood loss is under control (or at the discretion of the surgeon), the patient's blood is reinfused, resulting in an increase in the hematocrit. Other potential advantages include decreased likelihood of allogeneic transfusion and its associated morbidities. Additionally, clotting factors are preserved.

No adverse fetal effects have been described with this process. However, patients who might not tolerate an acute decrease in hematocrit are not candidates for ANH, as are those who are already anemic or have coronary artery disease, pulmonary disease, renal or hepatic insufficiency or evidence of fetal compromise.

SUGGESTED READING

Consensus Conference: Fresh-frozen plasma: indications and risks. *JAMA* 1985;253(4):551.

Consensus Conference: Perioperative red blood cell transfusion. *JAMA* 1988;260(18):2700.

Consensus Conference: Platelet transfusion therapy. *JAMA* 1987;257(13):1777.

Kruskall MS, Leonard S, Klapholz H: Autologous blood donation during pregnancy: analysis of safety and blood use. *Obstet Gynecol* 1987;70:938.

McVay PA, Hoag RW, Hoag SM, et al.: Safety and use of autologous blood donation during the third trimester of pregnancy. *Am J Obstet Gynecol* 1989;169:1479.

Miller RD. Transfusion therapy. In: Miller RD (ed) *Anesthesia*, 5th edn. New York: Churchill Livingstone, 2000.

Oberman HA: Transfusion therapy. In: Laros RK (ed), *Blood Disorders in Pregnancy*, (ed), 1st edn. Philadelphia: Lea and Febiger, 1986.

Placenta accreta. *ACOG Committee Opinion* No. 266, January 2002.

Transfusion Alert: Indications for the use of red blood cells, platelets and fresh-frozen plasma. *NIH Publication* No. 89-2974a, May 1989.

3 Postpartum Hemorrhage

Karrie Francois

INTRODUCTION

Postpartum hemorrhage is a leading cause of maternal morbidity and mortality throughout the world, contributing to nearly 30 percent of pregnancy-related deaths annually. In order to manage postpartum hemorrhage effectively, the obstetrician must have a thorough understanding of normal delivery-related blood loss, physiologic responses to hemorrhage, the most common etiologies of postpartum hemorrhage, and appropriate therapeutic interventions.

NORMAL BLOOD LOSS

Normal delivery-related blood loss depends upon delivery type. The average blood loss for a vaginal delivery, cesarean section, and cesarean hysterectomy is 500, 1000, and 1500 cc, respectively. These values are often underestimated and unappreciated clinically due to the significant blood volume expansion that accompanies pregnancy.

Postpartum hemorrhage has been defined in published literature. Definitions have included subjective assessments greater than the standard norms, a 10 percent decline in hematocrit, and need for blood transfusion. Because of these varied definitions, the exact incidence of postpartum hemorrhage is difficult to determine; however, rough estimates suggest that postpartum hemorrhage complicates 4 to 6 percent of all deliveries.

PHYSIOLOGIC RESPONSE TO HEMORRHAGE

The pregnant patient is able to adapt to hemorrhage more effectively than her nonpregnant counterpart due to hemodynamic changes that accompany pregnancy. These changes include increased red cell mass, increased plasma volume, and increased cardiac output. In the early phases of hemorrhage, the body compensates by raising systemic vascular resistance in order to maintain blood pressure and perfusion to vital organs. However, as bleeding continues, further vasoconstriction is impossible resulting in drops in blood pressure, cardiac output, and end-organ perfusion. Table 3-1 classifies the physiologic responses that occur with various stages of hemorrhage. It is important for the obstetrician to recognize these responses since the quantity of blood loss that occurs during a postpartum hemorrhage is often underestimated as stated previously.

ETIOLOGIES OF POSTPARTUM HEMORRHAGE

The etiologies of postpartum hemorrhage can be categorized as early—those occurring within 24 hours of delivery—and late—those occurring from 24 hours until 6 weeks postdelivery. Table 3-2 lists the most common causes of early and late postpartum hemorrhage. Since the obstetrician is faced with early postpartum hemorrhage more often than late, the remainder of this chapter will focus on its risk factors and therapy.

TABLE 3-1 Hemorrhage Classification and Physiologic Response

Hemorrhage class	Acute blood loss	% Lost	Physiologic response
1	900 cc	15	Asymptomatic
2	1200–1500 cc	20–25	Tachycardia and tachypnea Narrowed pulse pressure Orthostatic hypotension
3	1800–2100 cc	30–35	Worsening tachycardia and tachypnea Hypotension Cool extremities
4	>2400 cc	40	Shock Oliguria/Anuria

Source: Baker R.: Hemorrhage in obstetrics. *Obstet Gynecol Annu* 1977;6:295.

Uterine Atony

Uterine atony, or the inability of the uterine myometrium to contract effectively, is the most common cause of early postpartum hemorrhage. At term, blood flow through the placental site averages 600 cc/min. After placental delivery, the uterus controls bleeding by contracting its myometrial fibers in a tourniquet fashion around the spiral arterioles. If inadequate uterine contraction occurs, rapid blood loss will ensue.

Risk factors for uterine atony include uterine overdistension (multiple gestation, polyhydramnios, fetal macrosomia), prolonged oxytocin use, rapid or prolonged labor, grand multiparity, chorioamnionitis, placenta previa, and use of uterine-relaxing agents (tocolytic therapy, halogenated anesthetics, nitroglycerin).

Genitourinary Tract Lacerations

The second most common cause of postpartum hemorrhage is genitourinary tract lacerations. While operative vaginal delivery remains the most significant risk factor for a genitourinary tract laceration, other sources of obstetrical

TABLE 3-2 Causes of Postpartum Hemorrhage

Early
- Uterine atony
- Lower genital tract lacerations (perineal, vaginal, cervical, periclitoral, labial, periurethral, rectum)
- Upper genital tract lacerations (broad ligament)
- Lower urinary tract lacerations (bladder, urethra)
- Retained products of conception (placenta, membranes)
- Invasive placentation (placenta accreta, placenta increta, placenta percreta)
- Uterine rupture
- Uterine inversion
- Coagulopathy (hereditary, acquired)

Late
- Infection
- Retained products of conception
- Placental site subinvolution
- Coagulopathy

trauma can contribute to this cause of hemorrhage. These sources include fetal malpresentation, fetal macrosomia, episiotomy, precipitous delivery, prior cerclage placement, Duhrssen's incisions, and shoulder dystocia.

A genitourinary tract laceration should be suspected if bleeding persists after a delivery despite good uterine tone. Occasionally, the bleeding may be masked due to its location, i.e., broad ligament. In these circumstances, large amounts of blood loss may occur in an unrecognized hematoma. The astute obstetrician must be aware of the risk factors for this type of laceration as well as the patient's initial presenting symptoms of pain and physiological signs of shock.

Retained Products of Conception

Retained products of conception, namely, placental tissue and amniotic membranes, can inhibit the uterus from adequate contraction and result in hemorrhage. Risk factors for retained products of conception include midtrimester delivery, chorioamnionitis, and accessory placental lobes.

Invasive Placentation

Although uncommon, invasive placentation can result in massive postpartum hemorrhage. Placenta accreta represents the abnormal attachment of the placenta to the uterine lining due to an absence of the deciduas basalis and an incomplete development of the fibrinoid layer. Placenta increta and percreta represent attachments to and through the uterine myometrium, respectively. Attempts to remove a highly invasive placenta from its attachment site will result in rapid blood loss, often necessitating emergent surgical intervention.

Major risk factors for invasive placentation include prior curettage or hysterotomy, advanced maternal age, multiparity, placenta previa, and previous cesarean section. As exemplified in Table 3-3, the combination of placenta previa and previous cesarean section should alert the physician to a substantial risk of invasive placentation and subsequent hemorrhage. In these circumstances, an attempt for antepartum detection should be undertaken and scheduled cesarean hysterectomy performed at the time of delivery if no future fertility is desired.

Uterine Rupture

Despite an uncommon incidence of 1 in 2000 deliveries, uterine rupture represents a potential catastrophic event for both mother and fetus and may result in a significant hemorrhage if the placental implantation site is involved. While prior cesarean section remains the most common risk factor for uterine rupture,

TABLE 3-3 Risk of Invasive Placentation with Placenta Previa and Previous Cesarean Section

Number of cesarean sections	Invasive placentation risk (%)
0	5
1	24
2	47
3	40
≥4	67

Source: Clark SL, Koonings PP, Phelan JP.: Placenta previa/accreta and prior cesarean section. *Obstet Gynecol* 1985;66:89–91.

other risk factors include multiparity, fetal malpresentation, obstructed labor, multiple gestation, prior hysterotomy/myomectomy, uterine manipulation (e.g., internal podalic version), and mid- to high-operative vaginal delivery.

Uterine Inversion

Uterine inversion is a rare event, complicating approximately 1 in 2500 deliveries. Uterine inversion may be complete or incomplete. In complete uterine inversion, the internal lining of the fundus crosses through the cervical os, forming a rounded mass in the vagina with no palpable fundus abdominally. Incomplete uterine inversion represents a partial extrusion of the fundus to the cervix; however, no passage through the os occurs. Both types of uterine inversions signify need for rapid diagnosis and correction since large volume blood loss, often associated with symptoms of shock, may ensue.

The most commonly reported cause of uterine inversion is fundal placentation with excessive cord traction in the third stage of labor. Other associations include any clinical scenario with the potential for impaired uterine contraction after placental delivery, i.e., uterine overdistension secondary to fetal macrosomia and prolonged oxytocin use. Other risk factors include uterine malformations and invasive placentation.

Coagulopathy

Coagulopathy represents the final major etiology of postpartum hemorrhage. Coagulopathies may be hereditary or acquired in origin. Although rare, hereditary coagulopathies may present challenging clinical courses if appropriate therapy is unavailable. In general, most of these coagulopathies are effectively treated with replacement of coagulation factor products and/or additional agents, i.e., DDAVP, in the third stage of labor or at the time of cesarean section.

Acquired coagulopathies have numerous causes, including anticoagulant administration, sepsis, severe preeclampsia, amniotic fluid embolus, tissue necrosis (e.g., retained intrauterine fetal demise and trauma), placental abruption, and loss of clot-promoting factors due to massive hemorrhage. Figure 3-1 reviews the pathophysiology of acquired coagulopathy and its association with hemorrhage.

THERAPEUTIC INTERVENTIONS FOR POSTPARTUM HEMORRHAGE

When the obstetrician is faced with a postpartum hemorrhage, an organized care plan needs to be set in motion to minimize further bleeding and associated morbidity and mortality. Table 3-4 lists the components of such a care plan.

Blood Loss Needs

When faced with a postpartum hemorrhage, the first priority that a clinician should assess is his or her blood loss needs. Appropriate intravenous (IV) access is critical. This includes at minimum one or two large-bore IV catheters. In addition, the patient's blood type should be confirmed and held for possible cross matching needs. Finally, need for ancillary support should be assessed. This support may include additional nursing assistance, operating room staff, physician assistance, and an anesthesiology team.

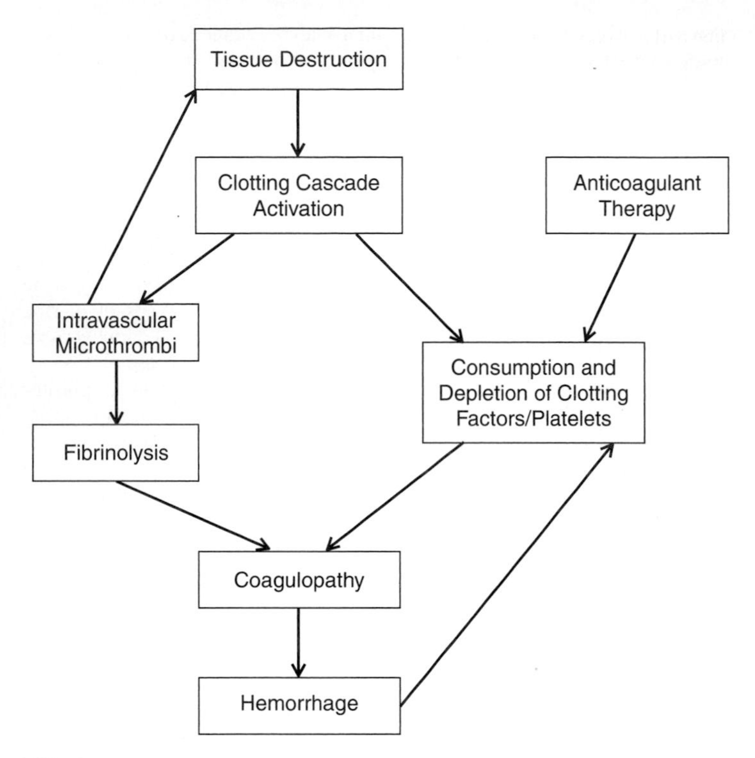

FIG. 3-1 Pathophysiology of acquired coagulopathy.

Loss Estimation

Many instances of hemorrhage result in compounded morbidity secondary to an inadequate blood loss estimation on the part of the obstetrician. At the onset of a postpartum hemorrhage, it is important for the clinician to realistically estimate the amount of blood loss that has occurred. At this time, baseline laboratory evaluations of hemoglobin, hematocrit, platelet count, fibrinogen, prothrombin time, and partial thromboplastin time should be taken. If rapid laboratory assessment cannot be obtained, drawing 5 cc of blood into an empty

TABLE 3-4 Postpartum Hemorrhage Care Plan

B	Blood loss needs
L	Loss estimation
E	Etiology
E	EBL replacement
D	Drug therapy
I	Intraoperative management
N	Nonobstetrical services
G	General complication assessment

tube and evaluating its clotting capability within 6 minutes will provide the clinician with a rough estimate of the degree of coagulopathy that exists.

Etiology

After assessing blood loss needs and estimation, a rapid yet thorough exploration for the hemorrhage etiology must be undertaken. A poorly cotractile uterus suggests uterine atony. If atony is not the source of bleeding, further exploration should occur. This exploration should begin with the most superior aspect of the genital tract and progress inferiorly since heavy downward blood flow may make visualization of the more inferior landmarks difficult.

Initial assessment should focus on the uterus. The most common uterine source of bleeding other than atony is retained products of conception. Figure 3-2 demonstrates proper manual exploration of the uterine cavity in order to remove retained products of conception. Wrapping the examination hand with

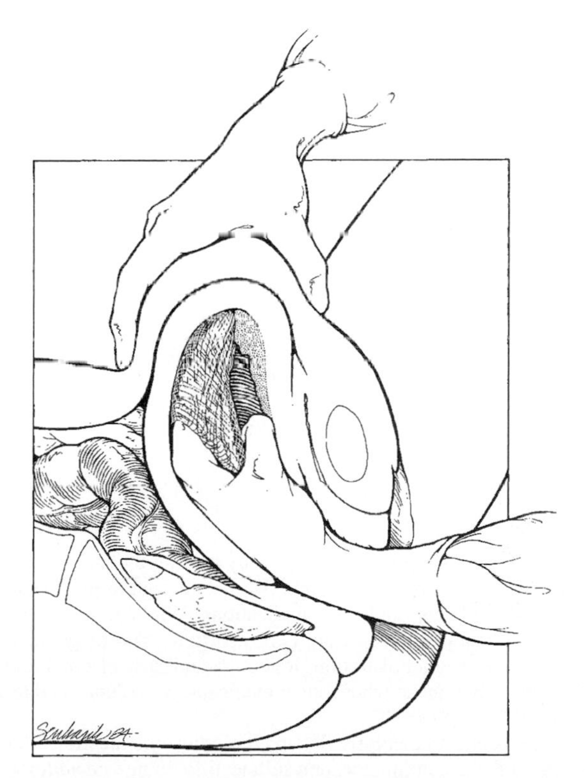

FIG. 3-2 Manual uterine exploration. (*Source: Benedetti TJ: Obstetric hemorrhage. In: Gabbe SG, Niebyl JR, Simpson JL (eds), Obstetrics: Normal and Problem Pregnancies, 3rd edn. New York: Churchill Livingstone, 1996; p. 499.*)

moist gauze can facilitate removal of retained amniotic membranes. If manual access to the uterine cavity is difficult or limited due to maternal body habitus or inadequate pain relief, transabdominal ultrasound may be used to assess for retained placental fragments. Once fragments are identified, appropriate removal may be undertaken via manual extraction and/or uterine curettage. Besides assessing for retained products of conception, a proper uterine examination can assess for evidence of invasive placentation, uterine rupture, and uterine inversion.

Once a uterine source has been excluded, attention should be focused on identifying a lower genitourinary tract laceration. Cervical and/or vaginal fornix lacerations are often difficult to repair due to their location. In these situations, it is best to have early assistance for retraction in order to visualize the laceration and provide adequate repair. In some instances, moving to an operating room to provide more adequate pain relief, pelvic relaxation, and visualization will save time and subsequent bleeding since a proper repair can be instituted more efficiently. In addition, lacerations that involve sites near the urethra and/or bowel may be challenging from the technical as well as visual perspectives. In these circumstances, employing additional instrumentation (e.g., transurethral catheter) may protect uninjured entities and allow for a better repair.

After the most common etiologies of postpartum hemorrhage are excluded, other sources of bleeding should be assessed. Being aware of the risk factors for these etiologies will decrease diagnostic time and allow for more timely intervention.

EBL Replacement

Understanding the patient's requirements for fluid and blood component therapy is critical to providing adequate care to the bleeding patient. Estimated blood loss (EBL) replacement begins with appropriate fluid resuscitation. Warmed crystalloid solution in a 3:1 ratio to EBL will provide the initial volume necessary to stabilize a bleeding patient. Once appropriate volume resuscitation has occurred, additional colloid and/or blood component therapy may be tailored to the individual patient's needs and blood loss. It is important for the clinician to understand the expected clinical response to the blood product therapy that is given (see Chap. 2).

Drug Therapy

Uterotonic medications represent the mainstay of drug therapy for postpartum hemorrhage due to uterine atony. Table 3-5 lists available uterotonic agents, their dosage, side effects, and contraindications. While recent reviews have questioned the efficacy of misoprostol in postpartum hemorrhage, its mild side effect profile, ease of administration, low cost, and lack of contraindications make it an attractive agent when other medications are unavailable or contraindicated.

When atony is due to tocolytic therapy, i.e., those medications that impair calcium entry into the cell (magnesium sulfate, nifedipine), an additional agent to employ is calcium gluconate. Given as an intravenous push, one ampule of calcium gluconate can effectively improve uterine tone and resolve bleeding due to atony.

TABLE 3-5 Uterotonic Medications

Agent	Dose	Route	Dosing frequency	Side effects	Contraindications
Oxytocin (Pitocin)	10–80 units in 1000 cc of crystalloid solution	First line: IV Second line: IM or IU	Continuous	Nausea, emesis, water intoxication	None
Methylergonovine (Methergine)	0.2 mg	First line: IM Second line: IU	Every 2–4 h	Hypertension, hypotension, nausea, emesis,	Hypertension, preeclampsia
Prostaglandin $F_{2\alpha}$ (Hemabate)	0.25 mg	First line: IM Second line: IU	Every 15–90 min (8 doses maximum)	Nausea, emesis, diarrhea, flushing, chills	Active cardiac, pulmonary, renal or hepatic disease
Prostaglandin E_2 (Dinoprostone)	20 mg	PR	Every 2 h	Nausea, emesis, diarrhea, fever, chills, headache	Hypotension
Misoprostol (Cytotec)	600–1000 μg	First line: PR Second line: PO	Single dose	Nausea, emesis, diarrhea, fever, chills	None

Abbreviations: IV, intravenous; IM, intramuscular; IU, intrauterine; PR, per rectum; PO, per oral.
Source: Adapted from Dildy GA, Clark SL.: Postpartum hemorrhage. *Contemp Obstet Gynecol* 1993;38:21–29.

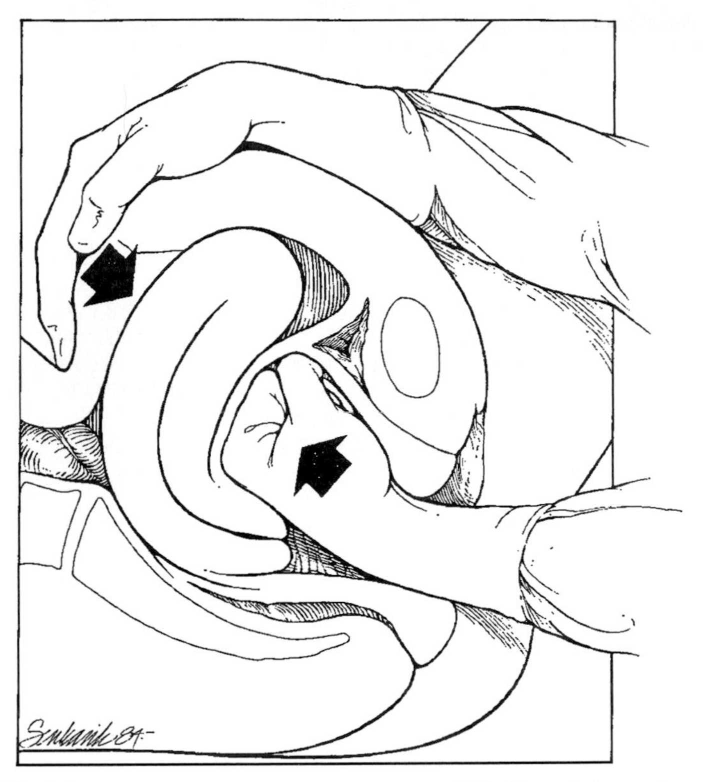

FIG. 3-3 Bimanual massage. (*Source: Benedetti TJ: Obstetric hemorrhage. In: Gabbe SG, Niebyl JR, Simpson JL (eds), Obstetrics: Normal and Problem Pregnancies, 3rd edn. New York: Churchill Livingstone, 1996; p. 499.*)

Intraoperative Management

Intraoperative management encompasses simple conservative techniques to hysterectomy. The main objective that a clinician must keep in mind when embarking upon an operative course is to proceed efficiently with those techniques that he or she finds simple and avoid those that are either technically difficult or excessively time consuming.

Along with concurrent drug therapy, uterine atony should initially be managed with gentle bimanual massage. Figure 3-3 demonstrates the proper technique for bimanual massage. Care must be taken to avoid aggressive massage that can injure the large vessels of the broad ligament.

If retained products of conception result in postpartum hemorrhage and manual extraction is unsuccessful, uterine curettage should be undertaken. While this may be performed in a delivery room, excessive bleeding mandates that an operating room be used for the procedure. Not only does moving the patient to the operating room remove potential distractions for efficient therapy, but it also allows for improved visualization, patient relaxation, ancillary support, and further operative management if the curettage is unsuccessful. A large Banjo curette should be employed with gentle traction in order to avoid uterine perforation. Transabdominal ultrasound guidance may be helpful in assisting the clinician with removal of retained placental fragments.

If uterine inversion is the source of bleeding, rapid replacement of the uterus to its proper orientation will resolve the hemorrhage. This is best accomplished in an operating room with the assistance of an anesthesiologist. The uterus and cervix should be initially relaxed with a tocolytic agent (e.g., magnesium sulfate, terbutaline), nitroglycerin, or a halogenated anesthetic. Once adequate relaxation is accomplished, gentle pressure should be applied to the uterine fundus in order to reinvert it back into its proper abdominal location. Once reinversion has occurred, uterotonic therapy should be given to assist with uterine contraction and prevent future inversion. On rare occasions, this conservative approach for uterine reinversion is unsuccessful and therefore surgical repair by laparotomy must be performed. The reader is referred to Benedetti[6] for further information on this topic.

When bleeding continues despite conservative therapy, surgical management via laparotomy must be performed. Interventions include arterial ligation, various uterine suturing techniques, packing, and hysterectomy.

The goal of arterial ligation is to decrease uterine perfusion and subsequent bleeding. Success rates have varied from 40 to 95 percent in published literature depending upon which arteries are ligated. Arterial ligation may be performed on the uterine and utero-ovarian vessels (Fig. 3-4) as well as the hypogastric arteries (Fig. 3-5). Hypogastric artery ligation can be technically challenging and is not recommended unless the obstetrician is extremely skilled in performing the procedure.

Uterine suturing techniques involve oversewing of a bleeding site, B-Lynch suture placement, and multiple square suturing. In cases of focal placental

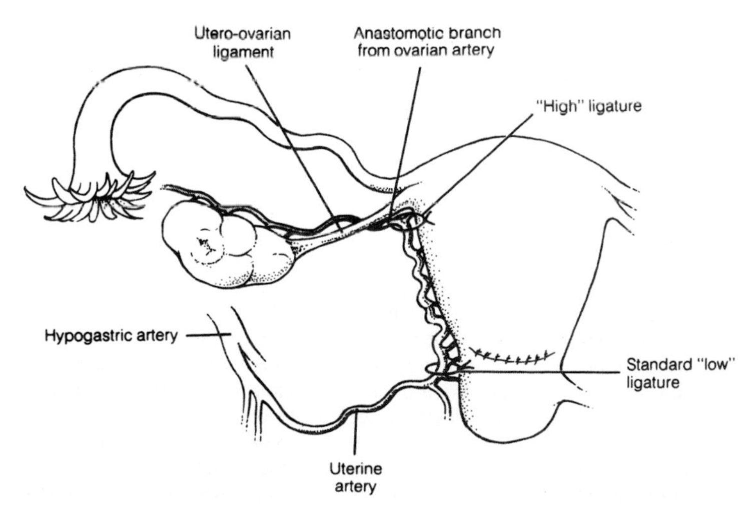

FIG. 3-4 Uterine artery ligation. (*Source: Clark SL, Koonings PP, Phelan JP: Placenta previa/accreta and prior cesarean section. Obstet Gynecol 1985;66:89–91.*)

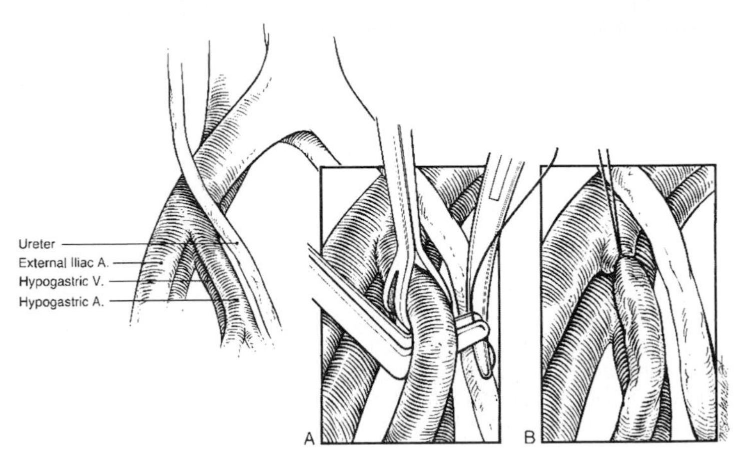

FIG. 3-5 Hypogastric artery ligation. (*Adapted from Breen J, Cregori CA, Kindzierski JA: Hemorrhage in gynecological surgery. Hagerstown, MD: Harper and Row, 1981; p. 438.*)

invasion and desire for future fertility, oversewing of the placental bed with absorbable suture may provide adequate hemostasis. If this technique fails or uterine atony remains a major bleeding source, consideration of a B-Lynch suture placement may be undertaken. In order to place a B-Lynch suture the patient should lie in a dorsal lithotomy position so that vaginal bleeding assessment can occur. A large absorbable suture is anchored within the uterine myometrium both anteriorly and posteriorly. It is passed in a continuous fashion around the external surface of the uterus and tied firmly so that adequate uterine compression occurs. Figure 3-6 demonstrates proper B-Lynch suture placement. In addition to the B-Lynch suture placement, a recent report demonstrated efficacy of multiple square sutures within the uterine wall to control hemorrhage. This technique involves the use of a large absorbable suture on a blunt straight needle. The needle is passed from the anterior to the posterior aspects of the uterus and back in the opposite directions to form a square. The suture is tied firmly to provide compression to the bleeding surfaces. Like the B-Lynch suture, this technique can be used for cases of invasive placentation and uterine atony.

Besides arterial ligation and uterine suturing techniques, packing of the uterus, vagina, and/or other bleeding surfaces remains an option for hemorrhage control. Packing provides a tamponade effect to the bleeding surfaces and allows time for replacement of clotting factors in situations involving coagulopathy. While techniques for packing vary, a few basic principles should be followed. The pack should be made of a long, continuous sterile gauze (e.g., Kerlex) rather than multiple small sponges. Placement of the gauze within a sterile plastic bag or glove can ease removal of the pack. Transurethral Foley catheter placement and prophylactic antibiotic use should be considered to prevent urinary retention and infection, respectively. Finally, prolonged packing should be avoided (not greater than 12 to 24 hours), and close attention to the patient's vital signs and hemoglobin/hematocrit should be paid while the pack is in place in order to minimize unrecognized ongoing bleeding.

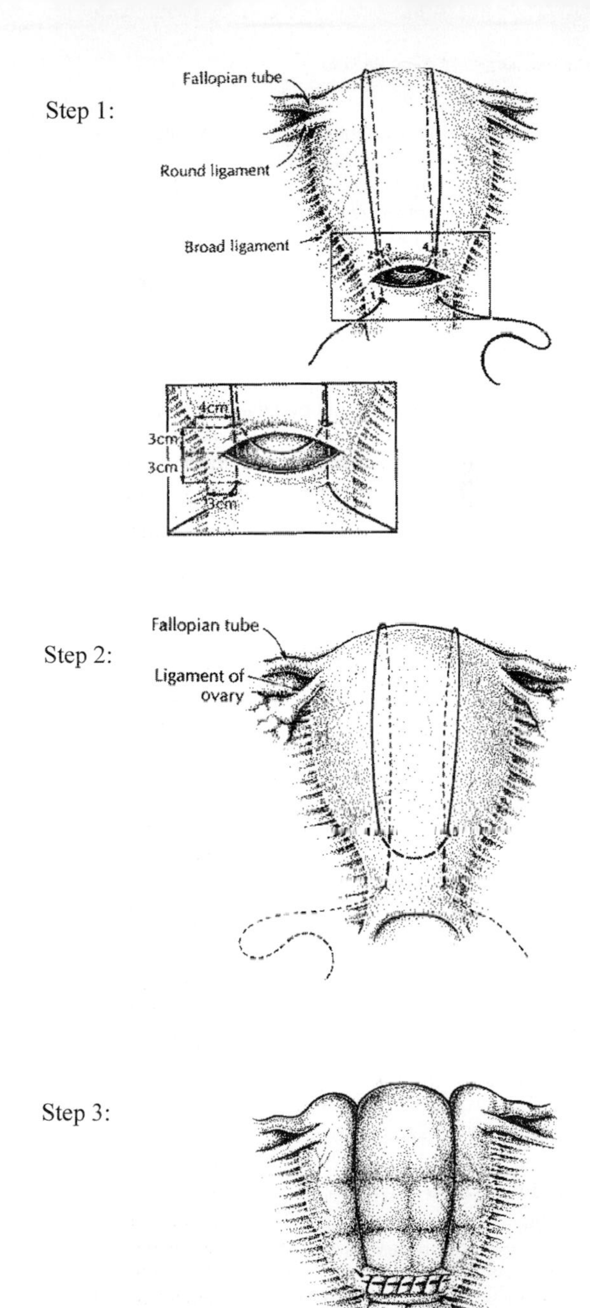

FIG. 3-6 B-Lynch suture. (*Source: B-Lynch C, Coker A, Lawal AH, et al. The B-Lynch surgical technique for control of massive postpartum hemorrhage: an alternative to hysterectomy? Five cases reported. Br J Obstet Gynecol 1997; 104:275–277.*)

The final surgical option available for postpartum hemorrhage is hysterectomy. Hysterectomy provides definitive therapy in cases of refractory bleeding. Since blood flow may be torrential, it is prudent for the clinician to consider performing a supracervical hysterectomy in some situations. This is especially important when the patient is unstable. Also, assistance from other surgical specialties may be necessary and a delay in consultation should be avoided.

Nonobstetrical Services

Nonobstetrical services that are particularly useful in postpartum hemorrhage management include interventional radiology and an intensive care team. In the past decade, the use of selective arterial embolization has gained success and popularity for postpartum hemorrhage management. The technique involves pelvic angiography to visualize the bleeding vessels and placement of Gelfoam (gelatin) pledgets into the vessels for occlusion.[15] Reported success rates have ranged from 85 to 95 percent.[16] Advantages to embolization include selectivity, uterine/fertility preservation, minimal morbidity, and ability to forego or delay surgical intervention. Reported disadvantages include postembolization fever, infection, ischemic pain, and tissue necrosis. In addition, a lack of rapid and widespread availability limits its usefulness.

In addition to interventional radiology, another nonobstetrical service that may be critical in successful postpartum hemorrhage management is an intensive care team. The patient who endures a severe postpartum hemorrhage is at risk of multiple comorbidities as noted in the following section. These comorbidities can often be avoided or dealt with more efficiently with the assistance of an intensive care team that is accustomed to the hemodynamic challenges of massive hemorrhage and transfusion.

General Complication Assessment

Once a postpartum hemorrhage has successfully been treated, the patient is still at risk of complications related to the blood loss, the therapy, or both. It is important for the obstetrician to critically assess the patient for general organ system complications. These complications include hypoperfusion injuries to the brain, heart, and kidneys, infection, coagulopathy, acute lung injury due to massive transfusion requirements, and pituitary necrosis. By being aware of these potential complications, the physician can ensure that proper posthemorrhage care and consultation is available in a timely fashion so that further morbidity can be avoided.

SUGGESTED READING

AbouZahr C, Royston E (eds): The global picture: the causes of maternal death. In: *Maternal Mortality: A Global Factbook.* Geneva: World Health Organization, 1991:7–11.

Baker R.: Hemorrhage in obstetrics. *Obstet Gynecol Annu* 1977;6:295.

Benedetti TJ. Obstetric hemorrhage. In: Gabbe SG, Niebyl JR, Simpson JL (eds), *Obstetrics: Normal and Problem Pregnancies*, 3rd edn. New York, Churchill Livingstone, 1996; p. 499.

B-Lynch C, Coker A, Lawal AH, et al.: The B-Lynch surgical technique for control of massive postpartum haemorrhage: an alternative to hysterectomy? Five cases reported. *Br J Obstet Gynaecol* 1997;104:275–277.

Bowes WA, Jr.: Clinical aspects of normal and abnormal labor. In: Creasy RK, Resnik R (eds). *Maternal-Fetal Medicine*, 4th edn. Philadelphia: W.B. Saunders, 1999; p. 541.

Brar HS, Greenspoon JS, Platt LD, et al.: Acute puerperal uterine inversion: new approaches to management. *J Reprod Med* 1989;34:173–177.

Cho JH, Jun HS, lee CN. Hemostatic suturing technique for uterine bleeding during cesarean delivery. *Obstet Gynecol* 2000;96:129–131.

Clark SL, Koonings PP, Phelan JP.: Placenta previa/accreta and prior cesarean section. *Obstet Gynecol* 1985;66:89–91.

Clark SL, Phelan JP.: Surgical control of obstetric hemorrhage. *Contemp Obstet Gynecol* 1984;24:70.

Combs CA, Murphy EL, Laros RK Jr.: Factors associated with hemorrhage in cesarean deliveries. *Obstet Gynecol* 1991;77:77–82.

Combs CA, Murphy EL, Laros RK, Jr.: Factors associated with postpartum hemorrhage with vaginal birth. *Obstet Gynecol* 1991;77:69–76.

Dildy GA, Clark SL.: Postpartum hemorrhage. *Contemp Obstet Gynecol* 1993;38:21–29.

Fuchs K, Peretz BA, Marcovici R, et al.: The "grand multipara"—is it a problem? A review of 5785 cases. *Int J Gynaecol Obstet* 1985;23;321–325.

Mousa HA, Walkinshaw S.: Major postpartum haemorrhage. *Curr Opin Obstet Gynecol* 2001;13:595–603.

Pahlavan P, Nezhat C.: Hemorrhage in obstetrics and gynecology. *Curr Opin Obstet Gynecol* 2001;13:419–424.

Pritchard JA, Baldwin RM, Dickey JC, et al.: Blood volume changes in pregnancy and the puerperium. II. Red blood cell loss and changes in apparent blood volume during and following vaginal delivery, cesarean section, and cesarean section plus total hysterectomy. *Am J Obstet Gynecol* 1962;84:1271–1282.

4 Disseminated Intravascular Coagulopathy and Thrombocytopenia Complicating Pregnancy: An Acute Care Approach

Philip Samuels

INTRODUCTION

Although uncommon, significant hemorrhage, coagulopathy and need for transfusion are encountered by every practicing obstetrician. Prevention is obviously superior to treatment. By understanding the pathophysiology and events that lead to these potentially catastrophic clinical situations, we can often prevent them from becoming critical situations. Even with meticulous care, we cannot prevent all such cases. Rapid, decisive, and knowledgeable action on the part of the obstetrician can usually avert a poor outcome. In this chapter, I cover the areas of clinical disseminated intravascular coagulopathy (DIC) and clinically significant thrombocytopenia. The best form of therapy is aimed at correcting the underlying pathophysiologic problem, as well as treating the acquired or inherent clotting problem. There are many ways to treat these clinical entities. This chapter outlines a practical approach to these patients.

DISSEMINATED INTRAVASCULAR COAGULOPATHY

Disseminated intravascular coagulopathy (DIC) describes a clinical scenario, but not a specific entity. It is characterized by accelerated formation of fibrin clots and breakdown of these same clots. It is, indeed, a consumptive coagulopathy. The body consumes clotting factors faster than they can be produced. Normally, our body is in a constant balance between fibrin generation and fibrinolysis. When this delicate balance is disturbed and the coagulation cascade and fibrinolytic systems go unchecked, DIC can result. DIC may arise from massive activation of the coagulation system that overwhelms control mechanisms. Also, DIC may be initiated by exposure of blood to tissue factor, which triggers the extrinsic clotting system. This may be the result of trauma or endotoxins damaging tissue. Also proteolytic enzyme release may trigger DIC and can occur in events such as placental abruption. This critical clinical picture, in other words, can have many etiologies. One must rapidly determine the etiology while initiating therapy.

Etiology

The most common obstetric causes of DIC are listed in Table 4-1. The most common underlying cause of mild DIC encountered by the obstetrician is probably underestimation of blood loss at the time of delivery with inadequate

TABLE 4-1 Causes of DIC

Common causes
- Massive hemorrhage, especially with adequate fluid replacement with crystalloid or colloid
- Placental abruption
- Severe preeclampsia/HELLP *NOT* isolated thrombocytopenia

Rare causes
- Sepsis
- Acute fatty liver of pregnancy
- Amniotic fluid embolus
- Adult respiratory distress syndrome
- Acute hemolytic transfusion reaction
- Autoimmune disease
- Malignancies
- Retained dead fetus

replacement by crystalloid or colloid. In these cases, vasospasm occurs with resultant endothelial damage and initiation of DIC. Also, in these instances, hypotension occurs which results in decreased tissue perfusion leading to local hypoxia and tissue acidosis, which can further exacerbate DIC by causing tissue release of cytokines. By keeping the patient's volume replete, DIC can often be avoided, even in the presence of profound anemia.

Following placental separation after a vaginal delivery, fibrinogen is activated to become a fibrin mesh, which covers the old placental site. This results in a 10 percent reduction in the concentration of clotable fibrinogen following a normal vaginal delivery. Placental abruption is a similar situation gone awry. In severe cases, the placenta partially detaches from the wall of the uterus and a retroplacental clot forms. As the clot expands, it consumes coagulation factors, which continually breakdown and this results in a consumptive coagulopathy. In these cases, the earliest laboratory sign of DIC is a significant fall in fibrinogen. It is important to note that the concentration of clotable fibrinogen is usually greatly increased during a normal pregnancy. Therefore, the clinician should not be lulled into a false sense of security when the fibrinogen concentration is normal. A low-normal fibrinogen concentration may actually be a huge drop for the individual patient, representing early DIC.

Severe preeclampsia and HELLP syndrome can result in DIC if delivery is not effected promptly. Often these patients show isolated thrombocytopenia, which should not be confused with DIC in the absence of clinical bleeding or other coagulation abnormalities. This isolated thrombocytopenia is due to increased platelet destruction by the reticuloendothelial system, and is not a consumptive coagulopathy. Clinical DIC in these cases is uncommon, unless the preeclampsia/HELLP is prolonged. Laboratory evidence of subclinical DIC, nevertheless, is common in preeclamptics.

There is a common misconception that a retained dead fetus commonly results in DIC. This only rarely occurs and usually takes several weeks to develop. With effective cervical ripening agents, there is no reason to expectantly manage the intrauterine demise for extended periods. If, however, an unsuspected demise is discovered and it appears that the fetus expired some time previously, a coagulation profile would be indicated.

Sepsis, for any reason, can be associated with DIC. Obviously, any infection should be treated aggressively with antibiotics. New medications such as

TABLE 4-2 Diagnosis DIC

Clinical
- Bleeding from venipuncture and IV sites, incision sites, mucous membranes
- Profuse vaginal bleeding (postpartum and firm uterus)
- Associated shock (may be out of proportion to observed blood loss)

Laboratory studies
- Decreased fibrinogen
- Increased fibrin degradation products
- Increased D-dimer
- Prolonged prothrombin time/INR
- Prolonged aPTT (occasionally)
- Decreased antithrombin III
- Falling hemoglobin/hematocrit
- Rising LDH
- Rising bilirubin
- Examination of peripheral smear for schistocystes
- Nonclotting tube of blood

drotrecogin alfa can greatly reduce mortality and DIC in sepsis. There is no experience, however, with the use of this medication in pregnancy.

Diagnosis of DIC

The presumptive diagnosis of DIC is usually made clinically, with confirmation made through laboratory studies. Table 4-2 shows readily available diagnostic tests. Other research-based tests are available, but are not readily accessible to the clinician at the bedside. In obstetrics, a falling fibrinogen concentration is usually the hallmark of DIC. It is important to remember that the prothrombin time (PT) is affected by disorders of the extrinsic clotting system (Factors II, VII, IX, X). The PT will often become prolonged before there is prolongation of the activated partial thromboplastin time (aPTT) in DIC. This is because the aPTT depends upon the intrinsic clotting system, which includes Factor VIII. Not only does Factor VIII normally increase during pregnancy, but it also increases early in the course of DIC, secondary to a release of Factor VIII/vonWillebrand's factor, from damaged endothelial cells. However, as the DIC becomes overwhelming, the aPTT will also become prolonged. Tests of fibrin degradation such as fibrin degradation products and d-dimer will also be elevated. However, in normal pregnancy, one can often find mildly elevated levels of these tests.

Treatment

The basic treatment for DIC is to reverse the inciting event. Simultaneously while correcting the inciting event, blood component therapy should also be initiated if needed. Therapies are outlined in Tables 4-3 and 4-4. It is crucial to realize that treatment is not linear in time, but that several forms of therapy should be occurring simultaneously. Therefore, if possible, two intravenous lines should be established and a Foley catheter should be in place. Aggressive fluid resuscitation can be accomplished while blood component therapy is given. In addition to the modalities listed in Table 4-4, it is important to note that vitamin K and folate should be administered, as patients with DIC often develop deficiencies in these vitamins. There is some evidence that antithrombin III concentrate may promote endothelial healing and decrease

TABLE 4-3 Treatment of DIC in Pregnancy

Treat inciting event

- Massive hemorrhage
  - Treat cause (uterotonic agents, repair lacerations,)
- Placental abruption
  - Delivery
    - Attempt vaginal delivery if fetus and mother stable
- Preeclampsia/HELLP
  - Delivery
- Acute fatty liver
  - Delivery
- Amniotic fluid embolus
  - Cardiovascular support
  - Steroids
- Sepsis
  - Broad spectrum intravenous antibiotics
- Adult respiratory distress syndrome
  - Ventilatory support
  - Cardiovascular support
- Retained dead fetus
  - Delivery
  - (Consider) antibiotics

Blood component therapy

- See Table 4-4

TABLE 4-4 Blood Component Therapy for DIC in Pregnancy

Fresh frozen plasma (FFP) (volume = 250 cc)

- Used to correct PT, aPTT, and fibrinogen. Usually use as 4 units initially and then use more as needed
- Use for clinical hemorrhage, if INR ≥ 2 with bleeding, if aPTT prolonged with bleeding
- Each unit of FFP increases the circulatory fibrinogen 5–10 mg/dL

Cryprecipitate (volume = 35–40 cc)

- Rich in fibrinogen and used to raise fibrinogen utilizing less volume than fresh frozen plasma
- Administer when fibrinogen <100 mg/dL or if clinical hemorrhage and fibrinogen <150 mg/dL
- Each unit of cryoprecipitate increases the circulatory fibrinogen 5–10 mg/dL

Platelets

- Transfuse if maternal platelets <20,000/mm^3 whether or not clinical bleeding
- Transfuse if maternal platelets <50,000/mm^3 in the presence of hemorrhage
- Each pack of pooled platelets increases the platelet count by 7,000–10,000/mm^3. In DIC, transfused platelets are consumed rapidly

Packed RBCs

- Increase oxygen carrying capacity (a primary priority)
- Transfuse rapidly to keep up with clinical bleeding, and try to keep hematocrit ≥25%
- Follow electrolytes as hemolysis and RBC transfusion can lead to elevated serum potassium.
- Give one ampule of calcium after each five units of packed RBCs since the anticoagulant in the packed units can chelate circulatory calcium.

fibrinolytic activity. Also, the fluid status (intake and output) must be monitored closely. It is very easy to underestimate blood loss or underestimate the volume of crystalloid/blood components administered. It is crucial to keep meticulous track of this. If the patient is not given enough volume, she could develop acute renal failure. Conversely, if an overabundance of fluid is administered, the patient can develop fluid overload and pulmonary edema.

THROMBOCYTOPENIA

Etiology

Thrombocytopenia (a platelet count <150,000/mm^3) coincides with approximately 4 percent of pregnancies and is the most common reason for hematology consultation during gestation. Before diagnosing thrombocytopenia, the obstetrician must make certain that the patient does not have a platelet clumping disorder, which can give a spurious impression of thrombocytopenia. In three per 1000 individuals, platelets will clump in EDTA, the diluent in lavender-topped tubes used to analyze complete blood counts (CBC). In this process, platelets clump together so that many platelets are counted as a single platelet in the automatic counters. Examination of a peripheral smear as well as checking a platelet count in a blue-topped tube, containing citrate, can distinguish this from true thrombocytopenia. Those with a clumping disorder are not truly thrombocytopenic and are not at risk for bleeding. This work-up is shown in Fig. 4-1. The causes for thrombocytopenia encountered during pregnancy are listed in Table 4-5.

The most common cause for true thrombocytopenia accompanying pregnancy is gestational thrombocytopenia. This disorder occurs in about

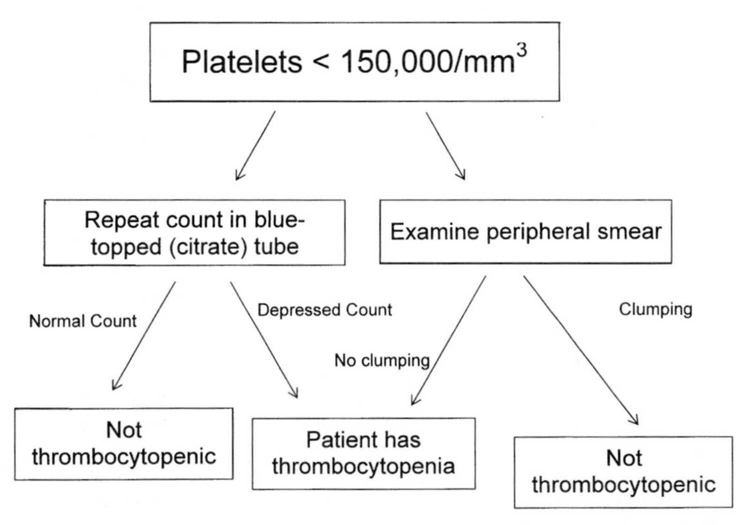

FIG. 4-1 The method for deciding whether a patient has true thrombocytopenia or a platelet clumping disorder which affects approximately three per 1000 individuals. Platelet clumping is an *in vitro* process and causes a spuriously low platelet count which may result in unnecessary anxiety, work-up, and treatment.

TABLE 4-5 Causes of Thrombocytopenia during Pregnancy

Major causes
1. Gestational thrombocytopenia
2. Severe preeclampsia
3. HELLP syndrome
4. Disseminated intravascular coagulopathy
5. Platelet clumping (spurious)

Uncommon causes
1. Immune thrombocytopenic purpura
2. Human immunodeficiency virus
3. Lupus inhibitor and antiphospholipid antibody syndrome
4. Systemic lupus erythematosus

Rare causes
1. Thrombotic thrombycytopenic purpura
2. Hemolytic uremic syndrome
3. Type IIB von Willebrand's disease
4. Hematologic malignancies
5. Folic acid deficiency
6. May-Heglin syndrome (congenital thrombocytopenia)

3 percent of pregnancies and is more frequent than all other causes of thrombocytopenia combined. It is generally characterized by mild, progressive thrombocytopenia detected incidentally on a routine CBC. Any invasive work-up or treatment for gestational thrombocytopenia may lead to more misadventure for the patient than the disease itself. To make this diagnosis, the patient must have no history of a bleeding diathesis outside of pregnancy. In general the platelet count should be >50,000/mm^3 and there should be no evidence of platelet clumping. Fewer than 1 percent of pregnant women have a platelet count below 100,000/mm^3. Therefore, the lower the maternal platelet count, the more likely the woman has an ongoing pathologic process. Pregnant women with a platelet count between 50,000/mm^3 and 100,000/mm^3 probably do not have a significant pathologic process. Platelet counts <100,000/mm^3 are infrequent, however, I feel these patients deserve a thorough evaluation. This point is illustrated in Fig. 4-2. Clearly, those with platelet counts <50,000/mm^3 must be evaluated by a hematologist or internist with a special interest in hematology.

Immune thrombocytopenic purpura (ITP) is an autoimmune disorder that results in increased platelet destruction by the reticuloendothelial system. This disorder complicates approximately three per 1000 pregnancies. There are two types of ITP, although they are rarely distinguished by physicians other than hematologists. Childhood ITP and adult-onset ITP have very different natural histories, and no observations have been made to ascertain whether or not they behave the same during pregnancy with regard to maternal and fetal/neonatal course. Childhood ITP, which also affects adolescents, usually follows an acute infection. It is characterized by an acute onset and has a rapid remission and rare relapses. Adult-onset ITP, conversely, is a chronic disorder that usually requires long-term steroid or immune globulin therapy and has frequent exacerbations and remissions.

Because it is an autoimmune disease, ITP is diagnosed in the laboratory by platelet antibody testing. The methodology of this testing is not uniform, so sensitivity and specificity vary with the laboratory used. Furthermore, traditional antibody testing cannot distinguish ITP from gestational thrombocytopenia.

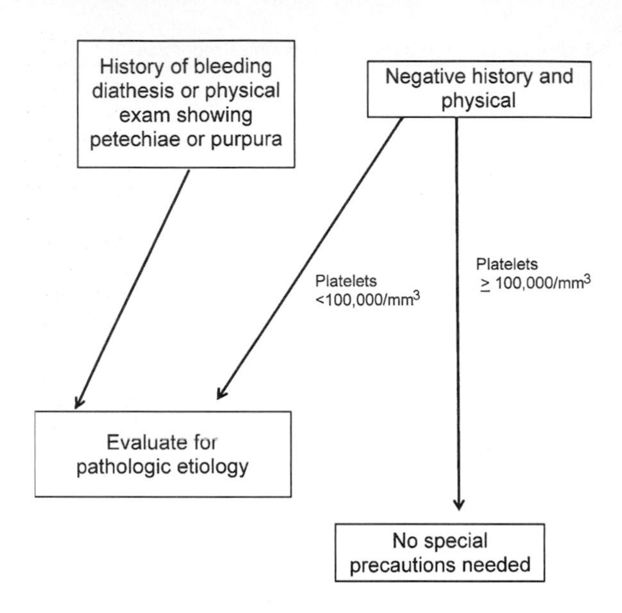

*After ruling out platelet clumping (Fig. 4-1)

FIG. 4-2 Evaluation of the patient after a diagnosis of thrombocytopenia has been established (Initial Evaluation of Thrombocytopenia* During Pregnancy).

During pregnancy, history and physical examination are more important than laboratory testing to distinguish the two disorders. Platelet antibodies can be platelet-associated (direct, platelet-bound) or circulating (free, indirect, serum). Unfortunately, neither of these antibody classes can be used to distinguish ITP from gestational thrombocytopenia. Circulating (indirect) antiplatelet antibodies have been associated with neonatal thrombocytopenia in women with ITP. In fact, 13 to 24 percent of women with true ITP will give birth to infants with platelet counts $<50{,}000/mm^3$. The presence of circulating antiplatelet IgG in the maternal serum can serve as a rough indicator that the pregnant woman is at risk of giving birth to a child with profound thrombocytopenia. The presence of these antibodies is only a rough indicator because their negative predictive value is excellent, but their positive predictive value is poor. This means that if these antibodies are absent, it is highly unlikely that the neonate will have a profoundly depressed platelet count at birth. The presence of these antibodies, however, indicates a risk, but not a high likelihood. Again, it is important to stress that the methodology of this testing varies between laboratories, and it is therefore safe to assume that the predictive values of these tests in predicting neonatal thrombocytopenia will also vary.

Most physicians feel that vaginal delivery is acceptable even in the case of an infant with an extremely low platelet count. Therefore, cordocentesis and scalp sampling for platelet count have fallen from favor in these patients. Nonetheless,

TABLE 4-6 Classic Findings in Thrombotic Thrombocytopenic Purpura[a]

- Microangiopathic, hemolytic anemia[b]
- Thrombocytopenia[b]
- Neurologic abnormalities[b]
  - Confusion
  - Headache
  - Paresis
  - Visual hallucinations
  - Seizures
- Fever
- Renal dysfunction

[a]The classic pentad is found in 40% of patients
[b]This triad is present in 75% of patients

I feel it is useful to know which patients are at risk of delivering a profoundly thrombocytopenic neonate. Therefore, I do look for circulating anitplatelet IgG in pregnant patients with true ITP. If present, I avoid operative vaginal delivery, and try to avoid scalp electrodes if possible. Furthermore, I am reticent about allowing these patients to have a prolonged second stage of labor. In any case of ITP, I notify the pediatric team so a neonatal platelet count can be obtained.

Thrombotic thrombocytopenic purpura (TTP) is a rare disorder, but one that must be considered when a pregnant patient's platelet count is severely depressed. Clinical ramifications are severe, and the disease is life-threatening. Pathologically, platelets aggregate, producing platelet thrombi that occlude arterioles and capillaries. This can produce ischemia and infarction in any organ system. It frequently affects those systems most dependent on microcirculation such as the brain and kidneys. The cause of TTP remains elusive, but probably includes the arachadonic acid/prostaglandin pathway as well as plasminogen and its activators.

TTP is a clinical diagnosis, and the disorder is characterized by a pentad of findings (Table 4-6). The classic pentad of signs/symptoms occurs in only about 40 percent of patients, whereas approximately 75 percent of patients experience the triad of microangiopathic hemolytic anemia, thrombocytopenia, and neurologic changes. When TTP occurs during pregnancy, it usually occurs antepartum, and possibly during the second trimester. It may be confused with HELLP (hemolysis, elevated liver transaminases, low platelets) syndrome. The degree of microangiopathic anemia is more severe in TTP and is usually readily evident on the peripheral smear. Occasionally a depressed antithrombin III level will be seen in HELLP syndrome and aid in the distinction between the two disorders. TTP is usually nonrecurring, but intermittent and chronic relapsing forms do exist, though rarely. See Chapter 15 for a more detailed discussion on this disorder and differential diagnosis.

Treatment

When does ITP require therapy? Spontaneous bleeding usually does not occur until the platelet count falls to around 20,000/mm^3, and surgical bleeding does not occur until the platelet count falls to about 50,000/mm^3. Many hematologists, therefore, do not empirically treat a patient until the platelet count approaches 20,000/mm^3 unless there is clinical bleeding. The commonly used modalities for treating ITP when it exacerbates during pregnancy

TABLE 4-7 Treatment Modalities for ITP During Pregnancy

Glucocorticoids
- Intravenous
  - Methylprednisolone 1.0–1.5 mg/kg daily in two or three divided doses
  - Prednisone 1.0 mg/kg/day
    - Then taper

Intravenous immunoglobulin
- 0.4–1.0 g/kg/day for 3–5 days
- May be repeated

Splenectomy
- Best carried out in second trimester

Platelet transfusion
- Reserved for severe active bleeding
- May cause more rapid platelet destruction
- Each unit of platelets raising count about 7,000–10,000/mm^3

are listed in Table 4-7. Glucocorticoid administration remains the initial line of therapy. If rapid response is needed, intravenous methylprenisolone is used. It has an advantage over hydrocortisone as it has much less mineralocortoicoid effect. Usually 1.0 to 1.5 mg/kg *total body weight* of methylprednisolone is administered daily in two or three divided doses. An initial response is usually seen within two days, but in refractory cases, it may take as long as 10 days to see a maximum response. After the anticipated response is obtained, the patient should be switched to oral prednisone and the dose should be tapered to keep the platelet count around 100,000/mm^3. If it is not emergent, therapy can be initiated with oral prednisone on an outpatient basis. The usual starting dose is 1 mg/kg *total body weight*/day in a single dose. One must watch for ulcer formation when large doses are administered over extended periods. After an appropriate response, tapering should be accomplished as previously mentioned. Approximately 70 percent of patients respond to glucocorticoid therapy. In order to avoid adrenal crisis, it is important not to wean off prednisone too quickly if the patient has been on glucocorticoids for over two weeks. Tips for tapering steroids are given in Table 4-8.

TABLE 4-8 Tips for Tapering Steroids

Tapering must be individualized and patients must be observed for symptoms
- Parameters that must be taken into account when tapering glucocorticoids in order to prevent adrenal crisis
- Age
  - Patients over 40 must be weaned very slowly
- Duration of therapy
  - No tapering needed for less than 1 week of therapy
  - Rapid tapering if 1–2 weeks of therapy
  - Slow taper if >2 weeks of therapy
- Dosage of prednisone used
  - Taper rapidly to 40 mg/day
  - Taper from 40 to 20 mg/day over several days
  - Taper from 20 mg/day to none over an extended period of 2–4 weeks, especially if duration of therapy has been >2 weeks

For pregnant patients who fail to respond to glucocorticoids, intravenous immunoglobulin (IVIG) should be administered. The usual dose is 0.4 to 1.0 gm/kg/day for three to five days. Occasionally, a higher dose will be required. The response usually begins in 2 to 3 days and usually peaks at about 5 days. This, however, is variable. The duration of response is variable, so if IVIG is being administered to raise the maternal platelet count before delivery, proper timing is essential. In general, if an adequate platelet count is needed for delivery, the course of therapy should be started five to eight days before the planned induction or cesarean delivery.

If there is inadequate response to IVIG, splenectomy can be performed safely during gestation. The best time for any type of surgery during pregnancy is during the second trimester. This is before the uterus enlarges enough to interfere with surgical exposure and before the risk of preterm labor rises. Splenectomy can be accomplished at the time of cesarean delivery if necessary, by extending a midline skin incision cephalad after uterine closure.

Platelet transfusion is indicated only for the profoundly thrombocytopenic patient who is experiencing clinically significant bleeding. The transfusions are given while awaiting the effect of other therapies or while preparing the patient for immediate surgery. Some advocate giving platelets at the time of surgery if the platelet count is <50,000/mm^3. At the very least, platelets should be available in the operating room for these patients. The same tenet holds for vaginal delivery in the patient with a platelet count approaching 20,000/mm^3. The viability of transfused platelets is extremely short because the same antibodies and reticuloendothelial cell clearance that affect the mother's endogenous platelets also destroy and sequester the transfused platelets. If a platelet transfusion is needed for surgery, therefore, it should be started at the time of the skin incision and not earlier. Each unit of platelets will increase the maternal platelet count by about 10,000/mm^3. A scheme for treating maternal ITP is outlined in Fig. 4-3. Certain technical surgical precautions should be taken when performing a cesarean delivery on a patient with severe thrombocytopenia or any other bleeding diathesis. These precautions are listed in Table 4-9.

Intensive plasma manipulation is the key for treating TTP. Therapy usually entails a combination of plasmapheresis and plasma exchange with platelet-poor fresh-frozen plasma (FFP, 3 to 4 L/day). Plasmapheresis removes

TABLE 4-9 Surgical Tips for Performing a Cesarean Delivery on a Patient with a Bleeding Diathesis

1. Use a midline incision if there is clinically significant bleeding. Otherwise a Pfannenstiel incision is acceptable
2. Use electrocautery liberally, especially in opening the subcutaneous tissue
3. Close the uterus meticulously from the start. The more needle holes you put in the uterus, the more it will bleed
4. Leave the bladder flap open to prevent hematoma formation that could later lead to abscess. Cauterize the edge of the bladder flap if necessary
5. Close the peritoneum in order to prevent bleeding from the edges. This also prevents subfascial bleeding from filling the peritoneal cavity and allows placement of subfascial drains
6. Place subfascial drains and leave them in place until they stop draining
7. Use skin staples, even in Pfannenstiel incisions. This allows partial opening of the incision if a subcutaneous hematoma or seroma forms
8. Place a pressure dressing over the incision and leave it in place until the danger of bleeding subsides.

platelet-aggregating substances, and plasma infusion provides some antiaggregating products that are deficient in the patient's plasma. If exchange plasmapheresis is not readily available, infusion of FFP (30 mL/kg/day) can be used as a temporizing measure. If this is done, the treating physician must be careful to watch for signs of volume overload and administer diuretics if necessary. If a patient responds to plasmapheresis, this procedure should be continued for at least five days. In patients who exhibit a partial response without clinical deterioration, plasmapheresis and plasma exchange should be continued for 3 to 4 weeks to achieve complete remission. Also, packed RBCs should be administered to keep the hemoglobin at an acceptable concentration.

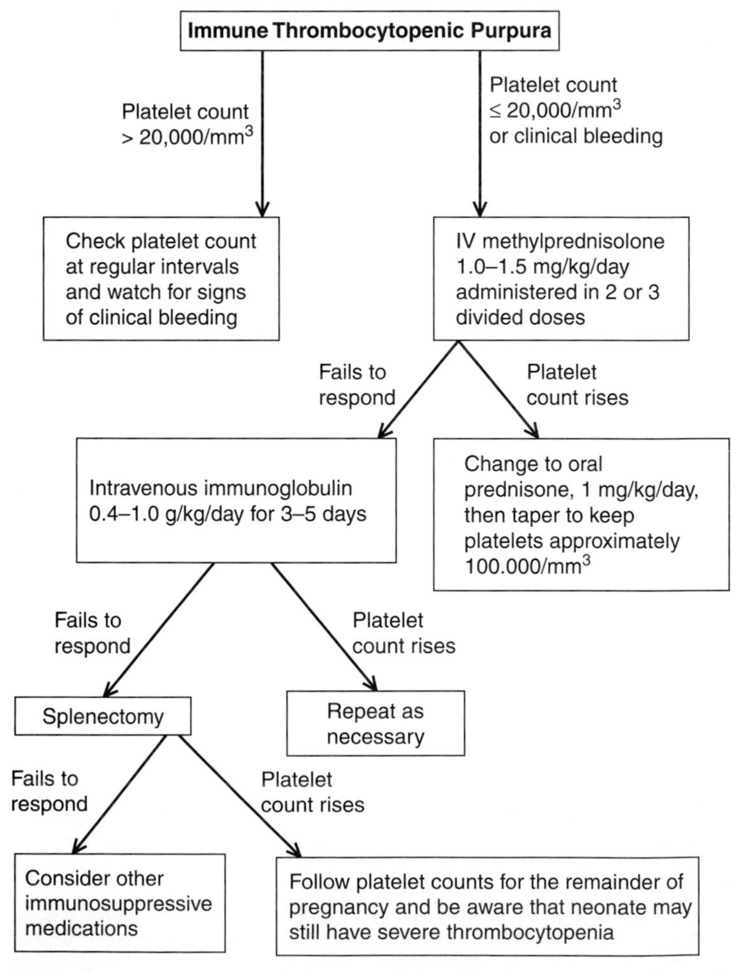

FIG. 4-3 Management of the pregnant woman with immune thrombocytopenic purpura.

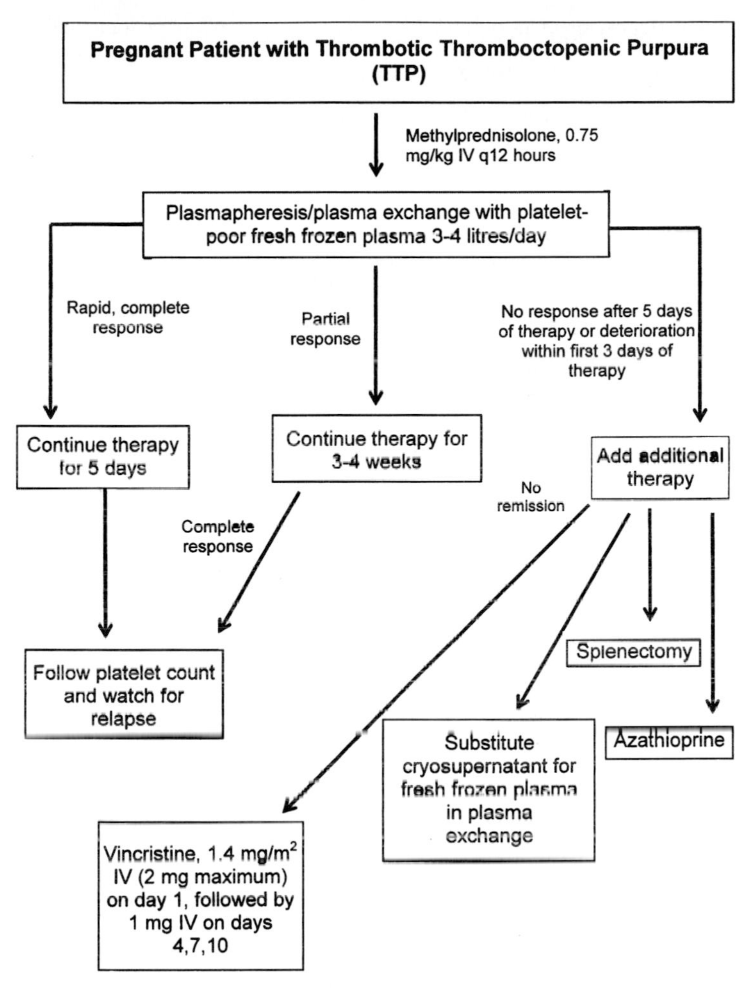

FIG. 4-4 Management of the gravida with TTP. Before adopting this approach, the treating physician must be certain of the diagnosis. TTP is a clinical diagnosis and can mimic severe preeclampsia. The criteria for diagnosing TTP are listed in Table 4-6.

Glucocortoicoids should be administered to all patients with TTP immediately after diagnosis. The usual dose is 0.75 mg/kg of intravenous methylprednisolone every 12 hours until the patient recovers. Then slow tapering should be performed.

If a patient does not begin to respond within five days of therapy, or if her condition deteriorates within the first three days, other therapies should be considered including vincristine, azathioprine, and splenectomy. In refractory cases, cryosupernatant may be substituted for FFP in the plasma exchange protocol. Treatment of the pregnant patient with TTP is outlined in Fig. 4-4.

SUGGESTED READING

Aster RH: Gestational thrombocytopenia. A plea for conservative management. *N Engl J Med* 1990;323:264.

Burrows RF, Kelton JG: Low fetal risks in pregnancies associated with idiopathic thrombocytopenic purpura. *Am J Obstet Gynecol* 1990;164:1147.

Burrows RF, Kelton JG: Fetal thrombocytopenia and its relation to maternal thrombocytopenia. *N Engl J Med* 1993;329:1463.

Cines DB, Dusak B, Tomaski A, et al.: Immune thrombocytopenic purpura and pregnancy. *N Engl J Med* 1982;306:826.

Gabbe SG, Neibyl JR, Simpson JL (eds), *Obstetrics: Normal and Problem Pregnancies,* 4th edn. New York: Churchill Livingstone, 2002;pp.1169–1176.

Hoffman R, Benz EJ, Jr, Shattil SJ, et al. (eds), *Hematology: Basic Principles and Practice.* New York: Churchill Livingstone, 1991;pp.1394–1405.

Hoffman R, Benz EJ, Jr. Shattil SJ, et al. (eds), *Hematology: Basic Principles and Practice.* New York: Churchill Livingstone, 1991;pp.1495–1500.

McCrae KR, Samuels P, Schreiber AD: Pregnancy-associated thrombocytopenia: pathogenesis and management. *Blood* 1992;80:2697.

Repke JT (ed), *Intrapartum Obstetrics.* New York: Churchill Livingstone, 1996; pp. 431–446.

Rousell RH, Good RA, Pirofsky B, et al.: Non-A non-B hepatitis and the safety of intravenous immunoglobulin pH 4.25; *A retrospective survey.* Vox sang 1988;54:6.

Samuels P, Bussel JB, Braitman LE, et al.: Estimation of the risk of thrombocytopenia in the offspring of pregnant women with presumed immune thrombocytopenic purpura. *N Engl J Med* 1990;323:229.

Weiner CP: Thrombotic microangiopathy in pregnancy and the postpartum period. *Semin Hematol* 1987;24:119.

5 Hypertensive Emergencies

Kristin H. Coppage   Baha M. Sibai

INTRODUCTION

Hypertensive disorders are the most common medical complications of pregnancy, affecting 5 to 10 percent of all pregnancies. Approximately 30 percent of hypertensive disorders in pregnancy are due to chronic hypertension and 70 percent are due to gestational hypertension-preeclampsia. The spectrum of the disease ranges from mildly elevated blood pressures with minimal clinical significance, to severe hypertension and multiorgan dysfunction. Understanding the disease process and its impact on pregnancy is of utmost importance, as hypertensive disorders remain a major cause of maternal and perinatal morbidity and mortality worldwide (Table 5-1).

DEFINITIONS AND CLASSIFICATIONS

Hypertension is defined as a systolic blood pressure ≥140 mmHg or a diastolic blood pressure ≥90 mmHg. These measurements must be made on at least two occasions, no less than 6 hours and no more than a week apart. It is important to note that choosing the appropriate cuff size will help to eliminate inaccurate blood pressure measurements. Abnormal proteinuria in pregnancy is defined as the excretion of ≥300 mg of protein in 24 hours. The most accurate measurement of total urinary excretion of protein is with the use of a 24-hour urine collection. However, in certain instances the use of semiquantitative dipstick analysis may be the only measurement available to assess urinary protein. Table 5-2 lists the classification of hypertension.

Gestational Hypertension

Gestational hypertension is the elevation of blood pressure during the second half of pregnancy or in the first 24 hours postpartum, without proteinuria and without symptoms. Normalization of blood pressure occurs in the postpartum period, usually within 10 days. Treatment is generally not warranted since most patients will have mild hypertension. Gestational hypertension in and of itself has little effect on maternal or perinatal morbidity or mortality. However, approximately 46 percent of patients diagnosed with preterm gestational hypertension will develop preeclampsia. Those with severe gestational hypertension are at risk for adverse maternal and perinatal outcomes and should be managed like those with severe preeclampsia. If a woman with gestational hypertension receives antihypertensive therapy, she should be considered to have severe disease. Therefore, antihypertensive drugs should not be used during ambulatory management of these women.

Preeclampsia and Eclampsia

The classic triad of hypertension, proteinuria and symptoms defines the syndrome of preeclampsia. Symptoms of preeclampsia include headache, visual changes, epigastric or right upper quadrant pain, and shortness of breath.

TABLE 5-1 Adverse Outcomes in Severe Hypertensive Disorders of Pregnancy

Maternal complications
- Abruptio placentae
- Disseminated intravascular coagulopathy
- Eclampsia
- Renal failure
- Liver hemorrhage or failure
- Intracerebral hemorrhage
- Hypertensive encephalopathy
- Pulmonary edema
- Death

Fetal-Neonatal complications
- Severe intrauterine growth retardation
- Oligohydramnios
- Preterm delivery
- Hypoxia-acidosis
- Neurologic injury
- Death

Preeclampsia may be subdivided into mild and severe forms. The distinction between the two is based on the severity of hypertension and proteinuria as well as the involvement of other organ systems (Table 5-2). Close surveillance of patients with preeclampsia is warranted, as either type may progress to fulminant disease. Therefore, all women with suspected or diagnosed

TABLE 5-2 Classification

I. Gestational hypertension
   Mild
   - Systolic < 160 mmHg or
   - Diastolic < 110 mmHg
   Severe
   - Systolic ≥ 160 mmHg or
   - Diastolic ≥110 mmHg

II. Gestational proteinuria
   Mild (≤1 + on dipstick and <5 g/24 h)
   Severe (≥5 g/24 h)

III. Preeclampsia (hypertension + proteinuria)
   Onset >20 weeks' gestation
   Mild
   - Mild hypertension and mild proteinuria
   Severe
   - Severe hypertension and proteinuria
   - Mild hypertension and severe proteinuria
   - Persistently severe cerebral symptoms
   - Thrombocytopenia
   - Pulmonary edema
   - Oliguria (<500 mL/24 h)

IV. Chronic hypertension
   Hypertension before pregnancy
   Hypertension before 20 weeks' gestation

V. Superimposed preeclampsia
   Exacerbation of hypertension and/or new-onset proteinuria

preeclampsia should be instructed to immediately report any of the symptoms listed below:

- Nausea and vomiting
- Persistent, severe headache
- Right upper quadrant or epigastric pain
- Scotomata
- Blurred vision
- Decreased fetal movement
- Rupture of membranes
- Vaginal bleeding
- Regular uterine contractions

A particularly severe form of preeclampsia is HELLP syndrome, which is an acronym for hemolysis (H), elevated liver enzymes (EL), and low platelet count (LP). The diagnosis may be deceptive because blood pressure measurements may be only marginally elevated. A patient diagnosed with HELLP syndrome is automatically classified as having severe preeclampsia. Another severe form of preeclampsia is eclampsia, which is the occurrence of seizures not attributable to other causes.

Chronic Hypertension

Hypertension complicating pregnancy is considered chronic if a patient is diagnosed with hypertension before pregnancy, if hypertension is present prior to 20 weeks' gestation or if it persists longer than six weeks after delivery. Women with chronic hypertension are at risk of developing superimposed preeclampsia. Superimposed preeclampsia is defined as an exacerbation of hypertension and new onset of proteinuria.

PREECLAMPSIA

The risk to the fetus in patients with preeclampsia relates largely to the gestational age at delivery. Risk to the mother can be significant and includes the possible development of disseminated intravascular coagulation, intracranial hemorrhage, renal failure, retinal detachment, pulmonary edema, liver rupture, abruptio placentae, and death. Therefore, astute and experienced clinicians should be in charge of the care of women with preeclampsia.

Etiology

The etiologic agent responsible for the development of preeclampsia remains unknown. The syndrome is characterized by vasoconstriction, hemoconcentration, and possible ischemic changes in the placenta, kidney, liver, and brain. These abnormalities are usually seen in women with severe preeclampsia.

Pathophysiology

Cardiovascular

The hypertensive changes seen in preeclampsia are attributable to intense vasoconstriction thought to be due to increased vascular reactivity. The underlying mechanism responsible for increased vascular reactivity is presumed to be dysfunction in the normal interactions of vasodilatory (prostacyclin, nitric oxide) and vasoconstrictive (thromboxane A2, endothelins) substances. Another hallmark of preeclampsia is hemoconcentration. Accordingly, patients with preeclampsia have lower intravascular volumes and have less tolerance for the blood loss associated with delivery.

Hematologic

The most common hematologic abnormality in preeclampsia is thrombocytopenia (platelet count <100,000/mm^3). The exact mechanism for thrombocytopenia is unknown. Another occasional hematologic abnormality is microangiopathic hemolysis, as seen in association with HELLP syndrome. It can be diagnosed by the presence of schistocytes on peripheral smear and by increased lactate dehydrogenase (LDH) or bilirubin levels. Interpretation of the baseline hematocrit level in a preeclamptic patient may be difficult. A low hematocrit may signify hemolysis and a high hematocrit may be due to hemoconcentration.

Renal

Vasoconstriction in preeclampsia leads to decreased renal perfusion and subsequent reductions in the glomerular filtration rate (GFR). In normal pregnancy the GFR increases by as much as 50 percent above prepregnancy levels. Because of this, serum creatinine levels in nonpreeclamptic patients rarely rise above normal pregnancy levels (0.8 mg/dL). Close monitoring of urine output is necessary in patients with preeclampsia, as oliguria (defined as <500 mL/24 h) may occur due to renal insufficiency. In rare cases profound renal insufficiency may lead to acute tubular necrosis. This is usually seen in the presence of abruptio placentae, HELLP syndrome, and unrecognized severe blood loss that is not corrected.

Hepatic

Hepatic damage in association with preeclampsia can range from mildly elevated liver enzyme levels to subcapsular liver hematomas and hepatic rupture. The latter two are usually associated with HELLP syndrome. Liver lesions seen on biopsy and at autopsy include periportal hemorrhages, ischemic lesions, and fibrin deposition.

Central Nervous System

Eclamptic convulsions are perhaps the most disturbing CNS manifestation of preeclampsia and remain a major cause of maternal mortality in the third world. The exact etiology of eclampsia is unknown, but may be attributable to hypertensive encephalopathy or ischemia from vasoconstriction. Radiologic studies may show evidence of cerebral edema and hemorrhagic lesions, particularly in the posterior hemispheres, which may explain the visual disturbances seen in preeclampsia. Other CNS abnormalities include headaches, altered mentation, scotomata, blurred vision, and, rarely, temporary blindness.

MANAGEMENT OF SEVERE PREECLAMPSIA

Any patient with severe preeclampsia should be admitted and initially observed in a labor and delivery unit. Initial workup should include assessment for fetal well being, monitoring of maternal blood pressure and symptomatology as well as laboratory evaluation. Laboratory assessment should include hematocrit, platelet count, serum creatinine, aspartate aminotransferase (AST), and 24-hour urine collection for total protein excretion. An ultrasound for fetal growth and amniotic fluid index should also be obtained

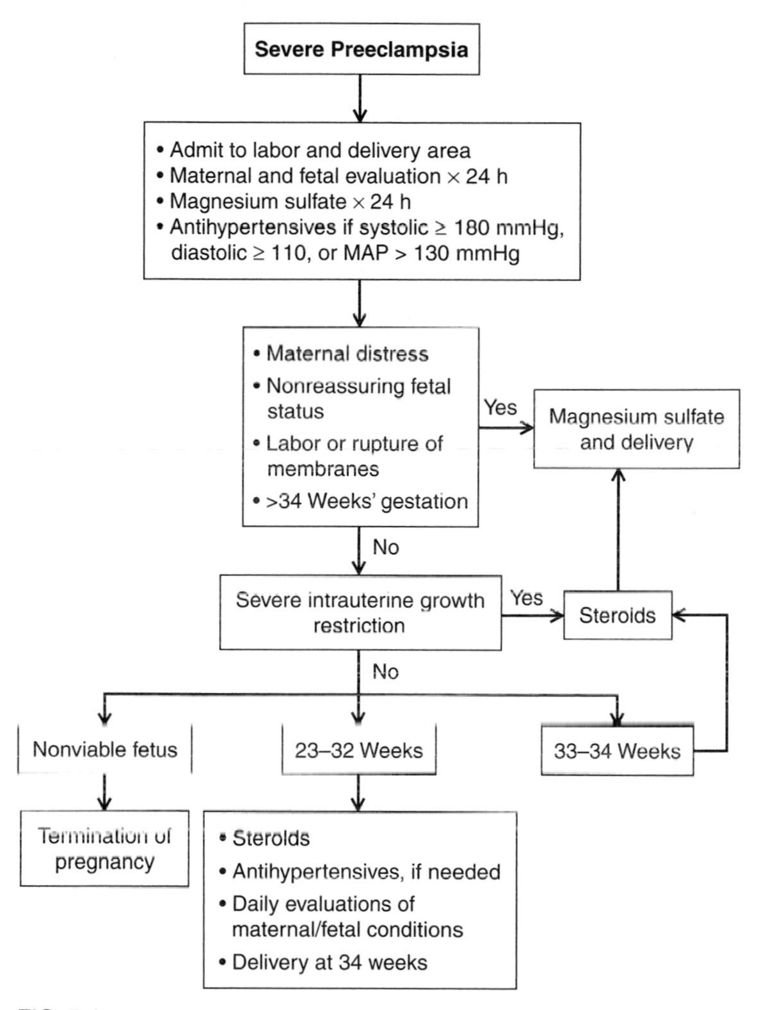

FIG. 5-1 Recommended management of severe preeclampsia.

(Fig. 5-1). Candidates for expectant management should be carefully selected. They should also be counseled regarding the risks and benefits of expectant management. Guidelines for expectant management are outlined in Table 5-3. Fetal well being should be assessed on a daily basis by nonstress testing and weekly amniotic fluid index determination. The patient should also be instructed on fetal movement assessment. An ultrasound for fetal growth should be performed every two to three weeks. Maternal laboratory evaluation should be done daily or every other day. If the patient maintains a stable maternal and fetal course, she may be expectantly managed until 34 weeks. Worsening maternal or fetal status warrants delivery, regardless of gestational age (Table 5-3). Women with a nonviable fetus should be presented with the option of pregnancy termination.

TABLE 5-3 Maternal/Fetal Guideline: Guidelines for Management of Severe Preeclampsia

	Maternal	Fetal
Expeditious delivery (within 72 h)	One or more of the following: • Uncontrolled severe hypertension[a] • Eclampsia • Platelet count <100,000/mm^3 • AST or ALT > 2 × upper limit of normal with RUQ or epigastric pain • Pulmonary edema • Compromised renal function[b] • Abruptio placentae • Persistent, severe headache or visual changes	One or more of the following: • Repetitive late or severe variable heart rate decelerations • Biophysical profile <4 on two occasions, 4 hours apart • Amniotic Fluid Index <2 cm • Ultrasound EFW <5th percentile • Reverse umbilical artery diastolic flow
Consider expectant management	One or more of the following: • Controlled hypertension • Urinary protein of any amount • Oliguria (<0.5 mL/kg/h) which resolves with hydration • AST/ALT > 2 × upper limit of normal without RUQ or epigastric pain	One or more of the following: • Biophysical profile >6 • Amniotic Fluid Index >2 cm • Ultrasound EFW >5th percentile

[a]Blood pressure persistently >160/110 despite maximum recommended doses of two antihypertensive medications.
[b]Rise in serum creatinine of at least 1 mg/dL over baseline levels.

TABLE 5-4 Acute Treatment of Hypertension

Medication	Onset of action (min)	Dose
Hydralazine	10–20	5–10 mg IV every 20 min up to maximum dose of 30 mg
Labetalol	10–15	10–20 mg IV, then 40–80 mg every 10 min up to maximum dose of 300 mg or continuous infusion- at 1–2 mg/min
Nifedipine	5–10	10 mg PO, repeated in 30 min, prn; then 10–20 mg every 4–6 hours up to maximum dose 240 mg/24 h
Sodium nitroprusside	0.5–5	0.25–5 μg/kg/min IV infusion Risk of fetal cyanide poisoning with prolonged treatment.

Maternal blood pressure control is essential with expectant management or during delivery. Medications can be given orally or intravenously as necessary to maintain blood pressure between 140 and 160 mmHg systolic and 90 and 110 mmHg diastolic. The most commonly used intravenous medications for this purpose are labetalol and hydralazine. The recommended dosages of medications for the acute treatment of hypertension are listed in Table 5-4. Care should be taken not to drop the blood pressure too rapidly so as to avoid reduced renal and placental perfusion.

A trial of labor is indicated in patients with severe preeclampsia. However, an appropriate time frame should be established regarding the achievement of active labor. Preeclamptic women receiving magnesium sulfate are also at risk for postpartum hemorrhage due to uterine atony. Patients should be closely monitored for at least 12 to 24 hours postpartum. Postpartum eclampsia occurs in 25 percent of patients; thus, $MgSO_4$ should be continued for 12 to 24 hours after delivery. There is usually no need for continued seizure prophylaxis beyond 24 hours postpartum.

HELLP Syndrome

The specific laboratory abnormalities demonstrating hemolysis, elevated liver enzymes and low platelets are shown in Table 5-5. The clinical presentation of patients with HELLP syndrome is highly variable. However, HELLP patients generally are multiparous, white females who present at less than 35 weeks' gestation. Sibai has noted that hypertension may be absent (20 percent), mild (30 percent), or severe (50 percent) in women diagnosed with HELLP syndrome. Therefore, the diagnosis of HELLP syndrome cannot necessarily

TABLE 5-5 Criteria for HELLP Syndrome

Hemolysis	• Abnormal peripheral smear • Lactate dehydrogenase >600 U/L • Total bilirubin ≥1.2 mg/dL
Elevated liver enzymes	• Serum aspartate aminotransferase >70 U/L • Lactate dehydrogenase >600 U/L
Low platelets	• <100,000/mm³

TABLE 5-6 Differential Diagnosis of HELLP

Acute fatty liver of pregnancy	Appendicitis
Cerebral hemorrhage	Diabetes insipidus
Gallbladder disease	Gastroenteritis
Glomerulonephritis	Hemolytic uremic syndrome
Hyperemesis gravidarum	Idiopathic thrombocytopenia
Pancreatitis	Pyelonephritis
Systemic lupus erythematosis	Thrombophilia
Thrombotic thrombocytopenic purpura	Viral hepatitis, including herpes

be ruled out in the normotensive patient who has other signs and symptoms that are consistent with preeclampsia.

Differential Diagnosis

HELLP may be confused with other medical conditions, particularly in the face of normotension. A list of the differential diagnoses is found in Table 5-6. HELLP can be confused with two other specific medical conditions, acute fatty liver of pregnancy and thrombotic thrombocytopenic purpura/hemolytic uremic syndrome (TTP/HUS). The differentiation among the three entities is based on specific laboratory findings (Table 5-7).

Management

The initial evaluation in women diagnosed with HELLP syndrome should be the same as that for severe preeclampsia. The patient should be cared for at a tertiary care center. Management initially should include maternal and fetal assessment, control of severe hypertension-(if present), initiation of magnesium sulfate infusion, correction of coagulopathy-(if present), and maternal stabilization. Immediate delivery should be performed in patients more than 34 weeks. In patients less than 34 weeks without proven lung maturity, corticosteroids should be given and delivery planned in 48 hours, provided there is no

TABLE 5-7 Clinical/ Laboratory Findings in HELLP/TTP/HUS/AFLP

	HELLP	TTP/HUS	AFLP
Ammonia	Normal	Normal	Elevated
Anemia	±	Severe	Normal
Antithrombin III	±	Normal	Decreased
AST	Elevated	Normal	Elevated
Bilirubin	Elevated, mostly indirect	Elevated	Elevated, mostly direct
Creatinine	±	Significantly elevated	Significantly Elevated
Fibrinogen	Normal	Normal	Decreased in all cases
Glucose	Normal	Normal	Decreased
Hypertension	Present	±	±
LDH	Elevated	Significantly elevated	Elevated
Proteinuria	Present	±	±
Thrombocytopenia	Present	Severe	±

HELLP, Hemolysis, elevated liver enzymes, low platelet count; TTP, Thrombotic thrombocytopenic purpura; HUS, Hemolytic uremic syndrome; AFLP, Acute fatty liver of pregnancy.

worsening of maternal or fetal status in the meantime. The use of steroids, volume expanders, plasmapheresis and antithrombotic agents in patients with HELLP have produced only marginal results, although some evidence suggests a benefit of steroid therapy for improvement in maternal condition: O'Brien and colleagues (2000) noted a dose-dependent prolongation in latency, reduction in liver enzyme abnormalities and improvement in platelet count with antepartum corticosteroids. Conservative management of HELLP syndrome poses a significant risk of abruptio placentae, pulmonary edema, adult respiratory distress syndrome (ARDS), ruptured liver hematoma, acute renal failure, disseminated intravascular coagulation, eclampsia, intracerebral hemorrhage, and maternal death. Therefore, expectant management past 48 hours is not warranted for the potential minimal fetal benefits, when weighed against the profound maternal risk.

Patients with a favorable cervix and a diagnosis of HELLP syndrome should undergo a trial of labor, particularly if they present in labor. An operative delivery in some situations may even be harmful. However, elective cesarean section should be considered in patients, at very early gestational ages, with unfavorable cervices. O'Brien et al. (2002) support the use of glucocorticoids to improve platelet counts so as to permit regional anesthesia in patients with HELLP syndrome. The anesthetist should be updated as to the trend in platelet count for patients with HELLP. Should such a patient require cesarean delivery, platelet transfusion of approximately 5 to 10 units should be initiated en route to the operating room in patients with severe thrombocytopenia. However, platelet consumption is rapid with a platelet transfusion in this setting. Intraoperative considerations should include drain placement (subfascial, subcutaneous, or both), due to generalized oozing. Postpartum management of the HELLP patient should include close hemodynamic monitoring for at least 48 hours. Serial laboratory evaluations should also be done to monitor for worsening abnormalities. Most patients should show reversal of laboratory parameters within 48 hours. Small uncontrolled studies have noted more rapid reversal of laboratory abnormalities with postpartum administration of steroids. However, we do not recommend such management at our center.

Another potential life-threatening complication of HELLP syndrome is subcapsular liver hematoma. Clinical findings consistent with this complication include phrenic nerve pain. Pain in the pericardium, peritoneum, pleura, shoulder, gallbladder, and esophagus are consistent with referred pain from the phrenic nerve. Confirmation of the diagnosis can be obtained via the computed tomography, ultrasonography or magnetic resonance imaging. Conservative management in a hemodynamically stable patient with an unruptured subcapsular hematoma is appropriate, provided that close hemodynamic monitoring, serial evaluations of coagulation profiles, and serial evaluation of the hematoma with radiologic studies are performed. Should the patient decompensate hemodynamically, the diagnosis of ruptured subcapsular hematoma should be entertained. If rupture of a subcapsular liver hematoma is suspected, immediate intervention is necessary. Liver hematoma rupture with hemodynamic shock is a life threatening surgical emergency. Management should involve general and vascular surgeons. Correction of coagulopathy and massive blood product transfusion is essential. Typically, rupture involves the right lobe of the liver. Maternal and fetal mortality is over 50 percent, even with immediate intervention. The current recommendation for treating rupture of subcapsular liver hematoma in pregnancy is packing and drainage.

ECLAMPSIA

The rate of eclampsia in the United States is 0.05 to 0.1 percent, and much higher in developing countries. Eclampsia continues to be a major cause of maternal and perinatal morbidity/mortality worldwide. The maternal mortality rate is approximately 4.2 percent. The perinatal mortality rate ranges from 13 to 30 percent. Eclampsia can occur antepartum (50 percent), intrapartum (25 percent) or postpartum (25 percent).

Management

During the eclamptic seizure, the main therapy is supportive care. Management of eclampsia is as follows:

1. Avoid injury—padded bed rails, restraints
2. Maintain oxygenation—O_2, pulse oximetry, arterial blood gas assessment
3. Minimize aspiration—lateral decubitis postion, suction
4. Initiate magnesium sulfate
5. Control blood pressure
6. Move toward delivery (corticosteroids if <34 weeks)

Most seizures are self-limited, lasting 1 to 2 minutes. Magnesium sulfate is the drug of choice for the prevention of eclampsia and should also be used for prevention of recurrent seizures. Approximately 10 percent of eclamptic women receiving magnesium sulfate will have more seizures. Immediately following an eclamptic seizure, it is common to see abnormalities in the fetal heart rate pattern. These include fetal bradycardia, decreased variability, late decelerations, and reflex tachycardia. They typically resolve within 5 to 10 minutes after the convulsion. It is important not to proceed directly to cesarean delivery after a seizure, if at all possible. Vaginal delivery is the preferred birth route, even after an eclamptic seizure. Cesarean delivery should be performed for obstetric indications only. Induction of labor may be performed with oxytocin or prostaglandins, with the patient maintained on magnesium sulfate throughout her labor course. Careful attention must be given to the overall fluid status of the patient. Patients with eclampsia may have profound hemoconcentration. Because of this, close hemodynamic monitoring is required in the setting of epidural anesthesia and/or of severe blood loss. Patients who are hypovolemic will not respond well to acute blood loss, yet it is also important to limit fluids, as these patients have capillary leakage and are predisposed to developing pulmonary edema. Magnesium sulfate should be continued for 24 hours postpartum. Intracranial imaging is typically not warranted unless coma or focal neurologic signs persist, or the diagnosis is uncertain. Postpartum eclampsia is a diagnostic dilemma. Any woman seizing in the postpartum period should be considered to have eclampsia; however, other disorders must be ruled out. Patients who develop postpartum eclampsia usually will have symptoms prior to seizure activity including severe, persistent headache, blurred vision, photophobia, epigastric pain, nausea and vomiting, and transient mental status changes. Therefore, it is important to educate patients to report these symptoms to health care providers so as to initiate preeclamptic evaluation. Eclamptics should receive $MgSO_4$ for at least 24 hours after seizure activity. If the patient has normal laboratory values and hypertension is controlled, she can be discharged after $MgSO_4$ treatment with instructions to return in one week for outpatient evaluation.

TABLE 5-8 Magnesium Sulfate-Dosages, Serum Levels and Associated Findings

Magnesium doses	
Loading dose:	6 g IV over 20–30 min (6 g of 50% solution diluted in 150 mL D_5W)
Maintenance dose:	2–3 g IV per hour (40 g in 1 L D_5LR at 50 mL/h)
Recurrent seizures:	Reload with 2 g over 5–10 min, 1–2 times and/or 250 mg sodium amobarbital IV
Magnesium levels and associated findings	
Loss of patellar reflexes	8–12 mg/dL
Feeling of warmth, flushing, double vision	9–12 mg/dL
Somnolence	10–12 mg/dL
Slurred speech	10–12 mg/dL
Muscular paralysis	15–17 mg/dL
Respiratory difficulty	15–17 mg/dL
Cardiac arrest	20–35 mg/dL

Magnesium Sulfate

The use of magnesium sulfate in the management of preeclamptic patients is for the prevention of eclamptic seizures. The exact mode of action of $MgSO_4$ for preventing seizures is unknown, although it has been in use since the early 1900s to prevent recurrent seizures and associated maternal/perinatal death. The recommended regimen is presented in Table 5-8. The intravenous route is the preferred method, as intramuscular injection of magnesium sulfate is very painful and occasionally can cause gluteal abscess formation. Magnesium sulfate is not a benign medication. Patients receiving $MgSO_4$ are at increased risk for postpartum hemorrhage due to uterine atony. This should be anticipated and steps should be taken to ensure availability of cross-matched blood, if the need arises. Monitoring patients for potential signs of magnesium toxicity should be done throughout the course of administration; this includes eliciting deep tendon reflexes, assessing mental status and checking respiratory rate. Table 5-8 lists the clinical findings associated with various serum magnesium levels. If a patient develops signs of magnesium toxicity, the infusion should be stopped immediately. The patient should then be evaluated for respiratory compromise by exam and pulse oximetry; oxygen should be administered and a serum magnesium level should be obtained. If magnesium toxicity is diagnosed, the patient should be treated with 10 mL of 10 percent calcium gluconate solution, infused over 3 minutes. Calcium competitively inhibits magnesium at the neuromuscular junction and decreases the toxic effects. The impact of calcium is transient and the patient should be closely monitored for continued magnesium toxicity. Should respiratory or cardiac arrest occur, immediate resuscitation including intubation and mechanical ventilation should be initiated.

ANTIHYPERTENSIVE AGENTS

Many agents are available for the control of hypertension. It is important to be familiar with the maternal and fetal side effects, as well as mode of action in order to choose the most effective agent for the gravida. Antihypertensive agents can exert an effect by decreasing cardiac output, peripheral vascular resistance, or central blood pressure, or by inhibiting angiotensin production.

Table 5-9 Indications for Antihypertensive Therapy

Indications for Antihypertensive Therapy
I. Antepartum and intrapartum
• Persistent elevations for at least 1 h
SBP ≥ 160 mmHg or
DBP ≥ 110 mmHg or
MAP ≥ 130 mmHg
• Persistent elevations for at least 30 min
SBP ≥ 200 mmHg or
DBP ≥ 120 mmHg or
MAP ≥ 140 mmHg
• Thrombocytopenia or congestive heart failure[a]
SBP ≥ 160 mmHg or
DBP ≥ 105 mmHg or
MAP ≥ 125 mmHg
II. Postpartum[b]
SBP ≥ 160 mmHg or
DBP ≥ 105 mmHg or
MAP ≥ 125 mmHg

[a]Persistent for at least 30 min.
[b]Persistent for at least 1 h.

Indications for therapy are listed in Table 5-9. Commonly used drugs in pregnancy are listed in Table 5-4.

HYPERTENSIVE EMERGENCIES

On rare occasions, pregnant women may present with life-threatening clinical conditions that require immediate control of blood pressure, such as hypertensive encephalopathy, acute left ventricular failure, acute aortic dissection or conditions characterized by increased levels of circulating catecholamines (pheochromocytoma, clonidine withdrawal, cocaine ingestion). Patients at the highest risk of these complications include those with underlying cardiac disease, chronic renal disease, hypertension requiring multiple drugs to achieve control, superimposed preeclampsia in the second trimester, and abruptio placentae in association with disseminated intravascular coagulation (DIC). Although a diastolic blood pressure of 115 mmHg, or greater, is usually considered a hypertensive emergency, this criterion is arbitrary; the rate of change of blood pressure may be more relevant than the absolute number. The combination of elevated blood pressure with evidence of new or progressive end-organ damage determines the seriousness of the clinical situation.

HYPERTENSIVE ENCEPHALOPATHY

Untreated essential hypertension progresses to a hypertensive crisis in up to 1 to 2 percent of cases. Hypertensive encephalopathy is usually seen in patients with systolic blood pressure above 250 mmHg or a diastolic above 150 mmHg. Patients with acute onset of hypertension may develop encephalopathy at lower pressure levels than those with chronic hypertension. Normally, cerebral blood flow is approximately 50 mL/100 g tissue per minute. To maintain this level of perfusion, cerebral arterioles dilate when blood pressure falls; the converse occurs when blood pressure rises. This mechanism usually remains operative between diastolic pressures of 60 and 120 mmHg. Hypertensive encephalopathy is considered to be a derangement of cerebral arteriolar autoregulation, which occurs when the upper limit of autoregulation is exceeded. Typically, hypertensive encephalopathy has subacute onset over 24 to 72 hours.

During a hypertensive crisis, other evidence of end-organ damage may also be present: cardiac, renal, or retinal dysfunction may arise, secondary to impaired organ perfusion, due to loss of vascular autoregulation. Ischemia of the retina (with flame-shaped retinal hemorrhages, retinal infarcts or papilledema) may occur, causing decreased visual acuity. Impaired regulation of coronary blood flow and marked increase in ventricular wall stress may result in angina, myocardial infarction, congestive heart failure, malignant ventricular arrhythmia, pulmonary edema, or dissecting aortic aneurysm. Necrosis of the afferent arterioles of the glomerulus results in hemorrhage of the cortex and medulla, fibrinoid necrosis, and proliferative endarteritis, resulting in serum creatinine >3 mg/dL, proteinuria, oliguria, hematuria, hyaline or red blood cell casts, and progressive azotemia. Severe hypertension may result in abruptio placentae with DIC. In addition, high levels of renin, angiotensin II, aldosterone, norepinephrine, and vasopressin accompany ongoing vascular damage. These circulating hormones increase relative efferent arteriolar tone, resulting in natriurisis and hypovolemia. The impact of these endocrine changes may be important in maintaining the hypertensive crisis.

Treatment of Hypertensive Encephalopathy

The goal of hypertensive therapy is to prevent the occurrence of a hypertensive emergency. Patients at risk for hypertensive crisis should receive intensive management during labor and for 48 hours after delivery. Although pregnancy may complicate the diagnosis, once life-threatening conditions are recognized, pregnancy should not slow or alter the mode of therapy. The only reliable clinical criterion for confirming the diagnosis of hypertensive encephalopathy is prompt response to antihypertensive therapy. Headache and sensorium often clear dramatically; sometimes within 1 to 2 hours after treatment. The overall recovery may be somewhat slower in patients with uremia and in whom the symptoms have been present for a prolonged period before therapy was initiated. Sustained cerebrovascular deficits should suggest other diagnoses.

Patients with hypertensive encephalopathy or other hypertensive crises should be hospitalized for bed rest. Intravenous lines should be inserted for the administration of fluids and medications. Although there is a tendency to restrict sodium intake in patients with a hypertensive emergency, volume contraction from natriuresis may be present. A marked drop in diastolic blood pressure with a concommittent rise in heart rate upon rising from the supine position is evidence of volume contraction. Infusion of normal saline solution during the first 24 to 48 hours to achieve volume expansion should be considered. Saline infusion may help decrease the activity of the renin-angiotensin-aldosterone axis and result in better blood pressure control. Simultaneous repletion of potassium losses with continuous monitoring of blood pressure, volume status, urinary output, electrocardiographic readings, and mental status is mandatory. An intraarterial line may provide the most accurate blood pressure readings. Laboratory studies include complete blood count with differential, reticulocyte count, platelet count, and blood chemistries. A urinalysis can be obtained to survey for protein, glucose, blood, casts, and bacteria. Assessment for end-organ damage in the central nervous system, retinas, kidneys, and cardiovascular system should be done periodically. Antepartum patients should undergo continuous electronic fetal heart rate monitoring.

Lowering Blood Pressure

The drug of choice in hypertensive crisis is sodium nitroprusside. Other drugs such as nitroglycerin, nifedipine, trimetaphan, labetalol, and hydralazine can also be used. There are risks associated with too rapid or excessive lowering of blood pressure. The aim of the therapy is to reduce the mean arterial pressure by no more than 15 to 25 percent. Small reduction in blood pressure in the first 60 minutes of therapy, working toward a diastolic level of 100 to 110 mmHg, is recommended. In chronic hypertensives, who have a rightward shift of the cerebral autoregulation secondary to medial hypertrophy of the cerebral vasculature, lowering blood pressure too rapidly may result in cerebral ischemia, stroke, or coma. Coronary blood flow, renal perfusion, and uteroplacental blood flow also may deteriorate, resulting in myocardial infarction, acute renal failure, fetal distress, or death. Hypertension that proves increasingly difficult to control is an indication for delivery. If the patient's outcome appears grave, consideration of and preparation for possible perimortem cesarean delivery should be made.

Sodium Nitroprusside

Sodium nitroprusside causes arterial and venous relaxation by interfering with both the influx and intracellular activation of calcium. It is given as an intravenous infusion at 0.25 to 5.0 μg/kg/min. The onset of action is immediate and its effect may last 3 to 5 minutes after discontinuation. Thus, hypotension caused by nitroprusside should subside within a few minutes of discontinuing the drip because of the short half-life. If it does not, other causes of low blood pressure should be considered. The effect of nitroprusside on uterine blood flow is unclear. Nitroprusside is metabolized into thiocyanate, which is excreted in the urine. Cyanide can accumulate as a result of large doses (>10 μg/kg/min) or prolonged administration (>48 h), if there is renal insufficiency or if there is decreased hepatic metabolism. Signs of toxicity include anorexia, disorientation, headache, fatigue, restlessness, tinnitus, delirium, hallucinations, nausea, vomiting, and metabolic acidosis. When infused at less than 2 μg/kg/min, however, cyanide toxicity is unlikely. A maximum rate of 10 μg/kg/min should never be continued for more than 10 minutes. The few published reports regarding nitroprusside use in pregnancy have stated that thiocyanate toxicity rarely occurs if used in standard doses. Indeed, tachyphylaxis generally occurs before toxicity. Whenever toxicity is suspected, however, therapy should be initiated with 3 percent sodium nitrite at a rate not to exceed 5 mL/min, up to a maximum of 15 mL. Next, administration of 12.5 g of sodium thiosulfate in 50 mL of 5 percent dextrose in water, infused over a 10-minute period, should be started.

Nitroglycerin

Nitroglycerin is an arterial, but mostly venous dilator. It is given as an intravenous infusion at an initial rate of 5 μg/min that is gradually increased every 3 to 5 minutes, titrated to blood pressure, to a maximum dose of 100 μg/min. It is the drug of choice in preeclampsia associated with pulmonary edema and for control of hypertension associated with tracheal manipulation. Side effects include a headache, tachycardia, and methemoglobinemia. It is contraindicated in hypertensive encephalopathy because it increases cerebral blood flow and intracranial pressure.

SUMMARY

Patients with severe preeclampsia, HELLP syndrome, and hypertensive emergencies are at risk of maternal and perinatal morbidity and mortality. Every effort should be made to optimize outcomes for both. The risk to the fetus relates largely to the gestational age at delivery. Risks to the mother can be significant and include development of disseminated intravascular coagulation, intracranial hemorrhage, renal failure, retinal detachment, pulmonary edema, liver rupture, abruptio placentae, and death. Therefore, astute and experienced clinicians should provide care for these women.

SUGGESTED READINGS

ACOG Practice Bulletin, No. 33: Diagnosis and management of preeclampsia and eclampsia. 2002;99:159–167.

Buckbinder A, Sibai BM, Caritis S, et al.: Adverse perinatal outcomes are significantly higher in severe gestational hypertension than in mild preeclampsia. *Am J Obstet Gynecol* 2002;186:66–71.

Chames MC, Livingston JC, Ivester T, et al.: Late postpartum eclampsia: A preventable disease? *AM J Obstet Gynecol* 2002;186:1174–1177.

Katz VL, Farmer R, Kuller JA: Preeclampsia into eclampsia: Toward a new paradigm. *Am J Obstet Gynecol* 2000;182:1389–1396.

Mabie BC, Gonzalez AR, Sibai BM, et al.: A comparative trial of labetalol and hydralazine in the acute management of severe hypertension complicating pregnancy. *Obstet Gynecol* 1987;70:328–333.

MacKay AP, Berg CJ, Atrash HI: Pregnancy related mortality from preeclampsia and eclampsia. *Obstet Gynecol* 2001;97:533–538.

O'Brien JM, Milligan DA, Barton JR: Impact of high-dose corticosteroids therapy for patients with HELLP (hemolysis, elevated liver enzymes, and low platelet count) syndrome. *Am J Obstet Gynecol* 2000;183(4):921–924.

O'Brien JM, Shumate SA, Satchwell SL, et al.: Maternal benefit of corticosteroids therapy in patients with HELLP (hemolysis, elevated liver enzymes, and low platelet count) syndrome: impact on the rate of regional anesthesia. *Am J Obstet Gynecol* 2002;186:475–479.

Report of the National High Blood Pressure Education Program Working Group on High Blood Pressure in Pregnancy: *Am J Obstet Gynecol* 2000;183:S1–S22.

Scardo JA, Vermillion ST, Newman RB, et al.: A randomized, double-blind, hemodynamic evaluation of nifedipine and labetalol in preeclamptic hypertensive emergencies. *Am J Obstet Gynecol* 1999;181(4):862–866.

Sibai B, Hnat M: Delayed delivery in severe preeclampsia remote from term. *OBG Management* 2002;14(5):92–108.

The Magpie Trial Collaborative Group: Do women with preeclampsia and their babies benefit from magnesium sulfate? The Magpie Trial. *Lancet* 2002;359:1877–1890.

Witlin AG, Mattar F, Sibai BM: Postpartum stroke: A twenty-year experience. *Am J Obstet Gynecol* 2000;183:83–88.

6 Obesity in the Obstetric Intensive Care Patient

Jordan H. Perlow

INTRODUCTION

A sedentary lifestyle and addiction to unhealthy foods has contributed significantly to an epidemic of obesity and the creation of a national health crisis. Each year, an estimated 300,000 adults die from complications of obesity. About half of the U.S. adult female population is either overweight or obese, with the highest prevalence in the non-Hispanic Black population. Recent data from 2001 indicate that despite the long-recognized morbidities and increased mortality associated with obesity, the prevalence of obesity in the United States has increased dramatically, by 74 percent over the past 10-year period. This constitutes an estimated current U.S. adult female obese population of 23 million individuals. Mississippi has the highest prevalence of obesity while Colorado's population is the leanest. The remarkably high prevalence of this condition and its significant negative impact on overall health makes its treatment a top priority for all healthcare disciplines. Obese women are at significantly increased risk for myriad medical complications, cancers, and premature sudden death (Table 6-1). Obesity coexisting with diabetes is a significant comorbidity which affects nearly 10 million U.S. obese women, with its prevalence having increased by 61 percent since 1991. Nearly 4 percent of the overall adult female population is both obese and diabetic.

Obesity should be of particular interest and importance to those providing health care to women because age-adjusted rates of obesity for females of all races significantly exceed those for males. It has been estimated that if the U.S. population was at ideal body weight, coronary heart disease, congestive heart failure, and stroke could be reduced by 25 to 35 percent and provide an additional average of three years of life expectancy. African-American women with severe obesity incur the greatest numbers of years of life lost to obesity-related premature mortality.

The complications of obesity and its relation to the obstetric intensive care patient cannot be overemphasized. Eighteen percent of obstetric causes of maternal death and 80 percent of anesthesia-related maternal mortality are associated with obesity as a risk factor. These patients are indeed at a high risk and deserving of intense efforts to minimize morbidity and mortality when possible, and thus improve perinatal outcome.

This chapter will serve to inform the reader of the various aspects of critical obstetric care for the obese gravida, reviewing antepartum, intrapartum, and postpartum considerations.

DEFINITION

Obesity has been defined and described in a variety of colorful ways. Terms such as severe, massive, morbid and grotesque appear in published literature to describe different degrees of obesity. Unfortunately, standardized definitions are lacking. The term *overweight* refers to an excess of body weight compared to set standards, with the excess weight coming from muscle, bone,

TABLE 6-1 Medical Complications of Obesity

Sudden death	Gout
Stroke	Osteoarthritis
Coronary artery disease	Digestive diseases
Hypertension	Cholelithiasis
Thromboembolic disease	Hiatal hernia
Diabetes mellitus	Pulmonary function impairment, obstructive sleep apnea/pulmonary hypertension, asthma
Dyslipidemias	Hepatic steatosis
Carcinoma	Endocrine abnormalities
Colon	Menstrual disorders
Gallbladder	Infertility
Ovary	Polycystic ovary disease
Endometrium	Psychosocial disorders
Breast	Depression, mood, and anxiety disorders
Cervix	
Compromised obstetric outcome	
Anesthetic complications	
Dermatologic diseases	
Acanthosis nigricans	
Gragilitas cutis inguinalis	

fat and/or body water. Obesity, however, is defined as an excess of body fat frequently resulting in impairment of health. Therefore, rarely, an individual (bodybuilder) could be overweight but not obese. Obesity is usually caused by an excess of caloric intake versus expenditure; however, its cause is primarily multifactorial accounting for 99 percent of all patients with obesity. A small percentage may be caused by a diverse group of neurologic and endocrine disorders (Table 6-2). Frequently, the body mass index (BMI) is used to measure obesity:

$$\text{Body mass index (BMI)} = \frac{\text{Patient weight (kg)}}{\text{Patient height (m}^2\text{)}}$$

Others have used percent of ideal body weight (%IBW) using actuarial tables. More sophisticated methods of quantifying percent body fat are available, though not utilized, for everyday clinical situation.

The National Institute of Health defines obesity as a BMI of ≥30 kg/m^2. This value approximates weight >120% IBW. Some studies, however, have shown adverse health consequences with IBW >110%. Patients twice IBW or 100 lb greater than ideal body weight have been described as morbidly obese and pregnant women ≥300 lb have been described as massively obese. The most severe degree of obesity, class 3 obesity (BMI ≥40) is increasing rapidly, now constituting nearly 5 percent of the adult population and 6 percent of Black women, and is associated with the most severe health complications.

TABLE 6-2 Obesity: Differential Diagnosis (<1% of Etiology)

Hypothyroidism	Insulinoma
Prader-Willi syndrome	Adiposogenital dystrophy
Lawrence-Moon-Biedl syndrome	Partial lipodystrophy
Hypothalamic pathology	Polycystic ovary disease
Craniopharyngioma	Cushing's syndrome
Hypogonadism	

More than 25 percent of patients were recently reported to be heavier than 200 lb. during pregnancy, with more than 7 percent heavier than 250 lb.

Given the health implications of obesity and the focus on body image being so prevalent in our society, bariatric surgery has become quite common and is seen not uncommonly among patients of reproductive age. Reports have shown an increased risk for gastric band complications during pregnancy and nutritional deficiencies have been reported. Gastrointestinal hemorrhage has also been reported during pregnancy due to erosion of the band. Pregnant patients with a history of gastric surgery for obesity should be counseled appropriately and surveillance during prenatal care heightened. Some devices can be adjusted to allow for the increased caloric needs of pregnancy and allow for appropriate weight gain and improved perinatal outcomes.

PATHOPHYSIOLOGY

Overview

Perinatal outcome is compromised among pregnancies complicated by obesity (Tables 6-3 and 6-4). The obese pregnant woman and fetus are at risk for a variety of complications during pregnancy. These include increased risks of hypertension, preeclampsia, diabetes (insulin-dependent and gestational), labor abnormalities, cesarean delivery, and congenital malformations. The neonate born to the obese mother has also been noted to be at significantly increased risk of adverse outcome including low Apgar scores, intrauterine growth restriction, preterm delivery, low birth weight, macrosomia/large for gestational age, and intensive care requirement.

Physiologic Changes in the Obese Pregnant Patient

In pregnancy, blood volume, and cardiac output increase by approximately 40 percent with further increases of cardiac output during labor and delivery,

TABLE 6-3 Obesity and Perinatal Outcome: Maternal Risks

Obstetric (direct) mortality
Aspiration
Hemorrhage
Thromboembolism
Stroke
Dysfunctional labor
Cesarean section—primary/repeat/emergent
Failed vaginal birth after cesarean (VBAC)
Cesarean section operative and anesthetic morbidities
Increased blood loss
Increased endometritis
Prolonged operative time
Failed epidural placement
Respiratory complications (atelectasis, pneumonia)
Wound infection/dehiscence
Thromboembolism
Medical complications (see Table 6-1)
Chronic hypertension
Diabetes—pregestational and gestation DM
Preeclampsia
Prolonged hospitalization
Urinary tract infection

TABLE 6-4 Obesity and Perinatal Outcome: Fetal/Neonatal Risks

Preterm birth
Increased perinatal mortality
Low Apgar scores
Intrauterine growth restriction
Low birth weight
Macrosomia/large for gestational age
Post dates
Shoulder dystocia/birth trauma
Intensive care nursery admission
Neonatal/childhood obesity
Congenital malformations
Spina bifida, omphalocele, heart defects, multiple anomalies (BMI >25–30)

reaching values 80 percent greater than prepregnancy values. Obesity accentuates these changes as blood volume and cardiac output expand in proportion to the increase in fat and tissue mass (see Table 6-5).

Obese patients have marked abnormal changes in respiratory physiology. In fact, obese gravidae have markedly diminished functional residual capacity, and except for residual volume, all lung volumes, vital capacity, and total lung capacity are reduced. Obese parturients have also been shown to have diminished Po_2 and chest wall/lung compliance. Total compliance in obesity diminishes by an average of 50 percent, which is equivalent to placing a 50-lb weight on the chest and abdomen of a nonobese patient. These respiratory changes in the obese parturient cause the work of breathing to be increased three times the normal. Morbid obesity may also be associated with obstructive sleep apnea, which can predispose to right-sided heart failure and secondary pulmonary hypertension. Given the increased mortality rate associated with pulmonary hypertension of any cause, appropriate evaluation of obese patients with a history of obstructive sleep apnea is recommended. Treatment with nasal continuous positive airway pressure (CPAP) may be helpful and improve the outcome.

INTRAPARTUM MANAGEMENT

The intrapartum management (Table 6-6) of the obese patient in labor is truly a team effort. The obstetrical physician, the labor and delivery nurse, and the obstetric anesthesiologist form the primary components of the team. Medical consultants who have evaluated the patient for given medical complications may be notified of the patient's admission to labor and delivery for additional management input.

TABLE 6-5 Physiology: Obesity and Cardiopulmonary Function

Diminished lung volumes and capacities
Decreased lung/chest wall compliance
Decreased breathing efficiency/gas exchange
Relative hypoxia
Pulmonary shunt→cardiac compensation
Blood/plasma volume ↑ cardiac work
Ischemia/infarction →↓ cardiac work
Cor pulmonale
Pulmonary hypertension←obesity/hypoventilation syndrome (Pickwickian syndrome)

TABLE 6-6 Obesity and Pregnancy: Intrapartum and Postpartum Management Challenges

Obesity-related problem/risk	Potential solutions/adjuncts
Increased respiratory work/ myocardial O_2 requirement	Epidural anesthesia, oxygen, left lateral laboring position
Difficult peripheral IV access	Central IV line
Inaccurate or difficult BP monitoring	Arterial line
Preexisting cardiopulmonary disease	Continuous ECG, ABG, CXR, pulse oximetry Prenatal echocardiography/cardiology, pulmonary consultations
Increased risks of general anesthesia	Anesthesia consultation/ prophylactic epidural catheter
Difficult emergent regional placement	Prophylactic epidural catheter
Difficult intubation probable	Capability for awake intubation/fiberoptics (see Chap. 20—Failed Intubation Drill)
Aspiration risks	Prophylactic epidural H_2 antagonist (ranitidine HCl 50 mg IV q 6–8 h, 45 min prior to surgery) or PPI pantoprazole 40 mg IV q.d. Sodium citrate with citric acid (Bictra) (30 mL of 0.3 M prior to anesthesia) Metoclopramide (10 mg IV over 1–2 min, 45 min prior to surgery) NPO status in labor
Thromboembolic risks	Low-dose heparin (5000–10,000 units SQ every 8–12 h) TED hose (thigh high) Sequential pneumatic compression device (thigh high) Early postoperative ambulation Minimize operative/immobilization times
Endometritis/wound infection	Prophylactic antibiotic (broad spectrum, prior to incision) Thorough skin preparation Pelvic/wound irrigation (consider placing antibiotics in the irrigant) Surgical drains Subcutaneous sutures

Given the marked physiologic changes occurring in the obese gravid patient and the high probability of coexisting medical complications, it is suggested that consideration be given to those patients at highest risk (greater degrees of obesity) to have an anesthesiology consultation; preferably during the antepartum period, but certainly at the time of admission to labor and delivery. In addition to careful evaluation of the patient's cardiovascular and pulmonary status, meticulous assessment of the patient's airway is critical. This cannot be overemphasized, as it has been reported that 80 percent of all anesthesia-related maternal mortality occurred among obese patients and the inability to accomplish endotracheal intubation was the principal cause. Securing intravenous access and accurate blood pressure monitoring may also prove challenging due to the obese body habitus. The use of central venous access and an arterial line may be helpful in individual cases.

Particular attention should be given to the obese gravida's laboring position with the left lateral position preferred to increase maternal oxygenation, uteroplacental blood flow and prevent aorto-caval compression. Obese patients may also benefit from elevation of the head and chest to prevent airway closure and improve oxygenation as well as overall comfort. Continuous pulse oximetry will provide the clinician with important information with respect to maternal oxygen saturation and allow for further evaluation of hypoxemia and the administration of oxygen as needed.

Another important aspect in labor management includes maximizing pulmonary function and decreasing myocardial oxygen requirements. Recall that the obese gravida's respiratory work requirement is approximately three times that for the gravida of ideal body weight. Epidural anesthesia decreases respiratory work, improves oxygenation, and by decreasing the perception of pain, can decrease the release of catecholamines which cause increased cardiac work (output).

Operative Management

Perhaps the most important aspect of epidural anesthesia lies in the fact that in an emergent situation, should cesarean section be required, a regional anesthetic can be administered through the existing catheter. It has been shown that neonatal outcome is not compromised by this approach. This is critically important as at least 90 percent of maternal deaths from anesthetic causes are attributed to general anesthesia, primarily due to complications of aspiration of gastric contents and failed endotracheal intubation.

The risks of general anesthesia for the obese parturient are intensified due to greater difficulty in intubation secondary to anatomic barriers, a greater gastric volume with lower pH and diminished barrier pressure (difference between lower esophageal sphincter tone minus intragastric pressure). Therefore, regional anesthesia should be considered the anesthetic of choice unless contraindications exist. Such contraindications may include coagulopathy, thrombocytopenia, maternal therapeutic anticoagulation, recent use of low molecular weight heparin, hemodynamic instability, acute hemorrhage and infection over the site of planned needle insertion. With increased utilization of regional anesthesia, one would anticipate a significant impact on the reduction of anesthetic-related maternal mortality. Therefore, the prophylactic placement of an epidural catheter nonemergently in the obese laboring patient should be strongly considered in the intrapartum management of these patients.

Other benefits of regional anesthesia include reduction in postoperative pulmonary complications in obese patients. Long acting intraspinal or epidural narcotics may be administered for postoperative analgesia, and their use reduces risks of respiratory depression from parenteral narcotics. Additionally, patients treated in this manner will ambulate earlier, which is likely to decrease risk of thromboembolic complications.

Patients undergoing cesarean section should receive 30 mL of 0.3 M sodium citrate with citric acid (Bicitra) just prior to anesthesia induction (general or regional) and have the dose repeated each hour if surgery continues beyond one hour for the patient with regional anesthesia. In patients at high risk for aspiration, the use of an H_2-receptor blocker (e.g., cimetidine, ranitidine, famotidine), proton-pump inhibitors [PPIs (e.g., pantoprazole)], and/or dopamine antagonists (metoclopramide) administered intravenously during labor may be helpful in reducing the sequela of aspiration should this potentially lethal complication occur. At least 60 minutes are required for H_2 antagonists to decrease gastric acidity to a safe pH if given parenterally. Therefore, its use is preferred on admission and during labor rather than in the acute situation. For scheduled cases or inductions of obese gravidae, ranitidine may be administered the night prior to surgery and then repeated on admission to the hospital and at appropriate intervals thereafter. Bicitra should also be administered in addition to an H_2-receptor blocker if cesarean section is required. These prophylactic measures will raise the gastric pH to approximately >3.0 in nearly 99 percent of patients. The importance of these measures cannot be overemphasized as pneumonitis and respiratory failure, resulting from aspiration of gastric contents, have been the most common causes of maternal mortality related to anesthetic causes accounting for 25 percent of 2700 maternal deaths from 1979 to 1986. In situations where evaluation of the patient's airway indicates the probability of difficult intubation, consideration of awake intubation and fiberoptic laryngoscopy should be considered. The environment of care should be capable of attending to these specialized needs or consideration for maternal transport to a fully equipped facility with specialists capable of managing these anesthetic challenges should be considered. Therefore, to decrease the risk of maternal morbidity and mortality associated with general anesthesia in the obese gravida, regional anesthesia should be considered the anesthesia of choice for the obese gravida undergoing cesarean delivery when not contraindicated.

Recent data indicate that obesity doubles the likelihood of cesarean section even among a low-risk obese population receiving midwifery care and that over the past 20 years, obesity related cesarean deliveries have tripled. The massively obese gravida (>300 lb) has been found to be at significantly increased risk of perioperative morbidity associated with cesarean section. These morbidities include the unsuccessful initial placement of the epidural catheter and the need for extended time periods to surgically deliver the fetus when compared to controls. These findings again emphasize the potential benefit of the prophylactic epidural. Other risks noted for the obese gravida undergoing cesarean section include increased blood loss, prolonged hospitalization, and a nearly 10-fold increase in postoperative endomyometritis and wound infection. Furthermore, the success rate for VBAC in the massively obese woman has been found to be just 15 percent with more than 50 percent of these VBAC attempts complicated by infectious morbidity. Given the potential need for urgent cesarean section in the course of VBAC and the potential for significant surgical and anesthetic morbidity for these women, counseling for VBAC in this population should be tailored to include these important unique issues.

Various adjuncts to perioperative care have been utilized to prevent morbidities associated with cesarean section in the obese population. These include H_2-receptor blockers, proton pump inhibitors and metoclopramide to prevent the risk of aspiration (discussed above), thromboembolic preventative stockings, intermittent sequential compression devices for the lower extremities and low-dose prophylactic unfractionated heparin to decrease thromboembolic complications and prophylactic antibiotics to decrease postoperative infectious morbidity. Unfortunately, these adjuncts have not been studied in the setting of randomized clinical trials. Therefore, there are little definitive data regarding the utility of these adjuncts, specifically in the obese obstetric population.

Nevertheless, while further study is encouraged, it would seem that the potential benefit of reducing significant life-threatening morbidities among the obese gravid population would outweigh the potential risks of these prophylactic interventions. Infectious complications of cesarean section are particularly common among the obese population undergoing cesarean section. Prophylactic antibiotics have been found to be the most significant protective factors in the reduction of postoperative wound infection and endometritis. Given that maternal obesity is a high-risk factor for maternal mortality and a large proportion of that mortality is related to thromboembolic complications, it would seem that a risk/benefit evaluation would favor the use of low-dose prophylactic heparin perioperatively in the obese population. Five thousand to 10 thousand units given subcutaneously every 8 to 12 hours beginning 6 to 8 hours prior to surgery and continuing until the patient is fully ambulatory is a suggested empiric protocol. Alternatively, an adjusted dose protocol to achieve subtherapeutic peak antifactor Xa heparin activity levels of 0.11 to 0.25 units/mL may be considered. This regimen has been used among obese patients undergoing gastric bypass surgery, and found to be effective and with minimal complications. Some reports would suggest that the concomitant use of both heparin prophylaxis with compression hose and pneumatic sequential compression of the lower extremities should be made to further reduce the occurrence of thromboembolic complications. It is suggested that these devices be applied to the lower extremities *prior to* surgery. Patients who may receive or who have received regional anesthesia *are not* candidates for low molecular weight heparin due to an increased risk of spinal and epidural hematoma formation. Table 6 6 reviews the intrapartum and postpartum management recommendations.

Incision Choice

While the incision of choice for cesarean section in obese patients is not entirely clear from the literature, it has been reported that 86 percent of massively obese patients had a transverse incision, 72 percent Pfannenstiel and 14 percent transverse periumbilical. Benefits of the transverse incision include a more secure closure, less fat transection, and less postoperative pain. Perhaps the most compelling reason to utilize a transverse incision is its association with a diminished risk for atelectasis and hypoxemia postoperatively and decreased pain leading to earlier ambulation and deep breathing, all critically important given the increased risk of pulmonary and thromboembolic complications. Criticisms of the Pfannenstiel incision include the placement of a surgical wound in the warm, moist intertriginous area beneath the panniculus, potentially increasing the risk of infection, more difficult surgical exposure, and the inability to explore the upper abdomen. It has been demonstrated, however, that the type of incision utilized is not independently related to operative morbidity and more recently a case-control study demonstrated no difference in postoperative morbidity among morbidly obese patients undergoing cesarean section with either a vertical supraumbilical skin incision with uterine fundal incision compared to a Pfannenstiel skin incision and low transverse uterine incision.

A suggested approach would include the retraction of the pannus utilizing Montgomery straps. This permits exposure of the lower abdomen, allowing the Pfannenstiel incision to be made through a minimum of adipose tissue (Fig. 6-1). At times, the pannus may be too large to accomplish retraction and doing so may lead to marked cardiorespiratory compromise in the patient with a massive panniculus or the retraction results in the pannus becoming a

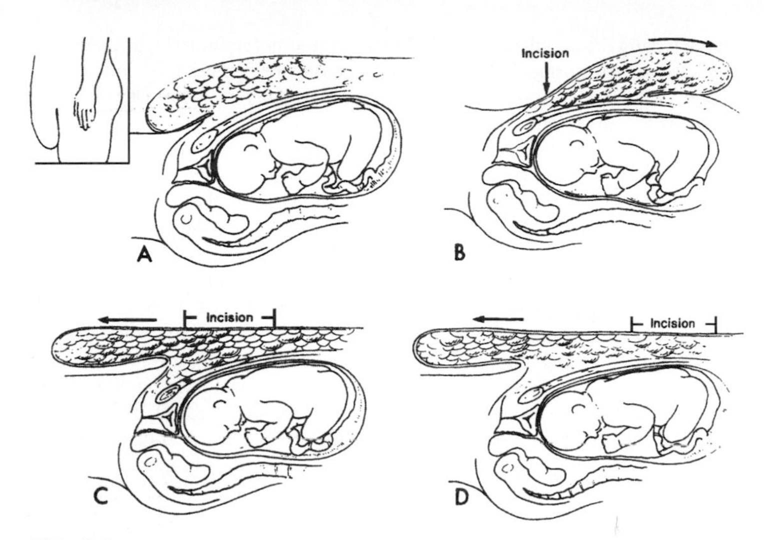

FIG. 6-1 Diagram of massive obese pregnant patient showing the following panniculus in place, **A**; placement of a Pfannensteil incision following retraction of the panniculus, **B**; location of a low midline vertical incision above the panniculus, **C**; and placement of a midline vertical incision higher in the abdomen or periumbilically, **D**; (*Source: Gross TL: Clin Perinatol 1983;10:411–421.*)

vertical wall of tissue prohibiting access to the lower abdomen. In this situation, or alternatively, a transverse or vertical periumbilical incision may be utilized. This allows for excellent exposure without pannus retraction and the potential for cardiorespiratory compromise (Fig. 6-2). The incision circumvents the intertriginous area beneath the pannus and avoids the thick and edematous portion of the panniculus transected in high Pfannenstiel or low vertical incisions. The supraumbilical vertical skin incision with a fundal uterine incision with breech extraction of the vertex fetus (in conjunction with bilateral tubal ligation) has been shown to have similar postoperative morbidity in morbidly obese patients when compared to a low transverse abdominal incision. Some have advocated the superiority of the surgical technique using less sharp dissection and greater use of manual manipulation of the tissues as in the Joel-Cohen incision and Misgav Ladach method for cesarean section. These techniques have yet to be studied specifically in the obese population, but in principle they are worthy of consideration for this high-risk group. At times it may be useful to use vacuum extraction assistance at the time of cesarean section on markedly obese patients. The forces, generated with fundal pressure as the vertex is typically delivered at cesarean section, will be dissipated throughout the large abdominal body mass of the patient and is therefore often times not helpful in assisting with delivery.

Uterine closure can be undertaken in the usual manner with close attention to hemostasis. Operative times are longer and blood loss greater in this population. Often, visualization of the operative field can be compromised and obviously, care must be taken with sharp instruments in a visually challenged surgical field. As needle-stick injuries occur commonly and given the risks for infectious disease transmission through these accidents, consideration for

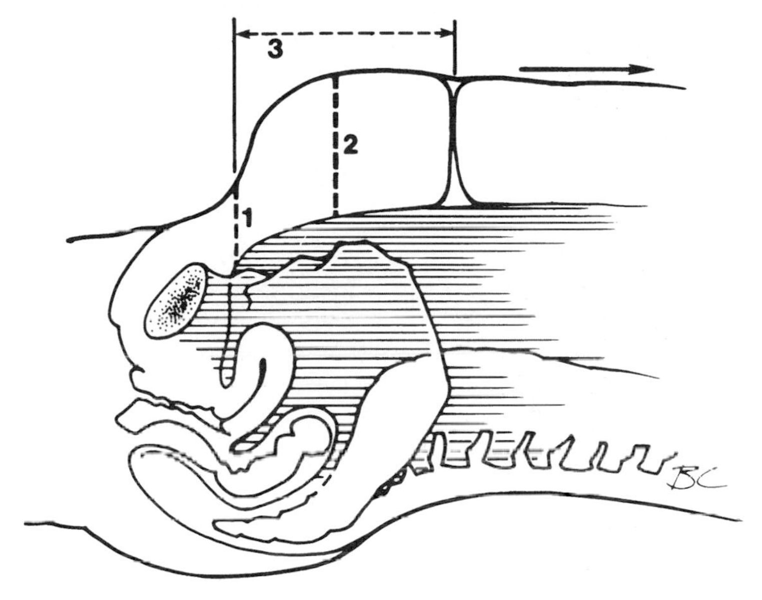

FIG. 6-2 Possible sites of abdominal incisions. The panniculus retracted in the direction of the solid arrow. **1** = low suprasymphyseal transverse abdominal incision; **2** = high suprasymphyseal transverse abdominal incision; **3** = low midline abdominal incision. (*Source: Krebs HB: Obstet Gynecol 1984;63:241–245.*)

blunt needle use should be given. These needles work well with cesarean section, and a recent survey study demonstrated their acceptance and efficacy. Fascial closure requires special attention. If a vertical incision is utilized, a Smead-Jones or modified Smead-Jones closure is preferred (Fig. 6-3). Transverse fascial incisions may be closed with a permanent (e.g., prolene) or delayed absorbable suture (e.g., 1 PDS, 1 Maxon, 1 Vicryl). The placement of closed surgical drains within the subcutaneous tissue has been studied in randomized fashion and while results have been conflicting, the preponderance of literature would suggest a decreased likelihood of wound complications with obliteration of the subcutaneous space with either sutures or closed suction drainage when the subcutaneous tissue is at least 2 cm in depth. An individualized surgical approach to the clinical situation is always appropriate.

Sterile skin staples may be used for skin closure; however, one should be careful not to remove them prematurely in the obese patient. With postcesarean patients being discharged as early as the second postoperative day, some patients may need to return as outpatients for staple removal several days postdischarge.

Finally, these patients should be given thorough discharge instructions including the signs and symptoms of wound infection and dehiscence, endomyometritis, thromboembolic complications (deep venous thrombosis and pulmonary embolism), and diligent follow-up with respect to the continued management of any existing medical complications.

In conclusion, the management and care of the obese gravida is extremely challenging and laden with significant risks. Our interventions and attention to

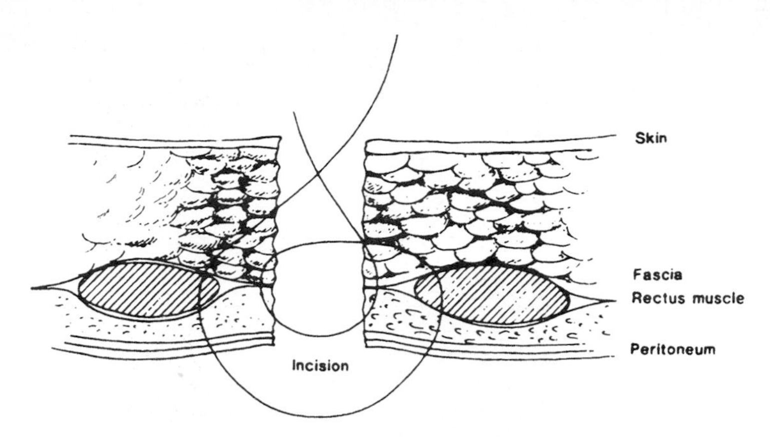

FIG. 6-3 Diagram showing placement of a Smead Jones suture. (*Source: Gross TL: Clinics in Perinatology 1983;10:411–421.*)

detail may allow us to markedly improve perinatal outcome and reduce maternal morbidity and mortality for this high-risk group of patients. Hopefully efforts in this regard will also allow for the development of a physician-patient relationship built upon mutual trust and rapport, contributing to a long-term influence of our care on the patient's obese condition. Truly, any impact made in this regard has the potential for tremendous health benefit over the patient's entire life and in a subsequent pregnancy.

SUGGESTED READING

Epidemiology

Dixon JP, Dixon ME, O'Brien PE: Pregnancy after Lap-Band surgery: management of the band to achieve healthy weight outcomes. *Obes Surg* 2001;11:59–65.

Ehrenberg HM, Dierker L, Milluzzi C, et al.: Prevalence of maternal obesity in an urban center. *Am J Obstet Gynecol* 2002;187:1189–1193.

Flegal KM, Carroll MD, Ogden CL, et al.: Prevalence and trends in obesity among US adults, 1999-2000. *JAMA* 2002;288(14):1723–1727.

Fontaine KR, Redden DT, Wang C, et al.: Years of life lost due to obesity. *JAMA* 2003; 289(2):187–193.

Garfinkel L: Overweight and cancer. *Ann Int Med* 1985;103:1034–1036.

Karlsson J, Taft C, Sjostrom L, et al.: Psychosocial functioning in the obese before and after weight reduction: construct validity and responsiveness of the obesity-related problems scale. *Int J Obes Relat Metab Disord* 2003;27(5):617–630.

King GA, Fitzhugh EC, Bassett DR Jr, et al.: Relationship of leisure-time physical activity and occupational activity to the prevalence of obesity. *Int J Obestet Relat Metab Disord* 2001;25(5):606–612.

Kral JG: Morbid obesity and related health risks. *Ann Int Med* 1985;103:1043–1047.

Mokdad AH, Ford ES, Bowman BA, et al.: Prevalence of obesity, diabetes, and obesity-related health risk factors, 2001. *JAMA* 2003;289:76–79.

Must A, Spadano J, Coakley EH, et al.: The disease burden associated with overweight and obesity. *JAMA* 1999;282(16):1523–1529.

Ogden CL, Flegal KM, Carroll MD, et al.: Prevalence and trends in overweight among US children and adolescents, 1999-2000. *JAMA* 2002;288(14):1728–1732.

Ramirez MM, Turrentine MA: Gastrointestinal hemorrhage during pregnancy in a patient with a history of vertical-banded gastroplasty. *Am J Obstet Gynecol* 1995; 173:1630–1631.

Weiss HG, Nehoda H, Labeck B, et al.: Pregnancies after adjustable gastric banding. *Obes Surg* 2001;11:303–306.

Obesity and Perinatal Outcome

Castro LC and Avina RL: Maternal obesity and pregnancy outcomes. *Curr Opin Obstet Gynecol* 2002;14:601–606.

Freedman MA, Preston LW, George WM: Grotesque obesity: a serious complication of labor and delivery. *S Med J* 1972;65:732–736.

Gross T, Sokol RJ, King K: Obesity in pregnancy: risks and outcome. *Obstet Gynecol.* 1980;56:446–450.

Johnson SR, Kolberg BH, Varner MW, et al.: Maternal obesity and pregnancy. *Surg Gynecol Obstet* 1987;164:431–437.

Lewis DF, Chesson AL, Edwards MS, et al.: Obstructive sleep apnea during pregnancy resulting in pulmonary hypertension. *S Med* 1998;91:761–762.

Lu GC, Rouse DJ, DuBard M, et al.: The effect of the increasing prevalence of maternal obesity on perinatal morbidity. *Am J Obstet Gynecol* 2001;185:845–849.

Naeye RL: Maternal body weight and pregnancy outcome. *Am J Clin Nutr* 1990; 52:273–279.

Perlow JH, Morgan MA, Montgomery DM, et al.: Perinatal outcome in pregnancy complicated by massive obesity. *Am J Obstet Gynecol* 1992;167:958–962.

Wolfe HM, Zador IE, Gross TL, et al.: The clinical utility of maternal body mass index in pregnancy. *Am J Obstet Gynecol* 1991;164:1306–1310.

Obesity and Surgical Risks, Cesarean Section

Allaire AD, Fisch J, McMahon MJ: Subcutaneous drain vs. suture in obese women undergoing cesarean delivery. A prospective, randomized trial. *J Reprod Med* 2000, 45:327–331.

Beattie PG, Rings TR, Hunter MF, et al.: Risk factors for wound infection following caesarean section. *Aust N Z J Obstet Gynaecol* 1994;34:398–402.

Chauhan SP, Magann EF, Carroll CS, et al.: Mode of delivery for the morbidly obese with prior cesarean delivery: Vaginal versus repeat cesarean section. *Am J Obstet Gynecol* 2001;185:349–354.

Chelmow D, Huang E, Strohbehn K: Closure of the subcutaneous dead space and wound disruption at cesarean delivery. *J Matern Fetal Neonatal Med* 2002;11: 403–408.

Del Valle GO, Combs P, Qualls C, et al.: Does closure of Camper fascia reduce the incidence of post-cesarean superficial wound disruption? *Obstet Gynecol* 1992;80:1013–1016.

Gallup DG: Modifications of celiotomy techniques to decrease morbidity in obese gynecologic patients. *Am J Obstet Gynecol* 1984;150:171–178.

Gross TL: Operative considerations in the obese pregnant patient. *Clin Perinatol* 1983;10:411–421.

Hema KR, Hohanson R: Techniques for performing caesarean section. *Best Pract Res Clin Obstet Gynaecol* 2001;15:17–47.

Holmgren G, Sjoholm L, Stark M: The Misgav Ladach method for cesarean section: method description. *Acta Obstet Gynecol Scand* 1999;78:615–621.

Houston MC and Raynor BD: Postoperative morbidity in the morbidly obese parturient woman: Supraumbilical and low transverse abdominal approaches. *Am J Obstet Gynecol* 2000;182:1033–1035.

Kaiser PS, Kirby RS: Obesity as a risk factor for cesarean in a low-risk population. *Obstet Gynecol* 2001;97:39–43.

Kamran SI, Downey D, Ruff RL: Pneumatic sequential compression reduces the risk of deep vein thrombosis in stroke patients. *Neurology* 1998;50(6):1683–1688.

Krebs HB, Helmkamp FB: Transverse periumbilical incision in the massively obese patient. *Obstet Gynecol* 1984;63:241–245.
Magann EF, Chauhan SP, Rodts-Palenik S, et al.: Subcutaneous stitch closure versus subcutaneous drain to prevent wound disruption after cesarean delivery: a randomized clinical trial. *Am J Obstet Gynecol* 2002;186:1119–1123.
Myles TD, Gooch J, Snatolaya J: Obesity as an independent risk factor for infectious morbidity in patients who undergo cesarean delivery. *Obstet Gynecol* 2002;100: 959–964.
Nielsen TF, Hokegard KH: Postoperative cesarean section morbidity: a prospective study. *Am J Obstet Gynecol* 1983;146:911–916.
Perlow JH, Barber C, Moorehead S: Blunt suture needle use in obstetrics: a survey of physician attitudes and experience with blunt needle use during cesarean. Abstract #163 *Am J Obstet Gynecol* 2002;187(6):105.
Perlow JH, Morgan MA: Massive obesity and perioperative cesarean morbidity. *Am J Obstet Gynecol* 1994;170:560–565.
Pisegna JR: Switching between intravenous and oral pantoprazole. *J Clin Gastroenterol* 2001;32:27–32.
Shepherd MF, Rosborough TK, Schwartz ML: Heparin thromboprophylaxis in gastric bypass surgery. *Obestet Surg* 2003;13(2):249–253.
Sicuranza BJ, Tisdall LH: Cesarean section in the massively obese. *J Reprod Med* 1975;14:10–11.
Wolfe HM, Gross TL, Sokol RJ, et al.: Determinants of morbidity in obese women delivered by cesarean. *Obstet Gynecol* 1988;71:691–696.

Obesity, Pregnancy and Anesthetic Morbidity and Mortality

Conklin KA: Can anesthetic-related maternal mortality be reduced? Letter: *Am J Obstet Gynecol* 1990;163:253–254.
Endler GC, Mariona FG, Sokol RJ, et al.: Anesthesia-related maternal mortality in Michigan, 1972 to 1984. *Am J Obstet Gynecol* 1988;159:187–193.
Endler GC: The risk of anesthesia in obese parturients. *J Perinatol* 1990;10:175–179.
Maeder EC, Barno A, Mecklenburg F: Obesity: a maternal high risk factor. *Obstet Gynecol* 1975;45:669–672.
May JW, Greiss FC Jr: Maternal mortality in North Carolina: A forty-year experience. *Am J Obstet Gynecol* 1989;161:555–561.

7 The Diagnosis and Treatment of Thromboembolic Disease in Pregnancy

Robert D. Auerbach   Charles J. Lockwood

INTRODUCTION

Hemorrhage and thrombosis are major contributors to both perinatal and maternal morbidity and mortality. That they do not occur more often is remarkable, given the paradoxical challenges presented to a woman's hemostatic system during the antepartum and postpartum period. During early placentation, syncytiotrophoblasts penetrate maternal uterine vessels to establish the primordial uteroplacental circulation. Subsequently, endovascular extravillous cytotrophoblasts invade uterine spiral arteries orchestrating a morphological transformation of these vessels to facilitate high volume, low resistance blood flow into the intervillous space. To ensure fetal survival these events must occur in the absence of either significant decidual hemorrhage (i.e., abruption) or intervillous thrombosis. To ensure maternal survival, decidual hemorrhage must be avoided throughout pregnancy. However, the greatest hemostatic challenge faced by the mother occurs during the third stage of labor. Following separation of the placenta from the uterine wall after delivery of the infant, hemostasis must be rapidly achieved to avoid potentially catastrophic hemorrhage. While local factors such as high decidual tissue factor (aka thromboplastin) expression contribute to this placental site hemostasis, dramatic changes in the mother's expression of clotting and anticlotting factors are also required to meet this hemostatic challenge. However, a high price is paid to prevent this hemorrhage since pregnancy and the puerperium are associated with a 10-fold increased risk of venous thromboembolic disease (VTE).

Virchow's classic triad of stasis, hypercoagulability, and vascular trauma is present during pregnancy. Pregnancy is a hypercoagulable state by virtue of the associated increases in coagulation factors, and decreases in anticlotting and antifibrinolytic factors. Stasis is increased due to venodilation and uterine compression of the inferior vena cava and iliac veins while trauma can result from cesarean delivery and/or endomyometritis.

Manifestations of VTE in pregnancy include superficial and deep vein thrombosis (DVT), pulmonary embolus (PE), septic pelvic thrombophlebitis, and ovarian vein thrombosis. A leading cause of maternal morbidity and mortality, the risk of VTE is 8.5 in 10,000 pregnancies with approximately 30 percent of events occurring in the antenatal period and 70 percent occurring in the postpartum period. If a DVT remains untreated, PE will occur in one quarter of the patients with a mortality rate of 15 percent. Two-thirds of these deaths occur within thirty minutes of the PE. In contrast, if promptly treated, less than 5 percent of patients with DVT will develop a PE and their mortality rate is less than one percent. Thus, prompt diagnosis and initiation of treatment is crucial to optimizing patient outcome. This chapter will define the regulation of hemostasis, changes initiated by pregnancy, and current methods to diagnose, treat, and prevent VTE.

THE REGULATION OF HEMOSTASIS

A detailed discussion of the clotting system, the anticoagulant system, and the fibrinolytic system is beyond the scope of this manual and can be found elsewhere in more comprehensive textbooks. A practical and user friendly version of the complex regulatory pathways of hemostasis and fibrinolysis is presented in Fig. 7-1.

Pregnancy and VTE: Risk Factors

Clinical Risk Factors

Cesarean delivery and postpartum endomyometritis lower the levels of protein S and cause tissue injury while increased parity promotes venous stasis. Not surprisingly each of these factors increases the risk of VTE. Cesarean delivery alone is associated with a ninefold increase in the risk of VTE compared to vaginal delivery. Other clinical risk factors unrelated to pregnancy include trauma, infection, obesity, nephrotic syndrome, age greater than 35, bed rest, orthopedic surgery, and a prior history of VTE. Smoking (odds ratio 2.4) and prior superficial venous thrombosis (odds ratio 9.4) are additional independent risk factors for VTE during pregnancy and the postpartum period.

Thrombophilia

Patients with inherited or acquired thrombophilia are at a particularly high risk for VTE in pregnancy (Table 7-1). The most common serious inherited thrombophilia is activated protein C resistance (APCR) which occurs in 5 percent of the Caucasian population but in up to 40 percent of patients with VTE. This condition is primarily inherited in an autosomal dominant fashion and is designated the factor V Leiden (FVL) mutation. The FVL mutation results in the substitution of a glutamine for an arginine at position 506 in the factor V polypeptide, preventing the inactivation of factor V by APC. Pregnancy-associated reductions in protein S levels and increases in factor VIII levels exacerbate FVL's prothrombotic tendency with the mutation increasing the risk of VTE in pregnancy from 0.07 percent to about 0.20 percent. Patients with a single mutation have a five- to 10-fold increased risk of VTE while the rare homozygote patient has a >100-fold risk (17 percent). While FVL is present in 40 percent of pregnant patients with VTE, the estimated risk of VTE among pregnant FVL heterozygotes is only 1 in 500. The presence of antiphospholipid antibodies, low protein S levels and elevated factor VIII levels (as occur in pregnancy) may cause false positive laboratory results. While clinical laboratories have the theoretical ability to screen for APCR in pregnancy, polymerase chain reaction (PCR) is the optimal method of confirming the presence of the FVL mutation in pregnancy.

A prothrombin gene promoter mutation (G20210A) is present in 2 to 3 percent of the European population and leads to increased circulating levels of prothrombin and an increased risk of VTE. However, while 17 percent of VTE events in pregnancy occur as a result of this mutation, the actual risk of clotting in an asymptomatic carrier is only 1/200, or 0.5 percent. Like FVL homozygotes, the rare prothrombin G20210A homozygote is at very high risk (15 to 20 percent) of VTE in pregnancy. In contrast, compound heterozygotes

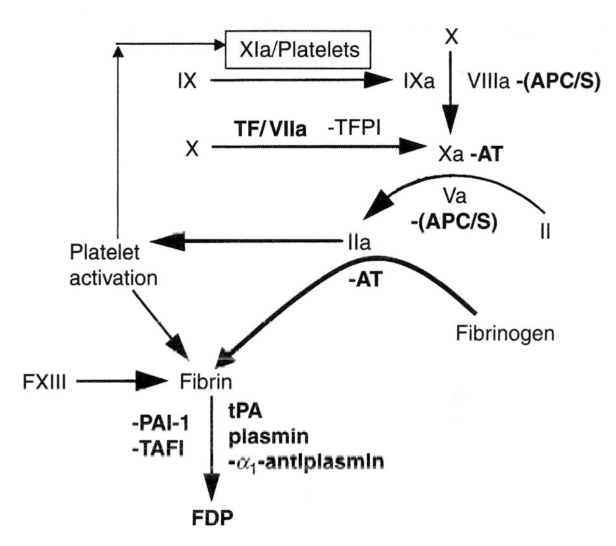

FIG. 7-1 Hemostatic and fibrinolytic pathways. The primary initiator of coagulation is tissue factor (TF) which is not normally expressed by cells in contact with the circulation (i.e., endothelial cells). Following vascular disruption, perivascular, cell membrane–bound TF complexes with plasma-derived factor VII or its more active form (VIIa) to directly convert factor X to Xa. TF/VIIa can also indirectly generate Xa by converting factor IX to IXa, which, in turn, complexes with factor VIIIa to convert X to Xa. Factor Xa, once generated, complexes with its co-factor, Va, to convert prothrombin (factor II) to thrombin (IIa). Thrombin activates platelets and cleaves fibrinogen to generate fibrin monomers, which spontaneously polymerize and are cross-linked by thrombin-activated factor XIIIa to form a stable clot. Clotting is restrained by a series of anticoagulant proteins. The initial anticoagulant response is by TF pathway inhibitor (TFPI) that binds to the TF/VIIa/Xa complex to rapidly stop TF-mediated clotting. However, thrombin-activated factor XIa maintains clotting by serving as an alternative activator of factor IX on the surface of platelets. Thus, effective inhibition of the clotting cascade requires prevention of factor IXa- and Xa-mediated clotting. Activated protein C and protein S (APC/S) complex serves this function by inactivating factors VIIIa and Va, respectively. However, the most crucial endogenous anticoagulant system involves antithrombin (AT) inactivation of thrombin and Xa directly. Finally, fibrinolysis breaks down the fibrin clot. Fibrinolysis is mediated by tissue-type plasminogen activator (tPA) that binds to fibrin where it activates plasmin. Plasmin, in turn, degrades fibrin but can be inactivated by alpha$_2$antiplasmin embedded in the fibrin clot. Fibinolysis is primarily inhibited by type-1 plasminogen activator inhibitor (PAI-1), the fast inactivator of tPA. Thrombin activatable fibrinolytic inhibitor (TAFI) is an alternative antifibrinolytic protein.

for the FVL and prothrombin gene mutations have a lower, 4.6 percent, risk of VTE.

Deficiencies of AT (aka ATIII), protein C, and protein S are rarer inherited thrombophilias. The most serious is AT deficiency which, though quite rare (1/3000), is associated with a >50 percent risk of antepartum and puerperal VTE and accounts for 2 to 20 percent of such cases in pregnancy. Protein C and protein S deficiencies are less rare (1/200 to 1/1500), are associated with a 4-percent

TABLE 7-1 The Risk of VTE in Pregnant Patients with a Thrombophilia

Condition	Inheritance	Risk of thrombosis
APA	None	~2%
Factor V Leiden	AD	0.20%
Prothrombin mutation	AD	0.50%
Antithrombin deficiency	AD	50%
Homozygote FVL	AR	20–50%
Homozygote prothrombin	AR	20–50%
Protein C deficiency	AD	~4%
Protein S deficiency	AD	~4%
Elevated factors VII, VIII & XI	AD	~0.1% each
Thrombocythemia	None	Moderate
Hyperhomocysteinemia	AD	0.20%

Risks extrapolated from general population and affected case frequencies assuming a risk of VTE in pregnancy of 0.67/1000.

risk of VTE in pregnancy, and account for 10 to 25 percent of pregnancy-associated VTE. Inherited increases in factors VII, VIII, and XI, as well as thrombocythemia and hyperhomocysteinemia each confer a minimally increased risk (two- to three-fold). It is unclear to what extent VTE risk is increased in homozygotes for the 4G/4G type-1 plasminogen activator inhibitor (PAI-1) allele, which causes increased PAI-1 levels.

The most common acquired thrombophilia results from antiphospholipid antibodies (APA) accounting for approximately 14 percent of VTE events in pregnancy. These antibodies also cause thrombocytopenia and adverse obstetrical outcomes including stillbirth, fetal growth restriction, and severe preeclampsia. At least two distinct classes of APA are closely linked to VTE. Lupus anticoagulants (LACs) were first described in patients with lupus, false positive serological tests for syphilis, and a plasma inhibitor of in vitro phospholipid-dependent clotting assays. Despite their name, LACs are associated with thrombosis. A second class of prothrombotic APAs react to the anionic phospholipid-binding protein β-2-glycoprotein-I (i.e., anticardiolipin (ACA) and anti-β2GPI antibodies). While these APAs often arise from conditions associated with VTE (e.g., SLE) they also directly promote vascular thrombosis by direct or indirect interference with a variety of anionic phospholipid-associated anticoagulant proteins (e.g., β2GPI, annexin V, antithrombin, thrombomodulin, protein C and S). The type and concentration of an APA predicts its pathogenicity with IgM ACA antibodies and low-positive IgG ACA antibodies seldom associated with medical complications, while LAC and IgG ACAs >19 GPL units are associated with a fourfold higher rate of medical complications. Thus, strict criteria are required to diagnose both LAC activity and ACA reactivity prior to initiating therapy.

Patients with newly diagnosed VTE or a personal or strong family history of VTE should be studied for the FVL and Prothrombin 20210A mutations, AT, protein C and protein S deficiencies, LAC, ACA, and anti-β2GPI antibodies.

DEEP VEIN THROMBOSIS (DVT)

An acutely erythematous, edematous, and tender lower extremity is the classic presentation of a DVT. Unfortunately, many of these same complaints are

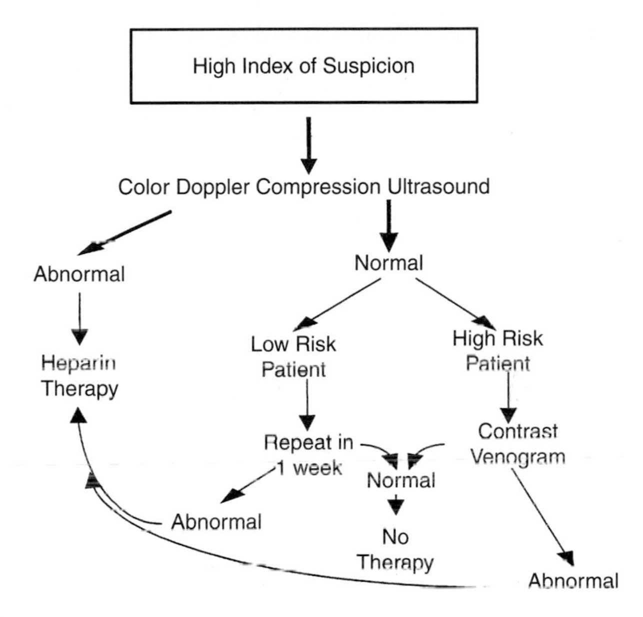

FIG. 7-2 Ruling out DVT in pregnant patients.

present in women with a normal pregnancy. Pain in the calf, when the foot is passively dorsiflexed (i.e., Homan's sign) may be demonstrated. However, >50 percent of patients with this classic presentation do not have a DVT. Therefore, all clinically suspicious cases require further study. Noninvasive testing has emerged as the initial step in the diagnostic management of these patients (Fig. 7-2).

Compression color Doppler ultrasound is both highly sensitive (92 percent) and specific (98 percent) for popliteal and femoral vein thrombosis but less effective for evaluating calf vein thrombosis with a sensitivity of only 50 percent. Isolated iliac vein thrombosis can sometimes be diagnosed by placing patients in the left lateral decubitus position, and assessing Doppler flow variations with respirations. If these sonographic findings are abnormal, venous thrombosis can be diagnosed and treatment started. Conversely, if the sonographic findings are normal and the patient has no other risk factors (e.g., history of VTE, thrombophilia, or clinical progression), the study can be repeated in a week and if negative, no treatment is required. However, contrast venography should be performed if the sonographic findings are normal but there is a high index of suspicion.

Contrast venography remains the gold standard for diagnosing DVT in pregnancy. When used with an abdominal lead shield it exposes the fetus to very low levels of radiation (0.0005 Gy). This exposure is below that associated with childhood cancers and teratogenicity. Contrast agents are injected into lower extremity veins and the venous system of the leg and pelvis are evaluated radiographically. Chemical phlebitis occurs in 3 percent of cases.

Magnetic resonance imaging (MRI) is useful for detecting thigh and pelvic vein thrombosis. Although the safety of MRI in pregnant women is yet to be proven, no adverse effects have been noted and it is likely to find increasing use in the obstetric population as clinical experience is gained.

In summary, compression color Doppler ultrasound is recommended as the initial test in pregnant women with suspected DVT. If this study proves positive for a DVT, treatment should be initiated. With equivocal test results, contrast venography or MRI (for pelvic thromboses) are performed as detailed in Fig. 7-2.

PULMONARY EMBOLISM (PE)

The classic clinical triad of dyspnea, pleuritic chest pain, and hemoptysis occurs in only 25 percent of patients with documented PE. Similarly, cyanosis, tachypnea, syncope, diaphoresis, fever, a pleural friction rub and a fixed S2 are insensitive and/or nonspecific signs and symptoms. Complicating 1/2500 pregnancies, PE results in obstruction to pulmonary arterial blood flow, vasoconstriction of small arterial vessels, and a progressive loss of alveolar surfactant. Although patients may display hypoxia, 17 percent patients will have a normal PaO_2. A decreased PaO_2 is also not overly specific, since the supine position may lower PaO_2 by as much as 15 mmHg in the third trimester. Echocardiographic findings include right ventricular dilation and hypokinesis, tricuspid regurgitation, and pulmonary artery dilation. An EKG may reveal right bundle branch block, right axis shift, Q wave in leads III and aVF, S wave in leads I and aVL >1.5 mm, T wave inversions in leads III and aVF or new onset of atrial fibrillation. However, these cardiac findings are insensitive predictors since they require large pulmonary artery occlusions.

The initial evaluation should be a ventilation/perfusion scan (V/Q scan). However, the scan must be interpreted in the context of clinical probability. Only negative and low probability scans in the setting of a low clinical risk, and high probability scans in the setting of high clinical risks are considered diagnostic. Nondiagnostic scans (i.e., intermediate probability) or low probability scans in high-risk patients (e.g., thrombophilia, suggestive ECG, or echocardiogram) should be followed up with a Color Doppler compression ultrasound study of the lower extremities. A DVT in conjunction with a nondiagnostic V/Q scan requires therapy. However, fewer than 30 percent of unselected patients with PE have sonographic/radiographic signs of a DVT at the time of presentation. Thus, a pulmonary angiography should be obtained in a high-risk patient with a negative compression ultrasound (Fig. 7-3).

Certain medical centers with experience may use MRI or spiral volumetric computed tomography pulmonary angiography (SVCT) as a noninvasive substitute. However, the reported sensitivities of SVCT compared with the *gold standard* pulmonary angiography vary widely (64 to 93 percent). While SVCT is relatively sensitive and specific for diagnosing central pulmonary artery thrombi, it is insensitive for diagnosing subsegmental clots. Therefore, SVCT appears to have a role as a rule-in test for large central emboli, but cannot exclude smaller peripheral lesions. Like compression ultrasonography, an equivocal V/Q scan in a high-risk patient with a positive spiral CT should require therapy, but a negative spiral CT should prompt pulmonary angiography.

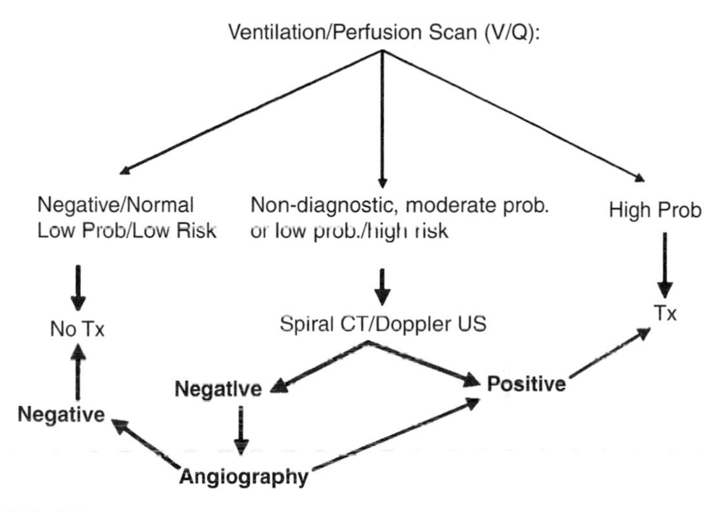

FIG. 7-3 Patient presents with a clinical history suspicious for PE.

Although the amount of radiation exposure from a V/Q scan is less than 0.005 Gy of radiation, in a 1998 survey, only 67 percent of respondents reported that they perform V/Q scans in pregnant patients. Since a normal perfusion study requires no further testing, radiation exposure may be reduced by performing this test first. Spiral CT scans and pulmonary angiography, with appropriate abdominal shielding and employing minimal fluoroscopy, expose the fetus to <50 mrad for the entire examination.

PELVIC THROMBOSES

Septic pelvic thrombophlebitis (SPT) is an uncommon and controversial complication of pelvic infection. It is more common after cesarean than vaginal delivery but has also been reported after gynecologic procedures. Thrombus formation in the pelvic veins is likely to result from inflammatory cytokine induction of tissue factor expression in the endothelium of pelvic vessels. Physical findings are nonspecific. Multiple infected emboli may result from fibrinolysis. The typical presentation is a patient who develops spiking fevers that persist despite adequate antibiotic coverage. MRI or CT imaging may aid in the diagnosis. Although these techniques may be specific, a nonocclusive thrombus in the iliofemoral veins may remain undetected. Traditional management was a course of therapeutic anticoagulation. Clinical response was considered both therapeutic and diagnostic with defervescence expected in 48 to 72 hours and the recommended duration of treatment ranging from 7 to 10 days to a full 6 weeks of anticoagulation. However, a recent study has called into question the role of anticoagulation in SPT. In a small study of 14 patients with CT documented SPT, eight received continued antibiotic therapy alone (ampicillin, gentamicin, and clindamycin) and six received a combination of heparin and antibiotic therapy. No difference was noted in the duration of fever between the two groups (Brown, 1999).

Ovarian vein thrombosis (OVT) typically presents with acute pain two to three days postpartum (with or without fever). It occasionally can be mistaken for appendicitis in a postpartum patient. Moreover, OVT can occur in the absence of infection and has been described in antepartum patients. The incidence of OVT is 1/4000 deliveries. Thrombosis can be diagnosed with CT or MRI and is most commonly noted in the right ovarian vein. Treatment for OVT is the same as outlined for SPT.

TREATMENT

Heparin anticoagulation is the therapy of choice for DVT with or without PE. In addition, leg elevation and application of warm moist heat may decrease swelling and provide some symptomatic relief. In the case of PE, attention should be focused on maintaining the maternal PaO_2 above 70 mmHg or O_2 saturation of >95 percent.

Heparin

Heparin does not cross the placenta nor enter breast milk. It enhances AT activity, increases factor Xa inhibitor activity and inhibits platelet aggregation. Side effects include hemorrhage, osteoporosis, and thrombocytopenia. Hemorrhage is more common with concomitant aspirin use, recent surgery, thrombocytopenia, and liver disease. Heparin-induced thrombocytopenia occurs in 3 percent of patients and has two forms: an early-onset, transient, heparin-induced platelet aggregation for which therapy need not be interrupted; and an IgG-mediated, heparin-induced thrombotic thrombocytopenia (HIT-2) occurring within two weeks of starting therapy and mandating cessation of therapy. The occurrence of heparin-associated and induced thrombocytopenia appears less with low molecular weight heparin. Platelet counts should be followed for the first three weeks of therapy. Heparin-induced osteoporosis is common when doses are greater than 15,000 U/day for more than six months. Again it seems less common with the use of low molecular weight heparin in pregnancy.

The goals of therapy for acute VTE are to maintain heparin levels of between 0.2 and 0.4 U/mL (protamine assay), or antifactor Xa activity between 0.6 and 1.2 U/mL or the aPTT between 1.5 and 2.5 times control. The dose required to achieve these goals will vary among different individuals because of variability in levels of heparin-binding proteins such as vitronectin, fibronectin, von-Willebrand factor, platelet factor 4, and histidine-rich glycoprotein, during pregnancy. Unfractionated heparin should be administered with an intravenous loading dose of 80 units/kg, followed by an infusion rate of 18 units/kg/h. Doses are adjusted until the target aPTT, heparin or antifactor Xa level is achieved. The aPTT, heparin or antifactor Xa level should be evaluated every 6 hours in the early stages of therapy. Figure 7-4 provides a practical weight based guideline for Heparin dosage. Because aPTT is not reliable in LAC patients, heparin or antifactor Xa activity concentrations should be followed in these patients. Intravenous therapeutic unfractionated heparin should be continued for at least 5 days or until clinical improvement is noted. Thereafter, administer unfractionated heparin subcutaneously 10,000 to 15,000 U every 8 to 12 hours titrating to an aPTT of 1.5 to 2 times control (or heparin level of at least 0.2 U/mL) six hours after injection.

Raschke's Protocol Orders

1. Make calculations using total body weight: __________ kg (see chart)
2. BOLUS HEPARIN 80 U/kg = __________ U IV.
3. IV HEPARIN infusion 18 U/kg/h = __________ U/h.
   (25,000 U heparin in 250 mL D_5W)
4. WARFARIN ________ mg PO qd; give first dose as soon as aPTT ≥ 50
   (nonpregnant or postpartum)

5. LABORATORY: aPTT, PT, CBC now
   CBC with platelet count q3d
   STAT aPTT 6 h after heparin bolus
   PT qd (start on third day of heparin)

6. ADJUST heparin infusion based on sliding scale below:
   PTT < 35 80 U/kg bolus, increase drip by 4 U/kg/h
   PTT 35–49 40 U/kg bolus, increase drip by 2 U/kg/h
   PTT 50–70 No change
   PTT 71–90 Reduce drip by 2 U/kg/h
   PTT > 90 Hold heparin for 1 h, reduce drip by 3 U/kg/h

2 U/kg/h		3 U/kg/h		4 U/kg/h	
Weight (kg)	Dose change (U/h)	Weight (kg)	Dose change (U/h)	Weight (kg)	Dose change (U/h)
40–74	100	40–50	100	40–60	200
75–124	200	51–80	200	61–87	300
125–170	300	81–115	300	88–112	400
		116–150	400	113–137	500
		151–170	500	138–162	600
				163–175	700

7. Order PTT 6 h after any dosage change, adjusting heparin infusion by the sliding scale until PTT is therapeutic (50–70 s). When two PTTs in a row are therapeutic, order PTT (and readjust heparin drip as needed) q24 h.

   Please make changes as promptly as possible, and round off doses to the nearest mL/h (nearest 100 U).

Signed______________________________Date_______/_______/_______

Note: This protocol provides management guidelines for full therapeutic anticoagulation. **It should not be used for prophylactic anticoagulation or after thrombolytic agents**.

FIG. 7-4 Raschke's protocol orders. APTT, activated partial thromboplastin time; CBC, complete blood count; PT, prothrombin time; PTT, partial thromboplastin time; PO, by mouth; q.d., every day; STAT, immediately.

(*Continued*)

The following chart gives the initial heparin bolus dose and infuslino rates (bolus of 80 U/kg infusion of 18 U/kg/h) rounded off.

Weight (kg)	IV Bolus (U)	Infusion (U/hr)
42–47	3500	800
48–52	4000	900
53–58	4500	1000
59–63	5000	1100
64–69	5300	1200
70–75	5700	1300
76–80	6300	1400
81–86	6700	1500
87–91	7100	1600
92–97	7500	1700
98–102	8000	1800
103–108	8400	1900
109–113	8900	2000
114–119	9300	2100
120–124	9800	2200
125–130	10,200	2300
131–136	10,600	2400
137–141	11,100	2500
148–152	12,000	2700

FIG. 7-4 *(continued)*.

Low molecular weight heparin (LMWH) has been shown to be safe and efficacious in pregnancy. Dalteparin sodium (Fragmin, Upjohn) is given as 100 antifactor Xa units/kg s.q., q 12 h. Alternatively enoxaparin (Lovenox, Aventis) is given at 1 mg/kg q 12 h. The dose of LMWH is titrated to maintain antifactor Xa levels of 0.6 to 1.0 U/mL, 4 hours after injection. Epidural and spinal anesthesia is contraindicated within 18 to 24 hours of LMWH administration to reduce the chance of a hematoma formation. For this reason, we recommend stopping LMWH therapy at 36 weeks, or earlier, if preterm delivery is anticipated and treating with therapeutic doses of unfractionated heparin until delivery.

Patients with AT deficiency, or those homozygous for the FVL or prothrombin mutation, require therapeutic heparin/LMWH throughout pregnancy regardless of their VTE history. However, after four months of either therapeutic unfractionated or LMWH therapy, most other patients with a VTE in pregnancy may be switched to a prophylactic dose of either unfractionated heparin (5000 to 10,000 U s.q., q 12 h) or LMWH (e.g., dalteparin 2500 to 5000 antifactor Xa units s.q., q.d. or enoxaparin 30 mg s.q., b.i.d) titrated to maintain antifactor Xa levels of 0.1 to 0.2 U/mL assessed 6 and 4 hours, for unfractionated and LMWH, respectively, after injection. As noted, we recommend stopping LMWH therapy at 36 weeks and initiating prophylactic unfractionated heparin to permit epidural and spinal anesthesia for delivery.

Vaginal or cesarean delivery should not be accompanied by treatment-related bleeding if the procedure occurs more than 4 hours after a prophylactic dose of unfractionated heparin. If the patient has been on therapeutic doses of unfractionated heparin, the aPTT should be checked preoperatively. If needed, protamine sulfate may be given to reverse a markedly prolonged aPTT at the time of vaginal or cesarean delivery. Similarly, vaginal or cesarean delivery should not be accompanied by treatment-related bleeding if it occurs more than 12 hours after a prophylactic dose of LMWH or more than 18 to 24 hours after a dose of therapeutic LMWH. Antithrombin concentrates can be used in AT deficient patients in the peripartum period. The clinician should restart heparin or LMWH 6 hours after a vaginal delivery and 8 to 12 hours after a cesarean delivery.

Prophylactic anticoagulant therapy should continue during the postpartum period. Six to 12 weeks is indicated following a DVT. Following a PE or complex iliofemoral DVT, four to six months of prophylaxis is indicated. Oral anticoagulant therapy can then begin postpartum by adjusting the Warfarin dose to maintain the patient's INR at approximately 2 to 2.5. Warfarin has a more rapid inhibitory effect on levels of protein C than on many of the clotting factors because of the former's shorter half-life (6 hours vs. 24 to 48 hours). Therefore, unfractionated heparin or LMWH should always be maintained during the initial *four* days of Warfarin therapy *and* until a therapeutic INR is achieved. This regimen will avoid Warfarin-induced paradoxical thromboembolism.

All patients treated with unfractionated heparin or LMWH during pregnancy should receive 1500 mg of calcium supplementation each day. In patients receiving over 15,000 U of unfractionated heparin for greater than six months, bone densitometry studies can be performed in the postpartum period. Osteoporosis should prompt referral to a reproductive or medical endocrinologist familiar with this condition in premenopausal women.

Warfarin

Warfarin inhibits the action of vitamin K which is a cofactor in the synthesis of the final molecular forms of factors VII, IX, X, and prothrombin. As a small molecule loosely bound to albumin, it readily crosses the placenta and carries with it a 33-percent risk of embryopathy when there is exposure between 7 and 12 weeks gestation. The classic stigmata include nasal hypoplasia, stippled epiphysis, and central nervous system abnormalities including: agenesis of the corpus callosum, Dandy-Walker malformation, midline cerebellar atrophy, and ventral midline dysplasia with optic atrophy. Fetal and placental hemorrhage is also a major complication with warfarin use during pregnancy. Vitamin K or fresh-frozen plasma can be used to reverse the effects of warfarin in the rare pregnant patient using this anticoagulant, with normalization of the PT within 6 hours of an oral or subcutaneous 5 mg dose of vitamin K.

Adequate controlled trials do not exist to guide therapy in pregnant patients with a mechanical heart valve. However, this may be one of the few clinical presentations in pregnancy in which the benefits of warfarin use outweigh the risks. Older studies using unfractionated heparin with predominantly older-generation prosthetic heart valves have shown an increase in thrombogenic complications, including fatal maternal valve thrombosis. No large clinical studies exist to guide in the use of LMWH in pregnant patients with mechanical heart valves; however, the manufacturer of Lovenox, Aventis, specifically recommends against its use in this setting, based on reports to the FDA of valvular thrombosis in pregnant women treated with Lovenox. The use of low dose aspirin as an adjunct to warfarin or heparin has been advocated, based on a study of antithrombotic therapy in high-risk patients with mechanical valves. The risk of fatal maternal valve thrombosis may outweigh the risks of warfarin to the fetus between 12 and 36 weeks gestation. A full discussion of these risks should precede conception in this select population. Women with mechanical heart valves who choose either unfractionated or LMWH during the first trimester should realize that they will be at higher risk for thrombosis. It may be prudent to maintain these women on therapeutic doses of unfractionated heparin or LMWH sufficient to prolong the aPTT two times control or to maintain a therapeutic anti-Xa level (0.6 to 1.2 U/mL), respectively, during trough periods (i.e., just prior to their next dose). After the first trimester and until the near term, these women can be switched to warfarin. Since warfarin does not accumulate in breast milk and does not induce an anticoagulant effect in the infant, it is not contraindicated in breast-feeding mothers.

Inferior Vena Cava (IVC) Filters

Inferior vena cava filters may be used in pregnant patients with recurrent PE despite adequate anticoagulation. Additionally, cases of PE or ileofemoral DVT in a patient with a contraindication to anticoagulation such as recent surgery, hemorrhagic stroke, or active bleeding may be an indication. They may be useful in women with allergies to both unfractionated heparin and LMWH. Finally, the development of serious hemorrhagic complications with anticoagulant therapy may warrant an IVC filter. Retrievable IVC filters may prove ideal for pregnant patients requiring this therapy. Currently they remain investigational.

Surgery and Thrombolytic Therapy

Surgical embolectomy should be reserved for life threatening settings. Massive PE with hemodynamic instability should be the only indication for thrombolytic therapy (i.e., tPA, urokinase, and streptokinase) in pregnancy given the high risk that these agents will induce abruption. However, no controlled studies exist examining the efficacy and safety of thrombolytic therapy in pregnancy. In a review of 172 pregnant patients treated with thrombolytic therapy, the maternal mortality rate was 1.2 percent, the fetal loss rate was 6 percent, and maternal complications from hemorrhage occurred in 8 percent (Turrentine et al., 1995).

New Anticoagulants

Recently, several new anticoagulants were approved for clinical use. Two broad categories define these agents: direct thrombin inhibitors (DTI) and specific factor Xa inhibitors. Minimal information exists to guide their use in the pregnant population. The following agents are all listed as category B in the 2002 PDR. Such listing is given to pharmaceuticals that animal studies show no risk or adverse fetal effects but controlled human first trimester studies are not available; no evidence of second or third trimester fetal harm exists; the safety in nursing infants is unknown. Despite the above listing, current use of these medications in pregnant or breastfeeding women is considered investigational and great caution should be exercised in this setting.

Direct Thrombin Inhibitors

As a class, DTIs offer several advantages over indirect inhibitors of thrombin (e.g., unfractionated heparin, LMWH, and heparinoids). They are not bound to plasma proteins and do not rely on levels of AT. Thus, their anticoagulant effect is more predictable. Other advantages stem from their ability to resist neutralization by platelet factor 4 and to inhibit fibrin-bound, as well as fluid phase thrombin. Since no antidote exists, emphasis must be placed on the metabolic clearance of these agents. A disadvantage of all DTIs is that they may also prolong the prothrombin time and pose problems with warfarin regulation.

Hirudin is a 65-amino-acid protein originally extracted from the medicinal leech (*Hirudo medicinalis*). The anticoagulant activity is monitored with the aPTT. However, it is very difficult to obtain large quantities of this protein from its natural source for pharmaceutical use. Lepirudin is a recombinant polypeptide structurally similar to Hirudin and is produced from yeast cells. Its clinical response is also measured by elevation of the aPTT. After an intravenous bolus and continuous infusion, it has a half-life of 40 to 60 minutes. Since this medication is primarily excreted by the kidney, careful attention should be placed on evaluation of renal function. Lepirudin was approved for the management of heparin induced thrombocytopenia type 2 (HIT-2). As previously noted, HIT-2 is a heparin-induced immune mediated syndrome characterized by thrombocytopenia and paradoxical thrombosis that may be life threatening. Although patients treated with Lepirudin may develop anti-hirudin antibodies, these antibodies enhance the drug's anticoagulant effect.

Argatroban is a synthetic, small molecule derived from arginine and is a competitive inhibitor of thrombin. It was also approved for prophylaxis and treatment of HIT-2. Argatroban has a short half-life (45 minutes) and is cleared by the liver. Thus, it would be the DTI of choice in a patient with renal impairment. The goal of the therapy is 1.5 to 3 times the baseline aPTT.

Bivalirudin is another DTI that has been used primarily for cardiac patients. It was approved, for use, by the FDA in December 2000, in patients with unstable angina undergoing percutaneous transluminal coronary angioplasty (with aspirin). Excretion is by renal and proteolytic pathways. Patients with HIT in need of percutaneous coronary angioplasty may benefit from Bivalirudin.

Factor Xa Inhibitors

Fondaparinux is the first of this new class of anticoagulants. Efficacy is based on the pentasaccharide-AT binding site of the heparin molecule. This conformational change allows for the specific binding of AT and the inactivation of factor Xa. As the complex binds, the pentasaccharide is released to further accelerate AT/Xa formation. In December 2001, Fondaparinux was approved for prophylaxis in orthopedic surgery. The drug is excreted in the kidney, has a half-life of 15 hours and is given as a once daily subcutaneous injection.

PREVENTION

Nonpharmacologic Prevention

Nonpharmacologic therapies aimed at preventing VTE in pregnancy include left-lateral decubitus positioning during the third trimester, graduated elastic compression stockings, and pneumatic compression stockings. Graduated elastic compression stockings have been shown to increase femoral vein flow velocity in late pregnancy but their role in decreasing VTE in pregnancy is yet to be defined. Pneumatic compression stockings improve blood flow, decrease stasis, increase blood flow in the femoral vessels by 240 percent, and increase fibrinolysis. In a meta-analysis of moderate-risk surgery, they were shown to decrease the incidence of DVT by 60 percent. Since pneumatic compression stockings have no hemorrhagic risk, and have been shown to be an effective means of DVT prophylaxis in gynecologic oncology surgery, they should be an ideal device for prophylaxis in high-risk pregnant patients (e.g., thrombophilic patients at prolonged bed rest or who are undergoing a cesarean delivery).

Pharmacologic Prevention

Among pregnant patients who have had a previous VTE during pregnancy, recurrence risks of 10 percent have been reported. However, Brill-Edwards and colleagues prospectively followed 125 pregnant women with a previous episode of VTE in whom heparin was withheld until the postpartum period and observed that only three of the women (2.4 percent) had a recurrent VTE event (95 percent CI: 0.2 to 6.9 percent). Moreover, there were no recurrences in the 44 women who had no evidence of thrombophilia and whose previous VTE was associated with a temporary risk factor (e.g., oral contraception, surgery and pregnancy). In contrast, among the 51 women with a thrombophilia or unexplained previous VTE episode, or both, three (5.9 percent) had a recurrent VTE (95 percent CI: 1.2 to 16.2 percent). Other authors have also observed that thrombophilic patients with a prior VTE, or in whom the VTE was unexplained (i.e., not associated with nonrecurring risk factors) have a substantially increased risk of recurrent VTE in pregnancy. We suggest that patients whose prior DVT was associated with a nonrecurring and *nonpregnant state* (e.g., high estrogen dose oral contraceptives or after orthopedic procedures or surgery) and who are without other risk factors (e.g., thrombophilia, need for prolonged bed rest, obesity, superficial thrombophlebitis) do not appear to need prophylactic heparin therapy during pregnancy. However, they *should receive postpartum prophylaxis* since 80 percent of pregnancy-associated fatal PEs occur in the postpartum period. Obviously thrombophilic patients or those with prior unexplained DVT or other major risk factors for VTE should have both antenatal and postpartum unfractionated heparin or LMWH prophylaxis. In contrast to the opinion of Brill-Edwards et al., we posit that a VTE occurring in a prior pregnancy should be included as an unexplained risk factor.

Mini-dose heparin has been effective in preventing DVT in patients at risk. As noted, the standard dose of unfractionated heparin is 5000 units administered subcutaneously every 12 hours. This dose can be increased by 2500 U in the second and third trimesters. However, some authors recommend following antifactor Xa levels to guide VTE prophylaxis during pregnancy. Barbour et al. noted that heparin doses appropriate for prophylaxis varied from patient to patient and from one trimester to the next and recommended following heparin levels to obtain adequate prophylaxis. Adequate antifactor Xa levels for prophylaxis have been defined as 0.1 to 0.2 U/mL. Studies also exist that document the safety and effectiveness of LMWH for thromboprophylaxis. An enoxaparin dose of 40 mg s.q., per day is adequate to prevent VTE in a prospective study of 69 pregnancies (61 women). However, most experts recommend employing enoxaparin at 30 mg s.q., b.i.d. LMWH should be switched to unfractionated heparin and postpartum therapy should be administered as discussed above. Also as noted previously, patients with AT deficiency or homozygotes for either the FVL or prothrombin mutations should receive therapeutic unfractionated heparin or LMWH therapy during pregnancy. In this population, full anticoagulation in the pueperium is indicated regardless of their history of prior VTE.

SUMMARY

Since the clinical signs and symptoms of DVT are frequently unreliable, compression ultrasonography should be employed with follow-up contrast venography if needed. The clinical diagnosis of PE is also frequently incorrect. Ventilation/perfusion scanning, spiral CT or lower extremity compression Color Doppler ultrasonography may detect a PE or DVT directly, although occasionally a pulmonary angiography is required. A documented VTE in pregnancy requires therapeutic anticoagulation with either unfractionated heparin or LMWH for at least four months, or the duration of pregnancy which ever comes first. Postpartum anticoagulant treatment is continued for six weeks to six months depending on the patient's clinical condition and thrombophilia status.

Patients with AT deficiency or those who are homozygotes for the prothrombin or FVL mutations require therapeutic unfractionated heparin or LMWH therapy during pregnancy and full anticoagulation in the puerperium regardless of their history of prior VTE. In women at increased risk for VTE in pregnancy due to prior history of VTE, the presence of other thrombophilias or absence of an identifiable risk factor at the time of their initial thrombosis mandates antenatal prophylaxis with unfractionated heparin or LMWH followed by postpartum anticoagulation. In contrast, patients with a prior VTE associated with a known, nonrecurring risk factor (e.g., surgery, estrogen-containing contraceptive) who are without a maternal thrombophilia do not appear to require antenatal prophylaxis, but should receive postpartum anticoagulation since this is the point of maximal risk for PE. It is our contention that if the patient's prior VTE occurred in a pregnancy, antenatal prophylaxis is required even in the absence of a known thrombophilia.

Graduated elastic stockings may be a useful adjuvant in preventing VTE in pregnant women. Consider pneumatic compression stockings in patients undergoing cesarean delivery who have risk factors for VTE including obesity, prolonged bed rest, and anticipated prolonged surgery. In order for compression stockings to be effective, they must remain on the patient until ambulation has been achieved.

SUGGESTED READING

Ahearn GS, Hadjiliadis D, Govert JA, et al.: Massive pulmonary embolism during pregnancy successfully treated with recombinant tissue plasminogen activator: a case report and review of treatment options. *Arch Int Med* 2002;162:1221.

Barbour LA: Current concepts of anticoagulation therapy in pregnancy. *Obstet Gynecol Clin North Am* 1997;24:499.

Barbour LA, Smith JM, et al.: Heparin levels to guide thromboembolism prophylaxis during pregnancy. *Am J Obstet Gynecol* 1995;173:1869–1873.

Barclay L: Fondaparinux prevents venous thromboembolism better than enoxaparin. *Arch Intern Med* 2002;162:1806–1808.

Boiselle PM, Reddy SS, Villas PA, et al.: Pulmonary embolus in pregnant patients: Survey of ventilation-perfusion imaging policies and practices. *Radiology* 1998; 207:201.

Brill-Edwards P, Ginsberg JS, et al.: Safety of withholding heparin in pregnant women with a history of venous thromboembolism. *N Eng J Med* 343;1439–1444.

Brown CE, Stettler RW, et al.: Puerperal septic pelvic thrombophlebitis: Incidence and response to heparin therapy. *Am J Obstet Gynecol* 1999;181:143–148.

Danilenko-Dixon DR, Heit JA, et al.: Risk factors for deep vein thrombosis and pulmonary embolism during pregnancy and postpartum: A population-based, case-control study. *Am J Obstet Gynecol* 2001;184:104–110.

Fejgin MD, Lourwood DL: Low molecular weight heparins and their use in obstetrics and gynecology. *Obstet Gynecol Surv* 1994;49:424–431.

Ginsberg JS, Greer I, Hirsh J: Use of antithrombotoc agents during pregnancy. *Chest* 2001; Jan 119 (1Suppl):122S.

Ginsberg JS, Hirsh J, Rainbow AJ, et al.: Risk to the fetus of radiologic procedures used in the diagnosis of maternal thromboembolic disease. *Thromb Haemost* 1989; 61:189–196.

Ginsberg JS: Management of venous thromboembolism. *N Eng J Med* 1996; 335:1816–1828.

Girling JC, de Swiet M: Thromboembolism in pregnancy; an overview. *Current Opin Obstet Gynecol* 1996;8:458–463.

Granddone E, Margaglione M, et al.: Genetic susceptibility to pregnancy-related venous thromboembolism: roles of factor V Leiden, Prothrombin G20210A, and Methylenetetrahydrofolate reductase mutations. *Am J Obstet Gynecol* 1998;179:1324–1328.

Heijboer H, Buller HR, Lensing AWA, et al.: A comparession of real-time compression ultrasonography with impedance plethysmography for the diagnosis of deep vein thrombosis in symptomatic patients. *N Engl J Med* 1993;329:1365–1369.

Hirsh J: Heparin. *N Engl J Med* 1991;324:1565–1574.

Hirsh J, Levine MN: Low molecular weight heparin. *Blood* 1992;79:1–17.

Kiss Joseph: New anticoagulants in clinical practice. *Transfusion Medicine Update* 2, 2002.

Kyrle PA, Minar E, Hirschl M, et al.: High plasma levels of factor VIII and the risk of recurrent thromboembolism. *N Engl J Med* 2000;343:457–462.

Laros RK: Thromboembolism in pregnancy. ACOG Educational Bulletin Number 234, March 1997.

Lee D, Warkentin T: Practical treatment guidelines: Heparin-induced thrombocytopenia. The Thrombosis Interest Group of Canada, May 2002.

Lepirudin (rDNA) Injection (Refludan TM) Product Information. Kansas City: March 1998.

Lockwood CJ, Bach R, Guha A, et al.: Amniotic fluid contains tissue factor, a potent initiator of coagulation. *Am J Obstet Gynecol* 1991;165:1335–1341.

Lockwood CJ, Krikun G, Schatz F: The decidua regulates hemostasis in human endometrium. *Semin Reprod Endocrinol* 1999;17:45–51.

Meaney JF, Weg JG, Chenevert TL, et al.: Diagnosis of pulmonary embolism with magnetic resonance angiography. *N Engl J Med* 1997;336:1422.

Nelson-Piercy C, Letsky EA, et al.: Low molecular-weight heparin for obstetric thromboprophylaxis: Experience of sixty-nine pregnancies in sixty-one women at high risk. *Am J Obstet Gynecol* 1997;176:1062–1068.

Oakley CM: Pregnancy and prosthetic heart valves. *Lancet* 1994;344:1643.

Pettila V, Leinonen P, Markkola A, et al.: Postpartum bone mineral density in women treated for thromboprophylaxis with unfractionated heparin or LMW heparin. *Thromb Haemost* 2002;87:182–186.

Raschke RA, Reilly BM, Guidry JR, et al.: The weight-based heparin dosing nomogram. *Ann Int Med* 1993;119:874–881.

Stein PD, Hull RD, Saltzman HA, et al.: Strategy for diagnosis of patients with suspected acute pulmonary embolism. *Chest* 1993;103:1553.

Turrentine MA, Braems G, Ramirez MM: Use of thrombolytics for the treatment of thromboembolic disease in pregnancy. *Obstet Gynecol Surv* 1995;50:534.

Warkenton TE: Heparin-induced thrombocytopenia: pathogenesis, frequency, avoidance, and management. *Drug Saf* 1997;17:325–341.

Wells PS, Brill-Edwards P, Stevens P, et al.: A novel and rapid whole-blood assay for D-dimer in patients with clinically suspected deep vein thrombosis. *Circulation* 1995;91:2184–2187.

Zwaan N, Lorch H, Kulke C, et al.: Clinical experience with tempory vena caval filters. *J Vac Interv Radiol* 1998;9:594.

8 Cardiac Disease in Pregnancy

Afshan B. Hameed   Michael R. Foley

INTRODUCTION

Cardiac disease complicates less than 1 percent of all pregnancies. Circulatory stress of pregnancy may unmask a previously unrecognized cardiac condition and can cause rapid deterioration. Understanding cardiovascular adaptations in pregnancy and postpartum are crucial in the management of such patients. Cardiovascular changes in pregnancy are summarized in Table 8-1. Incidence of cardiac defects in the offspring of a mother with congenital heart disease is 3.4 to 14.3 percent.

Cardiac lesions are classified into congenital and acquired categories and can be further divided into cyanotic and acyanotic groups. Cyanotic (right to left shunt) lesions are the most critical, and pregnancy is contraindicated in such patients due to high maternal mortality. In general, valvular stenosis patients worsen in pregnancy and patients with valvular regurgitation tolerate pregnancy well. In addition, group-3 patients should be advised against pregnancy (Table 8-2).

A prospective multicenter study of pregnancy outcomes in women with heart disease was recently published. In this study, four predictors of an ensuing cardiac event (heart failure, arrhythmia, TIA, or stroke) during pregnancy are identified. These predictors include

1. *N*ew York Heart Association Class II or greater
2. Left heart *O*bstruction (mitral valve <2 cm; aortic valve <1.5 cm; peak left ventricular outflow tract gradient >30 mmHg
3. *P*rior cardiac event before pregnancy
4. *E*jection fraction less that 40 percent

The acronym for these predictors reveals the answer to the question: "Should pregnancy be attempted?"—NOPE! The number of predictors present correlates with the risk of a cardiac event during pregnancy.

No. of predictors	Risk of cardiac event (%)
0	5
1	27
>1	75

This new information may offer great assistance with the counseling of patients who have preexisting cardiac disease and are contemplating pregnancy.

GENERAL PRINCIPLES OF MANAGEMENT

Specific management is described with each condition

Antepartum

- All cardiac patients require meticulous follow-up during pregnancy
- Attention should be paid to subtle changes in exercise capacity and symptoms

TABLE 8-1 Cardiovascular Changes in Pregnancy

Antepartum
- Blood volume increases by 50%
- Systemic vascular resistance decreases by 20%
- Blood pressure
  - Systolic BP decreases by 5–10 mmHg
  - Diastolic BP decreases by 10–15 mmHg
  - After 24 weeks BP increases to nonpregnant level by term
- Central venous pressure remains unchanged (10 cm H_2O)
- Heart rate increases by 10–15 bpm
- Stroke volume increases
- Cardiac output increases by 30–50% (4.5–6.0 L/min)
  - Increases as early as 5–10 weeks
  - Peaks at 20–24 weeks
- Left ventricular ejection fraction increases
- Blood is hypercoagulable
- *EKG changes*
  - Left axis deviation by 15°
  - Low voltage QRS may be present
  - T wave inversion in lead III
  - Q waves in lead III and aVF
  - Premature atrial and ventricular beats may be present
- *Chest x-ray changes*
  - Straightening of the left upper cardiac border
  - Horizontal position of heart
  - Increased lung markings
  - Small pleural effusions early postpartum

Intrapartum
- Cardiac output increases by 20–30% in active labor
- Each contraction squeezes 300–500 mL of blood out of uterus into circulation
- Blood pressure increases by 10–20 mmHg during a contraction
- Supine position may decrease cardiac output by 30%
- Oxygen consumption is 100% higher than measured prior to labor

Postpartum
- Cardiac output increases by 10–20% in the immediate postpartum period
- Increase in stroke volume
- Reflex bradycardia
- These changes persist for 1–2 weeks after delivery

- Fetal echocardiogram is indicated in the presence of congenital heart disease in mother
- Periodic fetal growth assessments
- Antepartum fetal surveillance starting at 30–34 weeks
- Consider prophylactic anticoagulation in patients with pulmonary hypertension and Eisenmenger's syndrome

Labor and Delivery

- Avoid fluid overload
- Labor in left lateral decubitus position
- Supplemental oxygen
- Epidural anesthesia may be used except in (CAT PIE) *C*oarctation of aorta, *A*ortic stenosis, *T*etralogy of Fallot (uncorrected), *P*ulmonary hypertension, *I*diopathic hypertrophic subaortic stenosis, and *E*isenmenger's syndrome

TABLE 8-2 Maternal Mortality Associated with Pregnancy

Group 1—Mortality <1%
Atrial septal defect
Ventricular septal defect
Patent ductus arteriosus
Mitral stenosis—NYHA class I & II
Pulmonic/tricuspid valve disease
Corrected tetralogy of Fallot
Bioprosthetic valve
Group 2—Mortality 5–15%
2A
Mitral stenosis—NYHA class III & IV
Aortic stenosis
Coarctation of aorta without valvular involvement
Uncorrected tetralogy of Fallot
Previous myocardial infarction
Marfan syndrome with normal aorta
2B
Mitral stenosis with atrial fibrillation
Artificial valve
Group 3—Mortality 25–50%
Pulmonary hypertension
Primary
Eisenmenger's
Coarctation of aorta with valvular involvement
Marfan syndrome with aortic involvement
Peripartum cardiomyopathy with persistent left ventricular dysfunction

Source: From Clark SL, Phelan JP, Cotton DB (eds): *Critical Care Obstetrics: Structural Cardiac Disease in Pregnancy.* Oradell, NJ: Medical Economics Company, 1987.

- Endocarditis prophylaxis is recommended in all except ASD, Marfan's syndrome without aortic valve involvement, and cardiomyopathy (Table 8-3)
- Multidisciplinary management in consultation with anesthesiologist and cardiologist

COMMON CONGENITAL CARDIAC LESIONS

Atrial Septal Defect (ASD)

- Secundum ASD is the most common defect seen in pregnancy
- Systolic ejection murmur at left sternal border and wide fixed split second heart sound
- *EKG.* Partial right bundle branch block, right axis deviation, and sometimes right ventricular hypertrophy
- Patients with a large defect and significant left to right shunt may develop atrial arrhythmias (atrial fibrillation) and congestive heart failure in pregnancy
- *Thromboembolism* leading to a paradoxical embolus may occur and, therefore, attention should be paid to DVT prophylaxis, especially at the time of delivery (compression stockings)

TABLE 8-3 Antibiotic Prophylaxis for Labor and Delivery

Drug	Dosage regimen
Standard regimen	
Ampicillin, gentamicin, and amoxacillin	Ampicillin 2 g, plus gentamicin 1.5 mg/kg IV or IM, 30 min before the procedure; followed by amoxacillin 1.5 g orally 6 h after the initial dose; alternatively, parenteral regimen may be repeated once 8 h after the initial dose
Ampicillin/amoxacillin/penicillin-Allergic patient regimen	
Vancomycin and gentamicin	Vancomycin 1 g IV over 1 h plus gentamicin 1.5 mg/kg IV or IM, 1 h before the procedure; may be repeated once 8 h after initial dose
Alternate low-risk patient regimen	
Amoxacillin	3 g orally 1 h before the procedure; then 1.5 g 6 h after the initial dose

[a]Antibiotic prophylaxis is not recommended for cesarean section and uncomplicated vaginal delivery in the absence of infection.
Source: Adapted from Dajani AS, Bisno AL, Chung KG: Prevention of bacterial endocarditis: Recommendations of the American Heart Association. *JAMA* 1990;264:2919.

- *Labor and delivery*
  - See general principles
- *Cautions*
  - See Box 8-1

Ventricular Septal Defect (VSD)

- Common in childhood, but most close spontaneously or are repaired by adulthood
- Pregnancy is well tolerated
- Holosystolic thrill and murmur at left sternal border
- *EKG.* Usually normal. Left ventricular hypertrophy suggests large left-to-right shunt and right ventricular hypertrophy suggests elevated pulmonary pressures

BOX 8-1 **AVOIDS** (ASD, VSD, & PDA)

1. Avoid hypertension (increase in systemic vascular resistance increases left-to-right shunt)
2. Avoid decrease in pulmonary vascular resistance (increases left-to-right shunt)
3. Avoid supraventricular arrhythmias, tachycardia (may increase left-to-right shunt)
4. If pulmonary hypertension is present, avoid increase in pulmonary vascular resistance (metabolic acidosis, excess catechomines, hypoxemia, nitrous oxide, hypercarbia, pharmacologic vasoconstrictors, and lung hyperinflation)

- Large defects may be associated with arrhythmias, congestive heart failure, and may lead to pulmonary hypertension, reversal of shunt (right to left), cyanosis, and thus Eisenmenger's syndrome
- *Labor and delivery*
  - See general principles of management
  - Epidural anesthesia may be used in the absence of Eisenmenger's syndrome
- *Cautions*
  - See Box 8-1

Patent Ductus Arteriosus (PDA)

- Most cases are diagnosed and corrected in childhood
- Uncommon lesion in pregnancy
- Most patients with small PDA tolerate pregnancy well
- Wide pulse pressure and a continuous murmur
- *EKG.* Normal or left ventricular hypertrophy
- If uncorrected, pulmonary hypertension may develop leading to Eisenmenger's syndrome
- *Labor and delivery*
  - See general management principles
- *Cautions*
  - See Box 8-1

Secondary Pulmonary Hypertension and Eisenmenger's Syndrome

Pulmonary hypertension of any etiology carries a grave prognosis for pregnancy. Despite improved technology and critical care delivery, the maternal mortality rate has remained at 36 percent for the last two decades.

- Eisenmenger's syndrome is the reversal of left-to-right shunt (ASD, VSD, PDA) due to progressive pulmonary hypertension. Right-to-left shunt leads to cyanosis and the degree is determined by the extent of pulmonary vascular obstructive disease
- Pulmonary pressures may reach systemic levels and even a minimal decrease in the systemic blood pressure may cause a decrease in the ventricular filling and massive right-to-left shunting. This may lead to worsening hypoxia, further vasoconstriction of the pulmonary vascular bed leading to rapid homodynamic deterioration
- Termination of pregnancy is advisable due to high maternal mortality (50 percent)
- High risk of fetal loss (75 percent)
- *Labor and delivery*
  - See general management principles
  - Pulmonary artery catheterization to monitor pulmonary pressures and cardiac output (controversial)
  - Continuous pulse oximetry and supplemental oxygen to keep oxygen saturations at or above 90 percent
  - Epidural anesthesia is contraindicated owing to the risk of systemic hypotension
  - Narcotic epidural may be used
  - Cesarean section and vaginal delivery carry similar mortality rates

BOX 8-2 **AVOIDS** (Pulmonary Hypertension & Eisenmenger's Syndrome)

1. Avoid hypotension (decrease in systemic vascular resistance causes massive right-to-left shunting and thus bypassing pulmonary circulation/oxygenation leading to severe hypoxia)
2. Avoid excessive blood loss (causes hypotension by decrease in venous return)
3. Avoid increase in pulmonary vascular resistance (see #4 avoids in Box 8-1).
4. Avoid myocardial depressant drugs

- High risk for thromboembolism due to hypercoagulability of pregnancy and polycythemia
- Prophylactic anticoagulation during pregnancy and full anticoagulation for 7 to 10 days after delivery should be strongly considered

- *Cautions*
  - See Box 8-2
  - See Figure 8-1 for a diagrammatic representation of Eisenmenger's syndrome

Coarctation of Aorta

- Rarely seen in pregnancy, as most are corrected in childhood
- Most common site is at the origin of the left subclavian artery
- Rare cause of secondary hypertension
- Common associated congenital malformations are bicuspid aortic valve and berry aneurysm of the circle of Willis
- Aortic dissection, rupture, congestive heart failure, cerebrovascular accident, or bacterial endocarditis may occur
- *Labor and delivery*
  - See general principles
  - Narcotic epidural anesthesia
  - Shortening of the second stage of labor
- *Cautions*
  - See Box 8-3

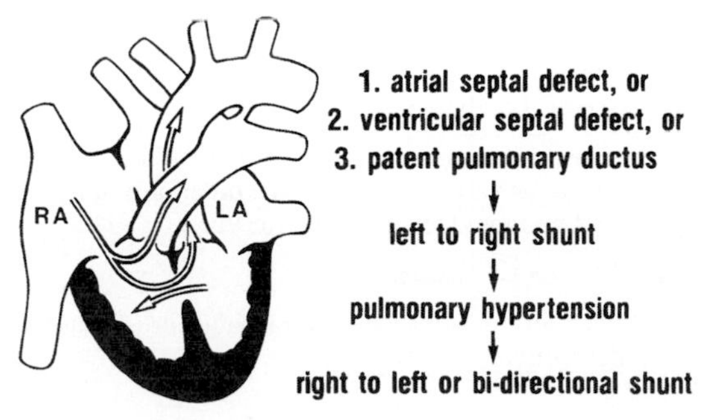

FIG. 8-1 Pathophysiology of Eisenmenger's syndrome. RA, right atrium; LA, left atrium. (*Adapted from Mangano DT: Anesthesia for the pregnant cardiac patient. In: Shnider SM, Levinson G (eds), Anesthesia for Obstetrics, 3rd edn. Baltimore: Williams & Wilkins, 1992.*)

BOX 8-3 **AVOIDS** (Coarctation, Pulmonary Stenosis, and Tetralogy of Fallot)

1. Avoid hypotension (decrease in systemic vascular resistance causes massive right-to-left shunting and thus bypassing pulmonary circulation/ oxygenation leading to severe hypoxia)
2. Avoid excessive blood loss (causes hypotension by decrease in venous return)
3. Avoid myocardial depressant drugs
4. Avoid bradycardia

Pulmonic Stenosis

- Well tolerated in pregnancy
- Valvular pressure gradient of >80 mmHg is severe and surgical correction should be considered
- Right ventricular failure may occur
- *Labor and delivery*
  - Left lateral decubitus position
  - Oxygen supplementation
  - Endocarditis prophylaxis is indicated
- *Cautions*
  - See Box 8-3

Tetralogy of Fallot

- Congenital anomaly consisting of VSD with an overriding aorta, right ventricular hypertrophy, and pulmonic stenosis
- Pregnancy associated decrease in systemic vascular resistance may result in right-to-left shunting
- Poor prognosis indicators are hematocrit >65 percent syncope, congestive heart failure, right ventricular hypertrophy, cardiomegaly, or peripheral oxygen saturations <90 percent
- *Labor and delivery*
  - See general principles
  - Maintain blood volume with replacement as needed
  - Narcotic epidural anesthesia
- *Cautions*
  - See Box 8-3

ACQUIRED CARDIAC LESIONS

Rheumatic heart disease accounts for 90 percent of cardiac disorders in pregnancy worldwide. Cardiac valves affected in the order of frequency are mitral, aortic, tricuspid, and pulmonic (Mary And Tim Play)

Pulmonic and Tricuspid Lesions

- Isolated right-sided lesions are seen in intravenous drug abusers secondary to bacterial endocarditis
- Well tolerated in pregnancy

Mitral Stenosis

- Stenosis of the mitral valve impedes flow of blood from left atrium to the left ventricle leading to elevated left atrial and pulmonary pressures

BOX 8-4 **AVOIDS** (Mitral Stenosis)

1. Avoid tachycardia (decreases diastolic ventricular filling time)
2. Avoid fluid overload (may cause atrial fibrillation, pulmonary edema, and right ventricular failure)
3. Avoid decrease in systemic vascular resistance/hypotension (decrease in cardiac output)
4. Avoid increase in pulmonary vascular resistance (#4 avoids for ASD, VSD, PDA)

- Most common valvular lesion in pregnancy
- Loud first heart sound, an opening snap and rumbling diastolic murmur
- *EKG.* Left atrial enlargement; right ventricular hypertrophy and right atrial enlargement in cases of pulmonary hypertension
- Mitral stenosis may cause arrhythmias (atrial fibrillation), thromboembolism, pulmonary edema, pulmonary hypertension, and right heart failure
- These patients require elevated left atrial pressures to maintain adequate left ventricular filling (pulmonary capillary wedge pressure of 14 to 16 mmHg)
- Diuretics and beta blockers are mainstays of therapy
- Patients refractory to medical therapy should be considered for mitral valvuloplasty or mitral valve replacement
- *Labor and delivery*
  - See general management principles
  - Tocolytic agents that cause tachycardia are contraindicated for premature labor
  - Hemodynamic monitoring for severe mitral stenosis
  - Shorten second stage of labor
- *Cautions*
  - See Box 8-4
  - See Figure 8-2 for diagrammatic representation of mitral stenosis

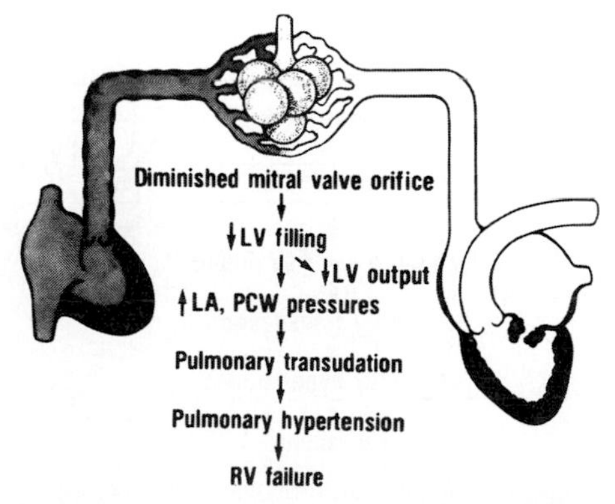

FIG. 8-2 Pathophysiology of mitral stenosis. LV, left ventricle; LA, left atrium; PCW, pulmonary capillary wedge; RV, right ventricle. (*Adapted from Mangano DT: Anesthesia for the pregnant cardiac patient. In: Shnider SM, Levinson G (eds), Anesthesia for Obstetrics, 3rd edn. Baltimore: Williams & Wilkins, 1992.*)

BOX 8-5 **AVOIDS** (Mitral Insufficiency, Aortic Insufficiency)

1. Avoid arrhythmia (immediate treatment, if occurs)
2. Avoid bradycardia (increases regurgitation)
3. Avoid increase in systemic vascular resistance (increases regurgitation)
4. Avoid myocardial depressant drugs

Mitral Insufficiency

- Well tolerated in pregnancy
- Severe cases associated with left atrial enlargement and atrial fibrillation
- *Labor and delivery*
  - See general management principles
- *Cautions*
  - See Box 8-5
  - See Figure 8-3 for diagrammatic representation of mitral insufficiency

Aortic Stenosis

- Aortic stenosis leads to a decreased fixed cardiac output
- Diminished carotid upstroke and harsh systolic ejection murmur in second right intercostal space
- *EKG.* Left ventricular hypertrophy and left atrial enlargement
- Symptoms are related to a decrease in coronary perfusion (angina), cerebral perfusion (syncope), and arrhythmias (sudden death)
- Limitation of physical activity is advisable

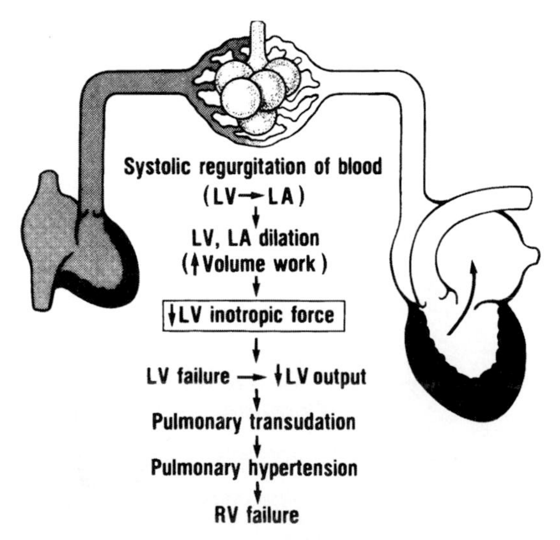

FIG. 8-3 Pathophysiology of mitral insufficiency. LV, left ventricle; LA, left atrium; RV right ventricle. (*Adapted from Mangano DT: Anesthesia for the pregnant cardiac patient. In: Shnider SM, Levinson G (eds), Anesthesia for Obstetrics, 3rd edn. Baltimore: Williams & Wilkins, 1992.*)

BOX 8-6 **AVOIDS** (Aortic Stenosis, IHSS)

1. Avoid hypotension (may be lethal due to decrease in coronary perfusion)
2. Avoid decrease in venous return (blood loss, valsalva)
3. Avoid bradycardia

- Poor prognosis if symptoms are present
- Treatment is primarily based on mechanical relief of obstruction
- *Labor and delivery*
  - See general principles
  - Avoid hypotension (may reduce coronary artery perfusion and cause sudden death)
  - Epidural anesthesia is contraindicated. Narcotic epidural may be used
  - Shorten second stage of labor
- *Cautions*
  - See Box 8-6
  - See Figure 8-4 for a diagrammatic representation of aortic stenosis

Aortic Insufficiency

- Tolerated well in pregnancy
- Significant long standing AI may lead to ventricular dilatation and failure
- *Labor and delivery*
  - See general principles
- *Cautions*
  - See Box 8-5
  - See Figure 8-5 for a diagrammatic representation of aortic insufficiency

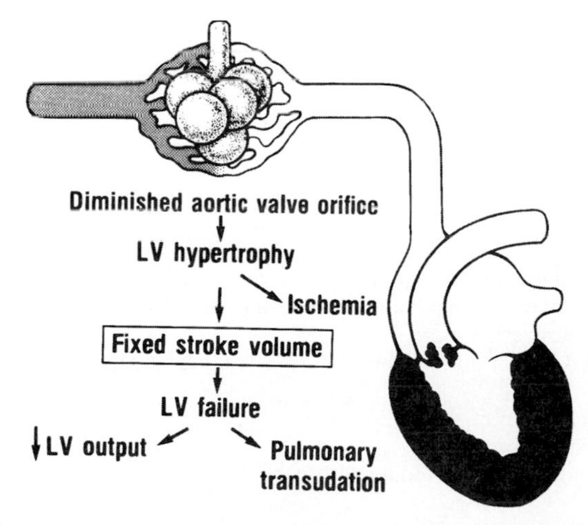

FIG. 8-4 Pathophysiology of aortic stenosis. LV, left ventricle. (*Adapted from Mangano DT: Anesthesia for the pregnant cardiac patient. In: Shnider SM, Levinson G (eds), Anesthesia for Obstetrics, 3rd edn. Baltimore: Williams & Wilkins, 1992.*)

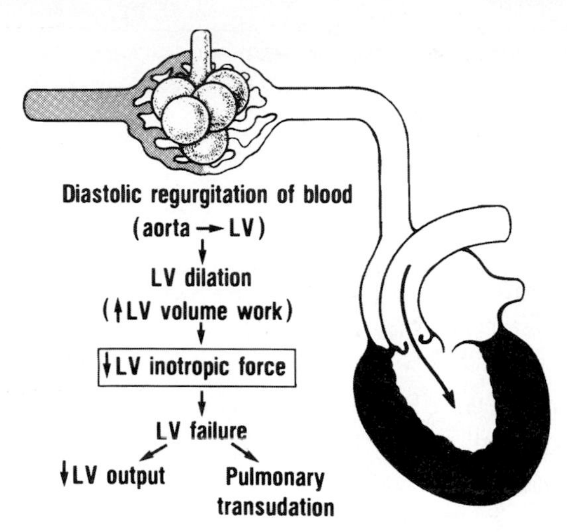

FIG. 8-5 Pathophysiology of aortic insufficiency. LV, left ventricle. (*Adapted from Mangano DT: Anesthesia for the pregnant cardiac patient. In: Shnider SM, Levinson G (eds), Anesthesia for Obstetrics, 3rd edn. Baltimore: Williams & Wilkins, 1992.*)

Primary Pulmonary Hypertension

- Mortality rate of up to 50 percent
- *EKG.* Right ventricular hypertrophy and right atrial enlargement
- *Labor and delivery*
  - See general principles
  - Avoid hypotension and maintain venous return
  - Left lateral decubitus position
  - Elastic support stockings
  - Prophylactic anticoagulation should be considered
- *Cautions*
  - See Box 8-2

Marfan's Syndrome

- Autosomal dominant condition
- Cystic medial necrosis of aorta may lead to dissecting aortic aneurysm and aortic regurgitation
- Increased risk of aortic rupture during pregnancy if aortic root diameter >4 cm
- *Labor and delivery*
  - See general principles
  - Prevention of tachycardia and excessive pulsatile pressure on the aortic wall
  - Beta blockers to reduce heart rate to <90 bpm
  - Shorten second stage of labor
  - Consider cesarean section to avoid valsalva

BOX 8-7 **AVOIDS** (Marfan's Syndrome)

1. Avoid hypertension
2. Avoid positive inotropic drugs

- *Cautions*
  - See Box 8-7

Idiopathic Hypertrophic Subaortic Stenosis (IHSS)

- Autosomal dominant inheritance
- Left ventricular outflow is impeded by asymmetric septal hypertrophy
- Hemodyanamics and management is very similar to valvular aortic stenosis
- *Labor and delivery*
  - See aortic stenosis
- *Cautions*
  - See Box 8-6

Peripartum Cardiomyopathy

- Cardiac failure during pregnancy or postpartum period without identifiable cause
- Mortality 5 to 60 percent
- 50 percent of survivors recover cardiac function
- *Labor and delivery*
  - Bed rest
  - Fluid restriction
  - Low sodium diet
  - Diuretic therapy
  - Vasodilators and digitalis may be used
  - Prophylactic heparinization during pregnancy with full anticoagulation for 7 to 10 days after delivery should be considered to decrease the risk of thromboembolism

Myocardial Infarction (MI)

- Acute MI occurs in 1:10,000 pregnancies
- In addition to atherosclerosis, thrombosis, coronary artery spasm, dissection, sickle cell disease, pheochromocytoma should be considered
- Maternal mortality varies from 20 to 30 percent
- 29 percent of pregnant women with MI have normal coronaries
- Diagnosis is based on angina, EKG changes and elevated cardiac enzymes (Troponin I)
- *Treatment.* Thrombolytics are the first line of therapy. Heparin, low dose ASA, nitrates, and beta blockers may be safely used in pregnancy
- *Labor and delivery*
  - Delivery should be postponed for two to three weeks after MI
  - Consider delivery at 32 to 34 weeks to minimize the cardiac stress due to hemodynamic changes
  - Cesarean section should be reserved for obstetrical indications or unstable patients

TABLE 8-4 Cardiovascular Drugs Commonly Used in the Obstetric Intensive Care Setting and their Effects on Uterine Blood Flow and the Fetus

Drug (safety in pregnancy)	Dose	Uterine blood flow (UBF)	Fetal effects
Inotropic agents			
Digoxin (C)	Loading dose 0.5 mg IV over 5 min, then 0.25 mg IV q 6 hr × 2. Maintenance 0.125–0.375 mg IV/PO q.d.	No change	Placental transfer Higher maternal maintenance dose required for fetal effect Not teratogenic
Dopamine (C)	Initiate with 5 μg/kg/min and titrate by 5–10 μg/kg/min to max. 50 μg/kg/min	Directly ↓ UBF May ↑ UBF with improved maternal hemodyanamics	No known adverse fetal effects
Dobutamine (B)	Initiate with 1.0 μg/kg/min and titrate up to 20 μg/kg/min		No known adverse fetal effects
Epinephrine (C)	Endotracheal, 0.5–1.0 mg q 5 min; IV 0.5 mg bolus and follow with 2–10 μg/kg/min infusion		Not teratogenic
Vasodilators			
Nitroprusside (C)	Initiate with 0.3 μg/kg/min and titrate to 10 μg/kg/min	↑ UBF unless significant ↓ in maternal BP	No known adverse fetal effects Potential for fetal cyanide toxicity Avoid prolonged use
Hydralazine (C)	5–10 mg IV q 15–30 min Total dose 30 mg		Not teratogenic
Nitroglycerin (B)	0.4–0.8 mg sublingual 1–2 in of dermal paste, IV infusion 10 μg/min, titrate up by 10–20 μg/min p.r.n.		Not teratogenic

Beta blockers			
Propranolol (C)	1 mg IV q 2 min as needed	May ↓ by ↑ uterine tone and/or ↓ maternal BP	Not teratogenic Readily crosses placenta Fetal bradycardia IUGR Category D if used in 2nd or 3rd trimester
Labetalol (C)	10–20 mg IV followed by 20–80 mg IV q 10 min to total dose of [illegible]50 mg		
Atenolol (D)	5 mg IV over 5 min, repeat in 5 min to a total dose of 15 mg		
Metoprolol (C)z	5 mg IV over 5 min; repeat in 10 min		
Esmolol (C)	500 ug/kg IV over 1 min with infusion rate of 50–200 μg/kg/min		No known adverse fetal effects Rapid metabolism (1/2 life 11 min) also occurs in the fetus
Calcium channel blockers			
Verapamil (C)	2.5–5 mg IV bolus over 2 min, repeat in 5 min and then q 30 min p.r.n. to a max dose 20 mg	Mild ↓ UBF	Not teratogenic
Nifedipine (C)	10 mg PO, repeat every 6 h		
Diltiazem (C)	20 mg IV bolus over 2 min, repeat in 15 min		

(continued)

TABLE 8-4 (*continued*) Cardiovascular Drugs Commonly Used in the Obstetric Intensive Care Setting and their Effects on Uterine Blood Flow and the Fetus

Drug (safety in pregnancy)	Dose	Uterine blood flow (UBF)	Fetal effects
		Vasoconstrictors	
Ephedrine sulphate (C)	10–25 mg slow IV bolus, repeat q 15 min p.r.n × 3	No effect	Not teratogenic 70% of maternal blood level in in the fetus
Metaraminol (C)	Initiate with 0.1 mg/min and titrate to 2 mg/min	Mild ↓ UBF	No data available
		Antiarrhythmic agents	
Lidocaine (B)	1 mg/kg bolus; repeat 1/2 bolus at 10 min as needed × 4; infusion at 1–4 mg/min; total dose 3 mg/kg	No effect	Not teratogenic Rapidly crosses placenta
Procainamide (C)	100 mg over 30 min, then 2–6 mg/min infusion; total dose 17 mg/kg		
Quinidine (C)	15 mg/kg over 60 min, then 0.02 mg/kg/min infusion		
Bretylium (C)	5 mg/kg IV bolus, then 1–2 mg/min infusion	↓ UBF	Unknown
Phenytoin (D)	300 mg IV, then 100 mg every 5 min to a total of 1000 mg	No effect	Teratogenic Fetal Hydantoin syndrome
Amiodarone (D)	5 mg/kg IV over 3 min, then 10 mg/kg/day		Teratogenic Transient bradycardia Prolonged QT

AV Node blocking agents			
Adenosine	6 mg IV bolus over 1–3 s, followed by 20 mL saline bolus; may repeat at 12 mg in 1–2 min × 2	↑ or ↓ UBF	No known adverse fetal effects
Verapamil	As stated above		
β-Blockers	As stated above		
Digoxin	As stated above		

Source: From McAnulty JH: Heart and other circulatory diseases. In: Bonica JJ, McDonald JS (eds), *Principles and Practice of Obstetric Analgesia and Anesthesia*, 2nd edn. Baltimore, MD: William & Wilkins, 1995; pp. 10[illegible]9–1020.

  - Second stage of labor should be shortened via vacuum or foreceps
- *Cautions*
  - Hypertension and tachycardia should be prevented

Pearls

The management of the critically ill obstetric patient with cardiac disease requires a specialized team approach. Developing a consistent team of care providers including: Perinatology, OB/critical care nursing, anesthesiology, cardiology, and intensive care medicine specialists will be important in order to meet the special challenges presented by this high risk group of patients.

- Stenotic valvular lesions are associated with a higher risk in pregnancy.
- Regurgitant lesions are well tolerated and mitral and aortic regurgitation improves due to the decreased systemic vascular resistance in pregnancy.
- Invasive hemodyanamic monitoring should be considered in severe aortic/mitral stenosis, pulmonary hypertension/Eisenmenger's syndrome, uncorrected tetralogy of Fallot and cardiomyopathy.
- In the conditions of: (CAT PIE) Coarctation of aorta, aortic stenosis, tetralogy of Fallot (uncorrected), pulmonary hypertension, idiopathic hypertrophic subaortic stenosis, and Eisenmenger's syndrome—only *narcotic* epidural should be considered.
- Endocarditis prophylaxis is indicated for vaginal delivery in all conditions except atrial septal defect, cardiomyopathy, and Marfan's without aortic insufficiency.
- Table 8-4 summarizes cardiovascular drugs commonly used in the obstetric intensive care setting and their effects on uterine blood flow and the fetus.

SUGGESTED READING

Burlew BS: Managing the pregnant patient with heart disease. *Clin Cardiol* 1990; 13:757–762.

Clark SL, Phelan JP, Cotton DB (eds): Critical Care Obstetrics: *Structural Cardiac Disease in Pregnancy*. Oradell, NJ: Medical Economics Company, 1987.

Elkayam U, Gleicher N (eds): *Cardiac Problems in Pregnancy,* 3rd edn. New York: Wiley-Liss, 1990.

Hameed A, Karaalp IS, Tummala PP, et al.: The effect of Valvular Heart Disease on maternal and fetal outcome of pregnancy. *JACC* 2001;37(3):893–809.

McAnulty JH: Heart and other circulating diseases. In: Bonica JJ, McDonald JS (eds), *Principles and Practice of Obstetric Analgesia and Anesthesia,* 2nd edn. Baltimore, MD: Williams & Wilkins, 1995.

Pitkin RM: Pregnancy and congenital heart disease. *Ann Internal Med* 1990;112:445–454.

Siu SC, Sermer M, Colman JM, et al.: Prospective multicenter study of pregnancy outcomes in women with heart disease. *Circulation* 2001;104:515–521.

9 Maternal Sepsis

George R. Saade

INTRODUCTION

Sepsis, severe sepsis, and septic shock are a continuum in the systemic response to infection. Sepsis is the leading cause of mortality in intensive care units and accounts for 10 percent of direct maternal deaths in North America. Most deaths in sepsis are due to multiple organ dysfunction syndrome (MODS), the final stage in the sepsis spectrum. The obstetric patient is particularly vulnerable to sepsis because of the association between pregnancy and infectious complications such as pyelonephritis, chorioamnionitis, endometritis, wound infection, necrotizing fascitis, and cholecystitis. Septic shock occurs in up to 4 percent of bacteremic patients, and 40 to 60 percent of patients in septic shock have bacteremia. The relationship between bacteremia and sepsis also depends on other contributing factors such as immune suppression, and associated medical conditions. Overall, gram-negative aerobic bacilli used to be the predominant organisms associated with sepsis. However, the incidence of infection with gram-positive organisms in patients with sepsis has increased and may now equal that of gram-negative infections.

DEFINITIONS

Sepsis is the development of systemic inflammatory response syndrome (SIRS, Table 9-1) in response to infection. Sepsis is called severe when there is evidence of end organ damage. Septic shock is defined as sepsis with hypotension (systolic blood pressure <90 mmHg or a reduction of ≥40 mmHg from baseline) despite volume replacement (or requirement for vasopressors) along with the presence of perfusion abnormalities that may include, but are not limited to, lactic acidosis, oliguria, or an acute alteration in mental status.

PATHOGENESIS

Sepsis has been viewed as an uncontrolled inflammatory response to infection. This hypothesis was based on animal studies as well as measures of immune response in humans, including cytokine levels. This view has been recently challenged by the failure to decrease mortality in clinical trials of anti-inflammatory agents, and by evidence of a severely compromised immune system that is unable to eradicate the infection. The immunological response in patients with sepsis may even be biphasic, with an anti-inflammatory phase following an initial overwhelming response. The cardiovascular manifestations of sepsis are the results of alterations in peripheral vascular tone and cardiac function. The decrease in vascular tone affects both the arterial and venous systems, and is believed to be due to an increase in smooth muscle relaxants such as nitric oxide. Microvascular changes such as endothelial cell swelling, fibrin deposition, and aggregation of circulating cells also contribute to the abnormal blood flow seen in patients with sepsis. Cardiac output depends on the intravascular volume status of the patient. In the early stages of septic shock, cardiac output may be decreased because of hypovolemia and low cardiac filling. Cardiac output increases after fluid replacement. Myocardial dysfunction is seen in most patients with septic shock and affects both the

TABLE 9-1 Definition of Systemic Inflammatory Response Syndrome (SIRS). At Least 2 of the Following are Required

- Temperature >38°C or <36°C
- Respiratory rate >20 breaths per minute or $PaCO_2$ <32 mmHg
- Pulse >90 bpm
- White blood cell count >12,000/cc, or <4000/cc, or bands >10%

right and left ventricles. Myocardial depressants include many of the cytokines as well as nitric oxide.

MANAGEMENT

The general management guidelines for a patient with sepsis are outlined in Table 9-2. The following discussion will concentrate on the overall principles for the management of sepsis, mostly septic shock. The details of each management option (central hemodynamic monitoring, drug pharmacology, fetal effects, etc.) are covered in the different chapters pertaining specifically to these issues.

During the initial evaluation, a search for the source of the infection should take into account the most common sources in a pregnant or postpartum woman (Table 9-3). Testing may include chest x ray to exclude pneumonia, abdomino-pelvic CT scan or MRI to search for abscesses, myometrial necrosis, and pyometria, as well as amniocentesis to exclude intraamniotic infection. Diagnosis of infection relies on clinical suspicion and a search for an infectious agent. Collections identified by radiology should be aspirated and drained under guidance, and samples sent for Gram and fungal staining and culture. Purulent wounds or those with spreading cellulitis should prompt swabbing for culture. When infection is suspected in contaminated or dirty abdominal wounds, anaerobic infections should be assumed irrespective of the culture results. Blood cultures should be taken as soon as possible after the onset of fever or chills. According to the recommendations of the International Sepsis Forum, blood for culture should be obtained by fresh venipuncture. The skin should be swabbed twice with either 70 percent isopropyl alcohol or iodine-containing solution. About 10 to 30 mL of blood should be inoculated in each culture bottle, and priority given to the aerobic bottle if the volume of blood obtained is insufficient. The needle used for venipuncture should be changed prior to inoculation of the blood into the culture bottles. About two to three sets of blood cultures should be obtained for each suspected episode of bacteremia. In critically ill patients, the source of sepsis is frequently iatrogenic such as caused by a central venous catheter (CVC), urinary indwelling

TABLE 9-2 General Treatment Guidelines for Sepsis

- Broad spectrum antibiotics
- Aggressive fluid replacement guided by CVP or pulmonary artery catheter (wedge pressure 12–18 mmHg)
- Blood products as needed (anemia, DIC)
- Vasopressors and inotropes
- Removal of infection source
- Ventilatory support
- Supportive care (DVT prophylaxis, nutritional support, stress ulcer prophylaxis, hemofiltration)
- Immunological therapy
- Delivery as last resort (unless chorioamnionitis)

TABLE 9-3 Most Common Sources for Infection in Obstetrical Patients

- Reproductive tract
- Urinary
- Wound infection
- Chorioamnionitis
- Cholecystitis
- Respiratory

catheter, or ventilator. Specific techniques and procedures should be followed to obtain and interpret cultures from these sources. These include culture of blood aspirated from the CVC, quantitative cultures of the CVC tip, and culture from the CVC insertion site. A sample of secretions aspirated via the endotracheal tube should be sent for Gram staining and for bacterial and fungal culture. Pleural effusions greater than 10 mm should be aspirated, cultured, and sent for Gram and fungal stainings. Unless contraindicated, bronchoscopy should be performed whenever ventilator-associated pneumonia is suspected. A policy of routine screening of hospitalized patients for *Candida* colonization is not recommended. Among septic patients, however, invasive fungal infection is more likely in those patients who are heavily colonized. Blood cultures should be obtained from septic patients colonized by *Candida* at two or more sites.

Early administration of antibiotics reduces mortality and morbidity in septic patients. The patient should be started empirically on broad-spectrum antibiotics. For pregnancy-related infection, a combination of penicillin, aminoglycoside, and either clindamycin or metronidazole for anaerobes should cover most possible organisms. Alternatively, a carbapenem or a third- or fourth-generation cephalosporin may be used in nonneutropenic patients. Aztreonam and fluoroquinolones do not have adequate activity against gram positive bacteria and therefore are not recommended for initial empirical treatment. Vancomycin should be used for suspected methicillin-resistant *Staphylococcus* infection (catheter-related infection, or centers where methicillin-resistant staphylococci predominate). Antifungal agents should not be used as routine empirical therapy. In situations where immune suppression, or other conditions conducive to fungal infection may have contributed to the initial inciting event, coverage with amphotericin or equivalent antimicrobials should be considered. Fluconazole is as effective as amphotericin B, and less toxic in nonneutropenic patients. However, amphotericin B should be used as first-line therapy in neutropenic septic patients until identification and susceptibility are determined. The initial and subsequent choice of antimicrobials, should always be predicated by allergy history, renal and liver function, culture results, and hospital- or community-specific microbial sensitivity testing. It is also important to remember that cultures may be falsely negative or yield incomplete information as some organisms may not be detected. This is especially true in obstetrically related infections which tend to be poly-microbial.

Hemodynamic support in sepsis is one of the central components of the management. The goal is to restore tissue perfusion and normalize cellular metabolism. Volume replacement, most often with fluid alone, is sometimes sufficient to reverse hypotension, restore hemodynamic stability, and improve oxygen delivery. Volume replacement should be titrated according to blood pressure (maintain a systolic blood pressure of at least 90 mmHg or a mean arterial pressure of 60 to 65 mmHg), heart rate, and urine output (≥0.5 mL/kg/h). Boluses of 250 to 1000 mL of crytalloids over 5 to 15 minutes are recommended.

Oncotic pressure decreases in pregnancy, with further decrease in malnourished or preeclamptic women. Combined with the propensity for capillary leak in sepsis, the gestational decrease in oncotic pressure predisposes pregnant or postpartum women for pulmonary edema. The initial fluid boluses can be guided by the overall subjective assessment of the patient's intravascular volume status (prior fluid replacements and losses), intravascular oncotic pressure (nutritional status, conditions decreasing oncotic pressure, etc.), and clinical measures of pulmonary function (oxygen saturation, auscultation, etc.). If hypotension persists despite the initial attempts, further volume expansion should be guided by central venous pressure (maintained at 8 to 12 mmHg) or pulmonary capillary wedge pressure (maintained at 12 to 16 mmHg), the latter being more appropriate than the former in cases where central venous pressure may not reflect left ventricular end diastolic pressures (e.g., preeclampsia) or when the central venous pressure is elevated. If central monitoring is indicated, then the use of a catheter with the capability to measure venous oxyhemoglobin saturation can be very useful in guiding further management. Systemic oxygen delivery depends on cardiac output and the oxygen-carrying capacity of the blood. Increases in cardiac output can be proportional to the degree of intravascular volume expansion, while increases in the oxygen-carrying capacity can be achieved by increasing the hemoglobin. The recommended hemoglobin concentration in patients with septic shock is 9 to 10 mg/dL.

Vasopressors are required when fluid and red blood cell replacement fail to restore adequate organ perfusion (Table 9-4). The choice between the different vasopressors depends on the balance between cardiac and peripheral vascular effects. Dopamine and epinephrine are more likely to increase heart rate than norepinephrine and phenylephrine. Dopamine and norepinephrine raise both blood pressure and cardiac index. Overall, recent data suggest that norepinephrine is the best choice for a vasopressor because of less tachycardia, no interference with the hypothalamic-pituitary axis, and a likely survival advantage over other vasopressors. In septic shock, norepinephrine is a more potent vasopressor than dopamine and increases cardiac output, renal blood flow, and urine output. Despite the negative effect of sepsis on cardiac function, most patients have increased cardiac output especially following intravascular volume expansion, with or without norepinephrine. If cardiac output remains low-normal or decreased, then inotropic support is required, with dobutamine being the most appropriate choice (start at 2.5 μg/kg/min and increase by 2.5 μg/kg/min every 30 minutes to achieve a cardiac index of 3 or more). In the presence of hypotension, dobutamine should be used in combination with a vasopressor, preferably norepinephrine. Finally, vasopressin can be added if organ perfusion remains abnormal despite high doses of vasopressors and inotropes. Doses should be limited to 0.01 to 0.04 units/min in order to prevent splanchnic and coronary artery ischemia, as well as decreased cardiac output. Routine intravenous bicarbonate therapy for anion gap acidosis, and supranormal oxygen delivery (increasing oxygen delivery to higher than

TABLE 9-4 Dose of Agents Used as Vasopressors in Septic Shock

Dopamine	10–25 μg/kg/min
Norepinephrine	1–50 μg/min
Epinephrine	1–10 μg/min
Phenylephrine	40–180 μg/min
Vasopressin	0.01–0.04 units/min

normal values) are no longer recommended. Early recognition of septic shock in patients with infection is critical in order to initiate aggressive and timely cardiovascular management since the response in the initial few hours has a tremendous bearing on outcome.

The source of infection should be eliminated as soon as the patient's condition permits. Debridement of infected and devitalized tissue is indicated in cases of wound infection or fasciitis. Ultrasound evaluation of the endometrial cavity can be used to determine the presence of retained products and need for curettage. If well defined and accessible, intraabdominal or pelvic abscesses detected on CT scan or MRI can be initially managed by percutaneous drainage, either for definitive treatment or as a temporizing measure while optimizing the patient's condition in preparation for laparotomy. Laparotomy should be reserved for not well-defined collections, presence of dead tissue that requires debridement, or failure of initial percutaneous drainage. In postpartum patients, the radiologist should be alerted to the possibility of myometrial necrosis, which can be detected on CT scan or MRI, and requires hysterectomy. Amniocentesis may be required to exclude chorioamnionitis in septic patients who are still pregnant, and who have no other obvious source as delivery would be required if intraamniotic infection is confirmed by low amniotic fluid glucose concentration and Gram staining. Since pregnant and postpartum women are prone to cholelithiasis, cholecystitis should be excluded and cholecystectomy be entertained if present. Similarly, pyelonephritis associated with urinary obstruction should be treated with stenting and drainage.

According to the recommendations of the International Sepsis Forum, early endotracheal intubation and mechanical ventilation should be used in severe sepsis or septic shock. Noninvasive positive-pressure ventilation should be avoided. Indications for mechanical ventilation include severe tachypnea (respiratory rate >40 bpm), muscular respiratory failure (use of accessory muscles), altered mental status, and severe hypoxemia despite supplemental oxygen. Permissive hypercapnia through reduced tidal volume ventilation (6 mL/kg ideal body weight to maintain end-inspiratory plateau pressures at <30 cm H_2O), and prone positioning are a few strategies that can be used in complicated cases. The respiratory management of patients with acute lung injury/acute respiratory distress syndrome (complicates 18 to 40 percent of cases) is discussed in detail in Chap. 12.

There are a number of therapies that fall into the supportive category in critically ill patients in general, and septic obstetrical patients in particular. Examples of such therapies include prophylaxis for thromboembolism, nutritional support, stress ulcer prophylaxis, and hemofiltration for renal insufficiency. Sepsis and pregnancy are predisposing factors for thromboembolism and deep vein thrombosis prophylaxis is recommended. Either low-dose unfractionated heparin (5000 U three times per day) or low molecular weight heparin can be used. If the patient has a contraindication to heparin (coagulopathy, active bleeding, allergy), then mechanical devices should be substituted. Nutritional support is recommended in septic patients. This topic is dealt with in more detail elsewhere. In summary, enteral nutrition is the preferred method, with parenteral nutrition as a second choice. The American College of Chest Physicians and the American Society of Parenteral and Enteral Nutrition have issued specific recommendations for septic patients (Table 9-5; not specific to obstetrical patients). The efficacy of antacids, sucralfate or histamine-2 receptor antagonists in prevention of stress ulcer bleeding has been confirmed in numerous trials of critically ill patients.

TABLE 9-5 Guidelines for Nutritional Support in Septic Patients

- Daily caloric intake: 25–30 kcal/kg usual body weight
- Protein: 1.3–2.0 g/kg/day
- Glucose: 30–70% of total nonprotein calories, to maintain serum glucose <225 mg/dL
- Lipids: 15–30% of total nonprotein calories (with reduction in polyunsaturated fatty acid)

(Established by the American College of Chest Physicians and the American Society of Parenteral and Enteral Nutrition consensus conferences.)

The popularity of certain additional therapies has waxed and waned over time, while others are still in the experimental phase. Corticosteroids are, currently, the favored immunological therapy. Corticosteroids should be reserved for refractory septic shock, and should not be used in sepsis without shock or with mild shock. Low dose (or stress dose) hydrocortisone (100 mg three times per day) for 5 to 10 days followed by tapering according to hemodynamic status is one treatment option. Corticosteroids should be started within the first few hours of septic shock and high doses should not be used. Recombinant activated protein C (rhAPC; drotrecogin alpha) was recently approved by the FDA for the treatment of patients in septic shock or those with severe sepsis at the highest risk for mortality (APACHE II ≥25). The anticoagulant and profibrinolytic effect of rhAPC targets the consumptive coagulopathy and the associated activation of inflammatory cascade in patients with sepsis. rhAPC also has direct anti-inflammatory properties. The benefits of rhAPC should be weighed against the risk of bleeding. Caution is advised in the use of rhAPC in patients with an INR >3 or platelet count <30,000 cells/mm^3. Intensive insulin therapy to maintain blood glucose between 80 and 100 mg/dL has been shown to reduce the death rate from multiple organ failure in patients with sepsis. If intensive insulin therapy is used, frequent monitoring of blood glucose is recommended to prevent hypoglycemic brain injury secondary to overzealous treatment. Granulocyte colony-stimulating factor should not be used in nonneutropenic patients, and hemofiltration should not be used without renal indications. Other therapies that have been tried, but which should not be used for the treatment of sepsis unless additional studies show a clear benefit, include ibuprofen, prostaglandins, pentoxifyilline, *N*-acetylcysteine, selenium, antithrombin III, immunoglobulins, and growth hormone.

The effect of pregnancy on the critically ill patient and vice versa, is discussed elsewhere. Pregnant septic patients are at risk for utero-placental insufficiency and preterm labor. The decision for continuous fetal heart rate monitoring and/or tocolysis should take into account the gestational age and the patient's condition. A nonreassuring fetal heart rate pattern or contractions frequently resolve with correction of maternal hypoxemia and acidosis of short-term duration. Longer periods of maternal hypoxemia and acidosis, however, may result in permanent fetal damage or progression into active labor and may require delivery. In the absence of chorioamnionitis, labor, or nonreassuring fetal status, the decision for delivery should also be based on gestational age and the patient's condition. If respiratory and cardiovascular functions continue to deteriorate despite aggressive management, then decompression of a gravid uterus after 28 weeks gestation may improve venous return and lung volumes.

SUGGESTED READING

Astiz ME, Rackow EC: Septic shock. *Lancet* 1998;351:1501–1505.

Bernard GR, Vincent JL, Laterre PF, et al.: Efficacy and safety of recombinant human activated protein C for severe sepsis. *N Engl J Med* 2001;344:699–709.

Bollaert PE, Bauer P, Audibert G, et al.: Effects of epinephrine on hemodynamics and oxygen metabolism in dopamine-resistant septic shock. *Chest* 1990;98:949.

Bone RC, Sibbald WJ, Sprung CL: The ACCP-SCCM consensus conference on sepsis and organ failure. *Chest* 1992;101:1481.

Brun-Buisson C, Doyon F, Carlet J, et al.: Incidence, risk factors, and outcome of severe sepsis and septic shock in adults. A multicenter prospective study in intensive care units. *JAMA* 1995;274:968.

Cook DJ, Reeve BK, Guyatt GH, et al.: Stress ulcer prophylaxis in critically ill patients: resolving discordant meta-analyses. *JAMA* 1996;275:308.

Cooper MS, Stewart PM: Corticosteroid insufficiency in acutely ill patients. *N Engl J Med* 2003;348–727.

Dellinger RP: Cardiovascular management of septic shock. *Crit Care Med* 2003; 31:946–955.

Hack CE, Zeerleder S: The endothelium in sepsis: source of and a target for inflammation. *Crit Care Med* 2001;29:S21.

Hinds C, Watson D: Manipulating hemodynamic and oxygen transport in critically ill patients. *N Engl J Med* 1995;333:1074.

Hotchkiss RS, Karl IE: The pathophysiology and treatment of sepsis. *N Engl J Med* 2003;348:138–150.

The Acute Respiratory Distress Syndrome Network: Ventilation with lower tidal volumes as compared with traditional tidal volumes for acute lung injury and the acute respiratory distress syndrome. *N Engl J Med* 2000;342:1301–1308.

The International Sepsis Forum: Recommendations for the management of patients with severe sepsis and septic shock. *Intensive Care Med* 2001;27:S1–S134.

Mabie WC, Barton JR, Sibai B: Septic shock in pregnancy. *Obstet Gynecol* 1997; 90:533–561.

Marshall JC: Inflammation, coagulopathy, and the pathogenesis of multiple organ dysfunction syndrome. *Crit Care Med* 2001;29(Suppl):S99–S106.

Martin C, Papazian L, Perrin G, et al.: Norepinephrine or dopamine for the treatment of hyperdynamic septic shock? *Chest* 1993;103:1826.

Martin GS, Mannino DM, Eaton S, et al.: The epidemiology of sepsis in the United States from 1979 through 2000. *N Eng J Med* 2003;348:1546–1554.

Rangel-Frausto MS, Pittet D, Costigan M, et al.: The natural history of the systemic inflammatory response syndrome (SIRS). *JAMA* 1995;273:117.

Rivers E, Nguyen B, Havstad S, et al.: Early goal-directed therapy in the treatment of severe sepsis and septic shock. *N Engl J Med* 2001;345:1368–1377.

Sharma S, Kumar A: Septic shock, multiple organ failure, and acute respiratory distress syndrome. *Curr Opin Pulm Med* 2003;9:199–209.

Vincent JL, de Carvalho FB, De Backer D: Management of septic shock. *Ann Med* 2002;34:606–613.

Wheeler AP, Bernard GR: Treating patients with severe sepsis. *N Engl J Med* 1999;340:207–214.

Wojnar MM, Hawkins WG, Lang CH: Nutritional support of the septic patient. *Crit Care Clin* 1995;11:717.

Yu M, Levy MM, Smith P, et al.: Effect of maximizing oxygen delivery on morbidity and mortality rates in critically ill patients: a prospective, randomized, controlled study. *Crit Care Med* 1993;21:830.

10 Thyroid and Other Endocrine Emergencies

Michael A. Belfort

THYROID AND OTHER ENDOCRINE EMERGENCIES

This chapter will address several common endocrine emergencies that may be seen in pregnant women. While most endocrine conditions can become emergencies if ignored or untreated, the intention of this chapter is not to exhaustively review endocrine complications in pregnancy; rather, the conditions that might realistically be faced in an ICU situation have been highlighted. These include thyrotoxicosis and thyroid storm, hypothyroidism and myxedema coma, Addisonian crisis, pheochromocytoma, primary hyperalderonism, and diabetes insipidus. Diabetes mellitus and ketoacidosis have been dealt with elsewhere.

Thyroid Disease

Thyroid disease is the second most common endocrine condition affecting women of reproductive age. It is now common for obstetricians to care for women who enter pregnancy with an established thyroid deficiency or overactivity state. Since pregnancy in and of itself affects thyroid function, even women who are well-controlled prepregnancy may become uncontrolled requiring continued monitoring and adjustment. In addition, it is important to remember that the developing fetus may be at significant risk from circulating maternal antibodies that are no longer an issue for the mother. Despite the fact that hyperthyroidism is uncommon during pregnancy (0.2 percent of pregnancies), and thyroid storm is considered rare, vigilance is important because of the potential for significant morbidity and mortality in these conditions.

Definitions

Thyrotoxicosis is a generic term referring to a clinical and biochemical state resulting from over production of, and exposure to, thyroid hormone. The most common cause of thyrotoxicosis in pregnancy is **Grave's disease**. This disorder is an autoimmune condition characterized by production of thyroid-stimulating immunoglobulin (TSI) and thyroid-stimulating hormone binding inhibitory immunoglobulin (TBII) that act on the thyroid stimulating hormone (TSH) receptor to mediate thyroid stimulation or inhibition, respectively.

Thyroid storm is characterized by an acute, severe exacerbation of hyperthyroidism.

Hypothyroidism results from inadequate thyroid hormone production and **myxedema coma** is an extreme form of hypothyroidism.

Thyroiditis is caused by an autoimmune inflammation of the thyroid gland and may occur for the first time postpartum. It is usually painless and may present as de novo hypothyroidism, transient thyrotoxicosis, or as initial hyperthyroidism followed by hypothyroidism within one year postpartum.

Physiology

Thyroxine (T_4) is the major secretory product of the thyroid. The majority of circulating T_4 is converted in the peripheral tissues to triiodothyronine (T_3), the biologically active form of this hormone. T_4 secretion is under the direct control of the pituitary thyroid-stimulating hormone (TSH). The cell surface receptor for TSH is similar to the receptors for luteinizing hormone (LH) and human chorionic gonadotrophin (hCG). T_4 and T_3 are transported in the peripheral circulation bound to thyroxine-binding globulin (TBG), transthyretin (formerly called prealbumin), and albumin. Less than 0.05 percent of plasma T_4 and less than 0.5 percent of plasma T_3 are unbound and able to interact with target tissues. Routine T_4 measurements reflect total serum concentration and may be factitiously altered by increases or decreases in concentrations of circulating proteins. Plasma concentrations of TBG increase 2.5-fold by 20 weeks' gestation, due to reduced hepatic clearance and an estrogen-induced change in the structure of TBG that prolongs the serum half-life. This TBG alteration causes significant changes in many of the thyroid test results in pregnancy. There is a 25 to 45 percent increase in serum total T_4 (TT_4) from a pregravid level of 5 to 12 mg% to 9 to 16 mg%. Total T_3 (TT_3) increases by about 30 percent in the first trimester and by 50 to 65 percent later. The increase in available protein binding induced by pregnancy causes a transient change in free T_4 and free thyroxine index (FTI) in the first trimester (possibly related to an increase in HCG). Increased concentrations of TSH stimulate restoration of the free serum T_4 level such that FT_4 and FTI levels are generally maintained within the normal nonpregnant range. Pregnancy affects other changes in the thyroid system and ultimately the interpretation of thyroid function tests (Table 10-1).

The fetal hypothalamic-pituitary-thyroid axis develops independently of the maternal thyroid function. The fetus begins concentrating iodine between 10 and 12 weeks of gestation. By 20 weeks gestation, the fetal pituitary TSH is functional. The human placenta acts as a significant barrier to circulating T_4, T_3, and TSH. Despite this, in cases of congenital hypothyroidism there is still sufficient passage of maternal thyroid hormones across the placenta (cord levels 25 to 50 percent of normal) to prevent overt hypothyroidism at birth. Immunoglobulin G (IgG) autoantibodies, iodine, thyrotropin-releasing hormone (TRH), and antithyroid medications (PTU, methimazole) can readily cross the placenta and interfere with fetal thyroid activity. Fetuses of women being treated with antithyroid drugs are at risk for hypothyroidism and goiter and should be closely monitored. Targeted ultrasound for fetal growth abnormalities and thyroid size should be performed serially. Antepartum fetal heart rate monitoring and occasionally percutaneous fetal blood sampling (if ultrasound reveals an obvious goiter) should also be entertained. Since IgG autoantibodies can cross

TABLE 10-1 Thyroid Function Changes During Pregnancy

Normal hypothalamic-pituitary-thyroid axis
First trimester TSH depression due to hCG, normalized thereafter
Increased renal iodide clearance (increased glomerular filtration rate)
Goiter-minimal in regions of iodine sufficiency; 30% increase in size in regions with dietary iodine deficiency
Increased serum TBG; decreased T_3 resin uptake
Increased total serum T_4 and total serum T_3
Normal serum free T_4 and free T_3

TABLE 10-2 Causes of Hyperthyroidism During Pregnancy

Grave's disease
Toxic multinodular goiter (rare in the reproductive age group)
Toxic adenoma
Hyperemesis gravidarum
Trophoblastic disease
Thyroiditis (chronic, subacute, viral)
Exogenous thyroid hormone

the placenta, it is important that women with a prior history of Grave's disease are tested for thyroid stimulating immunoglobulin (TSI) and thyroid stimulating hormone binding inhibitory immunoglobulin (TBII).

Hyperthyroidism

The causes of hyperthyroidism in pregnancy are listed in Table 10-2. Hyperthyroidism occurs in 0.2 percent of pregnancies and Grave's disease accounts for more than 90 percent of these cases. Autoantibodies (thyroid-stimulating antibody [TSAb]—formerly known as LATS [long-acting thyroid stimulator]) against TSH receptors act as TSH agonists, thereby stimulating increased production of thyroid hormone. The clinical presentation of mild hyperthyroidism is similar to the symptoms of normal pregnancy (fatigue, increased appetite, vomiting, palpitations, tachycardia, heat intolerance, increased urinary frequency, insomnia, emotional lability) and may confound the diagnosis. More specific symptoms highly suggestive of hyperthyroidism include tremor, nervousness, frequent stools, excessive sweating, brisk reflexes, muscle weakness, goiter, hypertension, and weight loss. Grave's ophthalmopathy (stare, lid lag and retraction, exophthalmos) and dermopathy (localized or pretibial myxedema) are diagnostic. The disease usually gets worse in the first trimester but moderates later in pregnancy. Untreated hyperthyroidism poses considerable maternal and fetal risks including preterm delivery, severe preeclampsia, and heart failure (Table 10-3).

Fetal and Neonatal Implications

Risks include IUGR, prematurity, cardiac dysrhythmias, and intrauterine death. Fetal thyrotoxicosis should be considered in any pregnancy with Grave's disease. Neonates of women with thyrotoxicosis are at risk for immune mediated hypothyroidism and hyperthyroidism secondary to autoantibodies that may cross the placenta (Grave's disease and chronic autoimmune thyroiditis). TBII can cause transient neonatal hypothyroidism and TSI can result in neonatal hyperthyroidism. The incidence is low (less than 5 percent) because of the balance between the stimulatory and inhibitory autoantibodies with thioamide treatment. Maternal autoantibodies are cleared slowly in the neonate sometimes resulting in delayed presentation of neonatal Grave's disease. Neonates of

TABLE 10-3 Fetal and Maternal Risks with Untreated Hyperthyroidism

Fetal	Maternal
Spontaneous abortion	Preeclampsia
Prematurity	Maternal heart failure
Low birth weight	Infection
Fetal/neonatal thyrotoxicosis	Anemia
	Thyroid storm

women with prior Grave's disease who have been treated with surgery or radioactive iodine and who do not need thioamide therapy during pregnancy remain at significant risk for neonatal Grave's disease.

Laboratory Diagnosis

Laboratory diagnosis of hyperthyroidism is confirmed with a suppressed serum TSH in the setting of elevated free T_4 levels (or FTI) without the presence of a nodular goiter or thyroid mass. In rare circumstances, the serum total T_3 may demonstrate greater (or earlier) elevation than T_4 (T_3 toxicosis).

Hyperthyroidism may also result from elevated serum levels of hCG, as seen with trophoblastic diseases and hyperemesis gravidarum. In these circumstances, treatment is seldom required, since the disease spontaneously resolves after the trophoblastic tissue is evacuated or vomiting resolves. Biochemical hyperthyroidism is seen in up to 66 percent of women with severe hyperemesis gravidarum (undetectable TSH level or elevated FTI, or both) but this usually resolves by 18 weeks. If therapy is needed, efforts should be directed towards uncovering an underlying thyroid condition since clinical hyperthyroidism (as opposed to biochemical hyperthyroidism) is extremely unusual with hyperemesis gravidarum. Cardiac decompensation in pregnancy usually occurs in poorly controlled hyperthyroid patients with anemia, infection, or hypertension. The hemodynamic changes associated with hyperthyroidism during pregnancy are outlined in Table 10-4.

A diastolic murmur, an apical systolic murmur, and a displaced pulse of maximal impulse suggest signs of clinical decompensation. β-adrenergic blockade is theoretically contraindicated with congestive heart failure, since adrenergic stimulation of the heart is the major compensating mechanism against cardiac failure. The negative inotropic effect imposed by β-adrenergic blockade may depress myocardial contractility. These drugs, however, are very effective for treating atrial fibrillation and supraventricular tachycardia that may accompany hyperthyroidism. Thus, cautious use of β-blocker therapy is recommended, since congestive heart failure during pregnancy is often rate related. Utilization of a pulmonary artery catheter is an important adjunct to the effective and safe use of β-blocker therapy in these critical situations. Other helpful therapeutic modalities include diuretic therapy, digoxin, and bed rest. Cardiac dysfunction may linger for months after restoration of normal thyroid function.

Treatment of Hyperthyroidism During Pregnancy

The primary objective of treatment is to effectively control thyroid dysfunction until after delivery. Protecting the fetus from the effects of the disease and the side effects of the medical regimen is a secondary yet important objective. Basic treatment options are outlined in Table 10-5.

TABLE 10-4 Hemodynamic Changes with Hyperthyroidism

Increased stroke volume and cardiac output
Increased pulse rate
Reduced peripheral vascular resistance
Increased blood volume
Impaired myocardial contractility
Electrocardiographic changes
Left ventricular hypertrophy (15 percent)
Atrial fibrillation (21 percent)
Wolff-Parkinson-White syndrome

TABLE 10-5 Treatment Options for Hyperthyroidism

Observation
Antithyroid medications
β-adrenergic blocking agents
Thyroid surgery

Observation alone may be a reasonable treatment plan for mild clinical disease without cardiovascular compromise. For overt disease, antithyroid medications are the mainstay of treatment. Propylthiouracil (PTU) and methimazole (Tapazole) are two of the thioamide agents currently available in the United States. In Europe, the methimazole derivative carbimazole is used. Since carbimazole is rapidly metabolized to methimazole, these drugs are essentially the same. Both methimazole and PTU effectively block intrathyroid hormone synthesis, but PTU also blocks extrathyroid conversion of T_4 to T_3. Both agents readily cross the placenta and may inhibit fetal thyroid function. Methimazole was believed to be approximately four times more bioavailable to fetal tissue than PTU and has also been associated with aplasia cutis in infancy. For these two reasons PTU has become the preferred medication for treating hyperthyroidism in pregnancy in the United States. Both of these beliefs have recently been disputed with studies showing no differences in mean umbilical cord TSH or FT_4 levels between PTU and methimazole treated neonates and no increased incidence of cutis aplasia.

Twice daily doses of 150 to 200 mg PTU or a dosage of 100 mg T.I.D will usually control hyperthyroidism within four to eight weeks. Lack of response is usually due to noncompliance and may require hospitalization. The goal of treatment is to use the smallest dose that maintains maternal free T_4 levels at or just above, the upper limit of normal. Clinical and laboratory follow-up (TSH, free T_4, free T_3) should occur every two to four weeks. Most women (90 percent) will have a significant improvement within two to four weeks. Rapid improvement necessitates a decrease in dosage. Improvement commonly occurs in the second trimester, and as many as 40 percent of mothers may discontinue therapy. It may, however, be reasonable to continue giving small doses to ameliorate the risks of fetal thyrotoxicosis imposed by transplacental passage of TSAb and to reduce the general overall incidence of thyroid storm during labor and delivery.

Baseline white blood cell (WBC) and liver function tests should be obtained before initiating antithyroid therapy, since hyperthyroidism itself may also cause liver enzyme elevations and leukopenia. The incidence of agranulocytosis with thioamides is about 0.1 to 0.4 percent. This is usually heralded by a fever and sore throat and these symptoms should precipitate immediate discontinuation of the drug and checking for leukopenia. Antithyroid medications should also be discontinued if liver function values become extremely abnormal. These medications may be restarted during the postpartum period as disease activity dictates but the clinician should be aware that treatment with other thioamides carries a high risk for cross reaction. Other major side effects of thioamides, which include a lupus-like syndrome, thrombocytopenia, hepatitis/hepatic infarction and vasculitis occur in less than 1 percent of patients. Minor side effects include rash, argthralgias, nausea, anorexia, fever, and a loss of taste or smell may occur in up to 5 percent of cases.

Breastfeeding is permissible while taking PTU because little is passed into breast milk with standard doses. Breastfeeding is also acceptable with methimazole therapy despite the fact that it is present in a higher ratio than PTU in breast milk.

β-adrenergic blockers may be used as adjunctive therapy to control the symptoms of tremor and palpitations until the thioamides decrease thyroid hormone levels. Propranolol is the most commonly used β-blocker for this purpose. Relative contraindications to the use of β-adrenergic blockers include obstructive lung disease, heart block, heart failure, and insulin use. Although unusual, there may be adverse fetal effects such as bradycardia, growth restriction, and neonatal hypoglycemia. It is advisable to minimize the duration of β-adrenergic blocker therapy during gestation.

Subtotal thyroidectomy is reserved for patients with severe antithyroid drug side effects or failed medical suppression of thyroid function. To minimize pregnancy complications, surgery is usually performed during the second trimester. Preoperatively, hyperthyroidism should be controlled with antithyroid medication for 7 to 10 days, a β-adrenergic blocker (propranolol, 20 mg times daily), and inorganic iodide (Lugol solution, three drops twice daily) for four to five days. The latter two can be discontinued 48 hours postoperatively. Iodide must be used cautiously to minimize the risk of severe fetal hypothyroidism and goiter.

Radioactive iodine administration is contraindicated during pregnancy because of the risk of fetal thyroid ablation. It is recommended that women avoid pregnancy or breastfeeding for four months after I-131 therapy. This agent readily crosses the placenta and may cause permanent damage to the fetal thyroid if used after 10 to 12 weeks of gestation. Inadvertent use of I-131 in very early pregnancy (up to 10 weeks) is usually not associated with any long-term fetal/neonatal thyroid side effects.

Thyroid Storm

Thyroid storm is a rare but potentially fatal hypermetabolic complication of hyperthyroidism characterized by cardiovascular compromise (tachycardia out of proportion to the fever, dysrhythmia, cardiac failure), hyperpyrexia, and central nervous system changes (restlessness, nervousness, changed mental status, confusion, and seizures) (Table 10-6). Thyroid storm is estimated to occur in 1 to 2 percent of pregnancies complicated by hyperthyroidism. This rare but devastating complication is usually seen in patients with poorly controlled hyperthyroidism complicated by additional physiologic stressors such as infection, surgery, thromboembolism, preeclampsia, and parturition. Precipitating events for thyroid storm are presented in Table 10-7. Diagnosis can be difficult and if delayed the patient may lapse into shock and/or coma. The laboratory profile of the mother with thyroid storm reveals leukocytosis, elevated hepatic enzymes, and occasionally hypercalcemia. Thyroid function test results are consistent with hyperthyroidism (elevated FT_4/FT_3 and depressed TSH) but do not always correlate with the severity of the thyroid storm. Treatment should, however, be initiated on the suspicion of the condition and the clinician should not wait to confirm the diagnosis before starting therapy. Management is best accomplished in an obstetric intensive care unit. Table 10-8 reviews basic supportive adjunctive care for patients in thyroid storm.

The basic goals of therapy are to:

1. reduce the synthesis and release of thyroid hormone,
2. remove thyroid hormone from the circulation and increase the concentration of TBG,

TABLE 10-6 Diagnosis of Thyroid Storm

Hypermetabolism
Fever above 100°F
Perspiration
Warm, flushed skin
Cardiovascular
Tachycardia
Atrial fibrillation
Congestive heart failure
Central nervous system
Irritability
Agitation
Tremor
Mental status change (delirium, psychosis, coma)
Gastrointestinal
Nausea, vomiting
Diarrhea
Jaundice
Supporting laboratory evidence
Leukocytosis
Elevated liver function values
Hypercalcemia
Low TSH, high free T_4 and/or T_3

TABLE 10-7 Common Precipitants of Thyroid Storm

Acute surgical emergency
Induction of anesthesia
Diabetic ketoacidosis
Pulmonary embolism
Noncompliance with antithyroid medications
Myocardial infarction
Infection
Hypertension/preeclampsia
Labor and delivery
Severe anemia

TABLE 10-8 Supportive Adjunctive Care for the Patient in Thyroid Storm

Intravenous fluids and electrolytes
Cardiac monitoring
Consideration of pulmonary artery catheterization (central hemodynamic monitoring to guide β-blocker therapy during hyperdynamic cardiac failure)
Cooling measure: blanket, sponge bath, acetaminophen
Oxygen therapy (consider arterial line to follow serial blood gases)
No salicylates (increased T_4)
Nasogastric tube if patient is unable to swallow (may be only avenue for PTU administration)

3. block the peripheral conversion of T_4 to T_3,
4. block the peripheral actions of thyroid hormone,
5. treat the complications of thyroid storm and provide support, and
6. identify and treat the potential precipitating conditions.

To these ends the following drugs are available: (1) propylthiouracil and methimazole, both of which inhibit iodination of tyrosine (leading to reduced synthesis of thyroid hormones), and block peripheral conversion of T_4 to T_3. These drugs alone can reduce the T_3 concentration by 75 percent. (2) For thyroid storm Lugol's iodine, SSKI (strong solution of potassium iodide), sodium iodide, orografin, and lithium carbonate. These drugs function by blocking the *release* of stored hormone by inhibiting the proteolysis of thyroglobulin. One of the side effects of such agents is to initially increase the *production* of thyroid hormone, and it is therefore very important to *start propylthiouracil prior to giving iodides.* The mainstay of therapy are glucocorticoids which should be started as soon as the condition is recognized and act by blocking the *release* of stored hormone (as do iodides), and by blocking *peripheral conversion* of T_4 to T_3 (as do the thioamides). Specifics of the medical therapy are detailed below:

1. Oral PTU (or by nasogastric tube if necessary) with a 300- to 600-mg loading dose followed by 150 to 200 mg orally every 4 to 6 hours.
2. Iodide initiated 1 to 2 hours after PTU administration:
   a. Oral saturated solution of potassium iodide (SSKI) to block T_4 release (two to five drops orally every 8 hours)
   b. Intravenous (IV) sodium iodide, 500 to 1000 mg every 8 hours
   c. Oral Lugol's iodine solution (eight drops every 6 hours)
   d. Oragrafin (62 percent iodine) can be used if other solutions are not available. Three grams given orally will suppress thyroid hormone release for two to three days.
   e. Oral lithium carbonate, 300 mg every 6 hours (therapeutic level = 1 meq/L)
3. Adrenal glucocorticoids: This may be in the form of dexamethasone, 2 mg intravenously or intramuscularly every 6 hours for four doses (or hydrocortisone, 300 mg per day IV or prednisone, 60 mg per day orally)
4. Propranolol (20 to 80 mg orally or by nasogastric tube every 4 to 6 hours or 1 to 2 mg per minute IV for 5 minutes for a total of 6 mg, followed by 1 to 10 mg every IV for 4 hours) is effective for controlling tachycardia. If the patient has a history of severe bronchospasm reserpine or guanethidine may be used:
   a. Reserpine, 1 to 5 mg IM every 4 to 6 hours
   b. Guanethidine, 1 mg/kg orally every 12 hours
5. Phenobarbital, 30 to 60 mg orally every 6 to 8 hours as needed to control restlessness.
6. Iodides and glucocorticoids may be discontinued after initial clinical improvement.
7. Plasmapheresis or peritoneal dialysis to remove circulating thyroid hormone is an extreme measure reserved for patients who do not respond to conventional therapy.
8. An algorithm for the management of thyroid storm is presented in Figure 10-1.

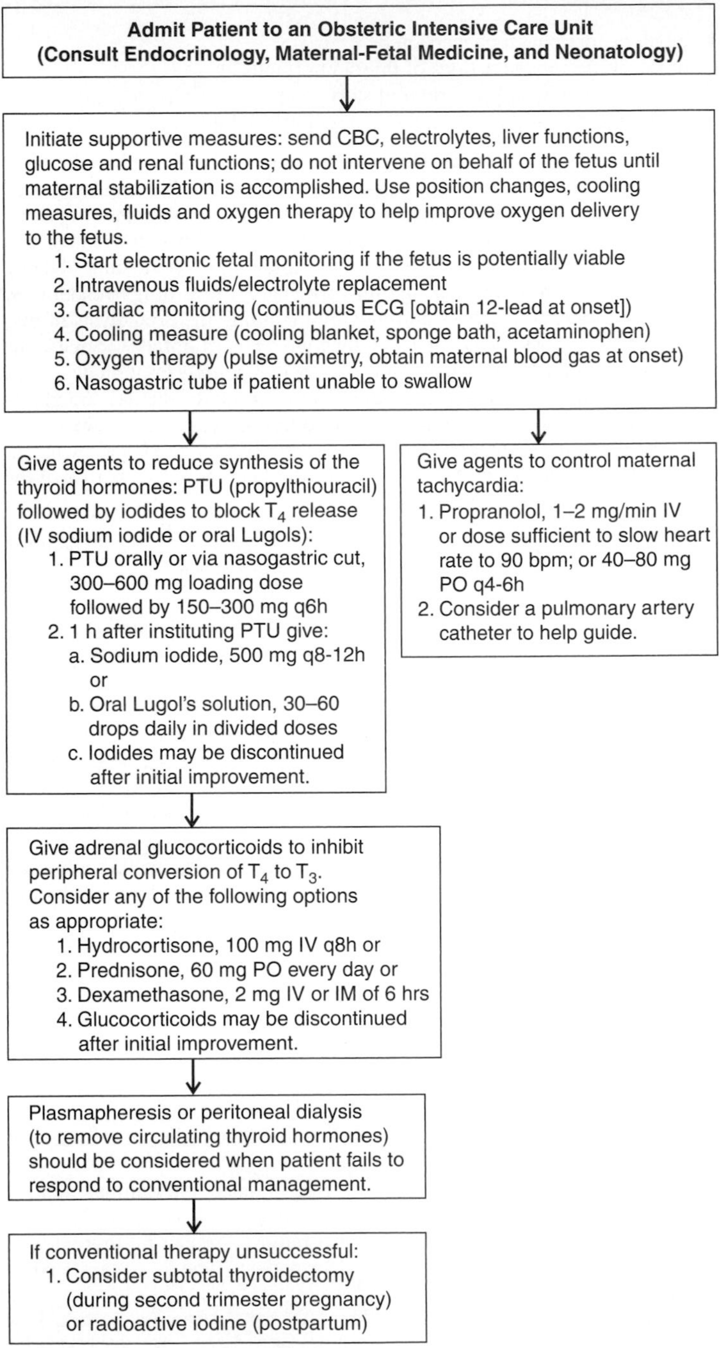

Admit Patient to an Obstetric Intensive Care Unit (Consult Endocrinology, Maternal-Fetal Medicine, and Neonatology)

↓

Initiate supportive measures: send CBC, electrolytes, liver functions, glucose and renal functions; do not intervene on behalf of the fetus until maternal stabilization is accomplished. Use position changes, cooling measures, fluids and oxygen therapy to help improve oxygen delivery to the fetus.

1. Start electronic fetal monitoring if the fetus is potentially viable
2. Intravenous fluids/electrolyte replacement
3. Cardiac monitoring (continuous ECG [obtain 12-lead at onset])
4. Cooling measure (cooling blanket, sponge bath, acetaminophen)
5. Oxygen therapy (pulse oximetry, obtain maternal blood gas at onset)
6. Nasogastric tube if patient unable to swallow

↓

Give agents to reduce synthesis of the thyroid hormones: PTU (propylthiouracil) followed by iodides to block T_4 release (IV sodium iodide or oral Lugols):

1. PTU orally or via nasogastric cut, 300–600 mg loading dose followed by 150–300 mg q6h
2. 1 h after instituting PTU give:
   a. Sodium iodide, 500 mg q8-12h or
   b. Oral Lugol's solution, 30–60 drops daily in divided doses
   c. Iodides may be discontinued after initial improvement.

Give agents to control maternal tachycardia:

1. Propranolol, 1–2 mg/min IV or dose sufficient to slow heart rate to 90 bpm; or 40–80 mg PO q4-6h
2. Consider a pulmonary artery catheter to help guide.

↓

Give adrenal glucocorticoids to inhibit peripheral conversion of T_4 to T_3. Consider any of the following options as appropriate:

1. Hydrocortisone, 100 mg IV q8h or
2. Prednisone, 60 mg PO every day or
3. Dexamethasone, 2 mg IV or IM of 6 hrs
4. Glucocorticoids may be discontinued after initial improvement.

↓

Plasmapheresis or peritoneal dialysis (to remove circulating thyroid hormones) should be considered when patient fails to respond to conventional management.

↓

If conventional therapy unsuccessful:

1. Consider subtotal thyroidectomy (during second trimester pregnancy) or radioactive iodine (postpartum)

FIG. 10-1 Management algorithm for thyroid storm.

Hypothyroidism

Most cases of hypothyroidism in pregnancy are the result of a primary thyroid dysfunction or are iatrogenic from prior thyroid surgery or radioactive iodine. A few cases are caused by hypothalamic abnormalities. The most common causes of hypothyroidism in pregnant or postpartum women are Hashimoto's disease (chronic thyroiditis or chronic autoimmune thyroiditis), subacute thyroiditis, thyroidectomy, radioactive iodine therapy and iodine deficiency, and drugs that interfere with thyroid function (Table 10-9). Hashimoto's disease is the most common etiology in developed countries and is characterized by production of antithyroid antibodies. These include thyroid antimicrosomal and antithyroglobulin antibodies. Hashimotos' disease may be associated with thyroid enlargement (as is iodine deficiency which is rare in the United States). Hashimoto's disease is more common in patients with diabetes mellitus; in one study of 100 diabetic women, 20 percent of patients with type-I diabetes also had Hashimoto's disease. Subacute thyroiditis is not associated with goiter. Goiter is generally thought to be a sign of compensatory TSH production in the face of low circulating thyroxine. On a worldwide basis the most common cause of hypothyroidism is iodine deficiency. Patients recently arrived in the United States from a region where iodine deficiency is endemic and who have features of hypothyroidism, as well as those with malnutrition, should be considered as candidates for iodine replacement.

The symptoms of hypothyroidism are common to all of the underlying etiologies (Table 10-10). Patients complain of constipation, cold intolerance, cool, dry skin, coarse hair, irritability, and inability to concentrate. Of note, however, is a significant overlap with complaints common to euthyroid pregnant women, making the clinical diagnosis difficult. The presence of paresthesias may be helpful, as it is an early symptom in approximately 75 percent of patients with hypothyroidism. The presence of delayed deep tendon reflexes is also suggestive of hypothyroidism. In addition, signs of gross myexedma, including a low body temperature, large tongue, hoarse voice, and periorbital edema, are not found in normal pregnancy, and their presence should prompt an immediate evaluation for hypothyroidism. Patients may complain of excessive fatigue. Gestational hypertension is common. Postpartum amenorrhea and galactorrhea associated with hyperprolactinemia may be indicative of hypothyroidism.

TABLE 10-9 Causes of Hypothyroidism during Pregnancy

Primary thyroid dysfunction
Hashimoto's disease (chronic thyroiditis, chronic autoimmune thyroiditis)
Subacute thyroiditis
Circulating TSH receptor blocking antibody
Hypothalamic dysfunction
Iatrogenic
Prior thyroid surgery (thyroidectomy)
Radioactive iodine therapy
Iodine deficiency[a]
Relative hypothyroidism and goitrogenesis

[a]Iodine deficiency does not usually cause overt hypothyroidism (unless very severe deficiency) and more commonly presents with compensatory goiter development and relative hypothyroidism.

TABLE 10-10 Symptoms and Signs of Severe Hypothyroidism

Hypometabolism
Cold intolerance and low body temperature
Failure to increase body temperature in the face of infection
Cool, dry skin
Coarse hair, loss of hair
Large tongue and hoarse voice
Periorbital edema and nonpitting edema of hands and feet
Postpartum amenorrhea and galactorrhea

Cardiovascular and respiratory
Gestational hypertension
Decreased pulse pressure with predominant increase in diastolic pressure
Slow heart rate and respiration
Enlarged tonsils, nasopharynx, and larynx
Lungs may be congested, consolidated and there may be pleural effusions
Pericardial effusion

Central nervous system
Parasthesias
Lethargy and fatigue
Irritability and inability to concentrate (may develop confusion, stupor, obtundation, seizures and coma in severe myxedema)
Delayed deep tendon reflexes

Gastrointestinal
Constipation
Distended abdomen associated with ileus or ascites

Supporting laboratory evidence
Increased TSH
Decreased T_4 and free T_4
Presence of antithyroid antibodies
Hyponatremia, low serum osmolality, elevated serum creatinine, hypoglycemia, elevated CK (skeletal muscle usually)
Electrocardiogram—Sinus bradycardia, low-amplitude QRS complexes, prolonged QT interval, flattened or inverted T waves

Fetal and Neonatal Implications

Laboratory Diagnosis An elevated TSH in association with a low serum free T_4 concentration is the most sensitive indicator of primary hypothyroidism. Because TBG is elevated in pregnancy, the total serum T_4 level may not be as low as would be expected, and may appear inappropriately high in the setting of an elevated TSH. Positive thyroid autoantibodies support the diagnosis of hypothyroidism, particularly in the absence of a past history of thyroidectomy or radioactive iodine therapy. Elevated serum cholesterol concentration is useful in nonpregnant patients but is not helpful in pregnancy since serum cholesterol concentrations increase by up to 60 percent above prepregnancy values during gestation.

Treatment of Hypothyroidism During Pregnancy

Once a diagnosis of hypothyroidism is made in a pregnant patient full replacement doses of T_4 should be instituted, regardless of the degree of thyroid function. This will minimize further fetal exposure to a hypothyroid environment. Therapy can be titrated rapidly in young pregnant women with no other comorbid conditions starting with 0.1 mg of T_4 daily for three to five weeks. Thereafter, dosage adjustments can be made depending on the thyroid function test results. Since T_4 has a long half-life it can be given once a day. With adequate treatment, the serum TSH concentration should decrease to values below 6 U/mL within four weeks, and the serum free T_4 concentration should increase to normal values for pregnancy in the same timespan. The optimal range for TSH during pregnancy is <3.0 U/mL. It is important to note that normal total serum T_4 concentrations in pregnancy are higher than the normal range for nonpregnant women due to an increase in thyroxine binding and increases in serum TBG concentration. The free T_4 concentration is ideally in the upper range of normal. If the values do not return to normal, the dose of T_4 should be increased by 0.05 mg increments. The serum TSH concentration may take longer to return to normal values.

MYXEDEMA COMA

Myxedema coma represents the extreme expression of severe hypothyroidism and is considered a medical emergency with a 20-percent mortality rate. It is very rare in pregnancy and usually affects older patients. It is characterized by hypothermia, hypotension, hypoventilation, hyponatremia, and bradycardia. Primary objectives in treating myxedema coma are restoration of normal thyroid hormone levels, correction of electrolyte disturbances, and identification and treatment of any underlying infection. Because of the inherently high mortality rate, treatment should be started immediately and should include appropriate supportive therapy and corticosteroids to prevent adrenal insufficiency (Table 10-11). Possible precipitating factors should also be identified and treated. Levothyroxine sodium may be given via a nasogastric tube, but the preferred route of administration is intravenous. A bolus dose of

TABLE 10-11 Treatment of Myxedema Coma

Endotracheal intubation and ventilation if there is hypercapnia or hypoxia
Ordinary warming (normal blankets)—avoid external rewarming devices
Intravenous fluids and electrolytes and inotropic supportive therapy if required
Intravenous sodium may be needed if serum sodium <120 meq/L
Cardiac monitoring
ECG
Troponin and CPK levels to rule out myocardial infarction
Blood pressure monitoring
Corticosteroids
Draw baseline cortisol level
100 mg hydrocortisone every 8 hours until baseline cortisol level is known, then titrate accordingly
Levothyroxine sodium (synthroid, levoxyl) intravenously (nasogastric tube if IV administration not possible—oral dose is 30–50% more than the IV dose)
Slow bolus IV dose 300–500 μg
Daily IV doses of 75–100 μg
Daily oral does of 50–200 μg once patient is ambulatory
Liothyronine (cytomel, triostat) T_3 replacement in young patients with low cardiovascular risk (more likely than T_4 to cause arrhythmias)
10 μg IV every 8 hours
Panculture and emperic antibiotic therapy until culture results are known

levothyroxine sodium is given as quickly as possible to increase the peripheral pool of T_4. This should usually be between 300 and 500 μg. Although such a dose is usually tolerated well, rapid intravenous administration of large doses of levothyroxine sodium should be cautiously undertaken in patients with cardiac compromise. Clinical judgment in this situation may dictate smaller intravenous doses of levothyroxine sodium. The initial dose is followed by daily intravenous doses of 75 to 100 μg until the patient is stable and oral administration is feasible. Normal T_4 levels are usually achieved within 24 hours, followed by progressive increases in T_3. Improvement in cardiac output, blood pressure, temperature, and mental status generally occur within 24 hours, with further improvement in the other manifestations of hypothyroidism in four to seven days.

ACUTE ADRENAL INSUFFICIENCY IN PREGNANCY

Acute adrenocortical insufficiency or Addisonian crisis can occur in pregnancy when a patient with chronic adrenal insufficiency is stressed, or in one who is undiagnosed. Normal levels of total and free cortisol, urinary free cortisol, and ACTH in pregnancy are shown in Table 10-12. It also may result from an obstetric complication that results in DIC, such as severe preeclampsia or eclampsia, abruptio placentae, amniotic fluid embolus, or postpartum hemorrhage. In such cases bilateral massive adrenal hemorrhage may occur and constitute an acute emergency. This condition usually presents with nausea, vomiting, abdominal pain, and shock, and is frequently fatal. Early recognition and treatment are paramount to avoiding a bad outcome. A similar presentation has been noted in the third trimester of pregnancy or in the postpartum period in association with acute pyelonephritis, gram-negative bacillemia, and fulminant meningococcal infection (Waterhouse-Friderichsen syndrome). Therapy for acute adrenocortical insufficiency in pregnancy should include an initial intravenous bolus of 200 mg hydrocortisone succinate (Solu-Cortef) followed by 100 mg in 1 L of normal saline solution given over 30 minutes. One hundred milligrams of hydrocortisone succinate should

TABLE 10-12 Normal Plasma Total and Free Cortisol, Urinary Free Cortisol and ACTH Levels in Normal Pregnancy

	Non pregnant	Third trimester
Total cortisol		
09.00 h	11.34 ± 3.5 mg/mL 324 ± 100 nmol/L	36.0 ± 7 mg/mL 1029 ± 200 nmol/L
24.00 h	3.6 ± 2.6 mg/mL 103 ± 76 nmol/L	23.5 ± 4.34 mg/mL 470 ± 124 nmol/L
Plasma free cortisol		
09.00 h	0.63 ± 0.3 mg/mL 18 ± 9 nmol/L	1.33 ± 0.4 mg/mL 32 ± 12 nmol/L
24.00 h	0.2 ± 0.14 mg/mL 6 ± 4 nmol/L	0.59 ± 0.17 mg/mL 17 ± 5 nmol/L
Urinary free cortisol	4.7–9.5 mg/day 13–256 nmol/day	82.4–244.8 mg/day 229–680 nmol/day
Plasma ACTH	15–70 pg/mL 3.3–15.4 pmol/L	20–120 pg/mL 4.4–26.4 pmol/L

be placed in each subsequent liter of normal saline infused, until the patient is adequately hydrated. This may take up to 5 L. Hypoglycemia may be prevented by instituting a 50-gm glucose infusion. Since the patient will receive up to 600 mg of hydrocortisone succinate with this protocol, no added mineralocorticoid is required.

Pheochromocytoma in Pregnancy

Pheochromocytoma is a rare endocrine tumor. When associated with pregnancy, it can be very dangerous for both the mother and the fetus. The main sign of the disease is hypertension, which is common in pregnancy, and can be easily mistaken for pregnancy-induced hypertension. Differentiation from preeclampsia should, however, be straightforward since the edema, proteinuria, and hyperuricemia found in preeclampsia are absent in pheochromocytoma. Plasma and urinary catecholamines may be modestly elevated in preeclampsia and other serious pregnancy complications requiring hospitalization, though they remain normal in mild preeclampsia and pregnancy-induced hypertension. Catecholamine levels may, however, be two to four times the normal level after an eclamptic seizure and this can be confusing.

An unrecognized pheochromocytoma can be lethal because a fatal hypertensive crisis may be precipitated by anesthesia or even normal delivery. As the uterus enlarges and an actively moving fetus compresses the adrenal neoplasm, maternal complications such as severe hypertension, hemorrhage into the neoplasm, hemodynamic collapse, myocardial infarction, cardiac arrhythmias, congestive heart failure, and cerebral hemorrhage may occur. Extra-adrenal tumors, which occur in 10 percent, such as in the organ of Zuckerkandl at the aortic bifurcation, are particularly prone to hypertensive episodes with changes in position, uterine contractions, fetal movement, and Valsalva maneuvers. Unrecognized pheochromocytoma is associated with a maternal mortality rate of 50 percent at induction of anesthesia or during labor. A recent review of 41 pregnant women with known pheochromocytoma by Ahlawat et al., however, showed a much lower maternal mortality rate of 4 percent and a fetal mortality rate of 11 percent. Antenatal diagnosis of pheochromocytoma reduced the maternal mortality rate to 2 percent. These mortality rates are significantly lower than those of prior studies and can be attributed to increased awareness of the condition and more reliable testing modalities (Table 10-13).

There is minimal placental transfer of catecholamines. Adverse fetal effects, such as hypoxia, are a result of catecholamine-induced uteroplacental

TABLE 10-13 Symptoms and Signs of Pheochromocytoma

Symptomatic hypertension
Severe and fluctuating
Dyspnea
Dizzyness
Severe headache
Perspiration
Palpitations and tachycardia
Arrhythmias
Postural hypotension
Chest or abdominal pain
Visual disturbances
Convulsions
Cardiovascular collapse

vasoconstriction and placental insufficiency, as well as maternal hypertension, hypotension, or vascular collapse. Pheochromocytoma can also occur as part of multiple endocrine neoplasia type 2 (MEN 2) in association with medullary carcinoma of the thyroid gland and parathyroid adenomas. Identification of the *RET* protooncogene mutations that cause MEN 2 can be used to screen family members of MEN 2 kindred and to monitor those who are at risk. The women at risk should be monitored very closely during pregnancy. Patients with MEN 2A are more likely to have paroxysmal hypertension and have higher rates of bilateral neoplasms than those with sporadic pheochromocytoma. Examination for associated evidence for MEN 2 may be difficult in pregnancy, with the expected pregnancy alterations in calcium, PTH, and calcitonin. Clinical thyroid examination should be assisted by fine needle aspiration of any suspicious nodules so that overt medullary carcinoma can be treated immediately.

Most pregnant patients with pheochromocytoma will initially complain of symptomatic hypertension that is severe and fluctuating, and which is often associated with severe headache, perspiration, palpitation, and tachycardia (Table 10-13). Other possible signs and symptoms include arrhythmias, postural hypotension, chest or abdominal pain, visual disturbance, convulsions, or sudden collapse. Symptoms may occur or worsen during pregnancy because of the increased vascularity of the tumor and mechanical factors such as pressure from the expanding uterus or fetal movement.

The coexistence of diabetes mellitus, possible hyperthyroidism, and myocardial infarction are important and should prompt a search for pheochromocytoma. Individuals with neurofibromatosis, von Hipple–Lindau disease, or retinal angiomatosis should also be screened for pheochromocytomas prior to pregnancy since these conditions are associated with an increased risk of pheochromocytoma.

The diagnosis is confirmed by an accurate 24-hour urine collection for both epinephrine, norepinephrine, and their metabolites. The assays should preferably be performed on specimens collected during or after a hypertensive episode. Laboratory diagnosis of pheochromocytoma is unchanged from the nonpregnant state since calecholamine metabolism is not altered by pregnancy per se. If possible, methyldopa and labetalol should be discontinued prior to the investigation as these agents may interfere with the quantification of the catecholamines and VMA. Provocative testing should be avoided because of the increased risk of maternal and fetal mortality.

Efforts to localize the tumor should be made once a biochemical diagnosis is made. MRI and ultrasound are the preferred methods for localization of tumors in pregnant patients because they avoid exposing the fetus to ionizing radiation. Metaiodobenzylguanidine scans are contraindicated in pregnancy, but may be necessary if other tumor localization methods fail.

Initial medical management involves an α-blockade with phenoxybenzamine, phentolamine, prazocin, or labetalol (Table 10-14). All of these agents are well tolerated by the fetus, but phenoxybenzamine is considered the preferred agent as it provides long-acting, stable, noncompetitive blockade. Placental transfer of phenoxybenzamine occurs, but is generally safe. If hypertension remains inadequately controlled, metyrosine has also been used successfully to reduce catecholamine synthesis in a pregnancy complicated by malignant pheochromocytoma, but may potentially adversely affect the fetus. β-blockade is reserved for treating maternal tachycardia or arrhythmias

TABLE 10-14 Management of Pheochromocytoma

Pharmacologic control of hypertension and tachycardia

α adrenergic receptor blockade

Phenoxybenzamine

- Start at 10 mg b.i.d and gradually increase (10 mg every other day) to maximum dosage (20–40 mg b.i.d./t.i.d.) or until patient develops orthostatic hypotension

Phentolamine

- Only given parenterally (5–10 mg IM or IV) and is reserved for emergency or preoperative situations

Prazosin

- Start at 1 mg PO b.i.d./t.i.d. and increase to a maximum daily dose of 6–15 mg given in divided doses (b.i.d/t.i.d.)

Labetalol

- Start 100 mg PO b.i.d. and increase by 100 mg b.i.d. every two weeks until blood pressure controlled; maximum dose is 2400 mg per day. When discontinuing labetalol taper dose over 1–2 weeks
- In an emergency labetalol can be given IV start with 20 mg IV over 2 minutes and increase by 20 mg every 10 minutes until blood pressure is controlled or a maximum dose of 300 mg is reached
- Labetalol can also be given as a continuous infusion of 2 mg/min until blood pressure is controlled and then switched to oral dosing with 200–400 mg every 6–12 h

Nitroprusside

- Start at 0.25 μg/kg/min IV infusion and titrate to control blood pressure. The maximum recommended infusion rate is 10 μg/kg/min

Metyrosine may be used if hypertension is still uncontrolled

Beta blockade

- Reserved for tachycradia or arrythmia, and predominantly adrenaline-secreting tumors. Selective and short acting agents are preferred:
- Metoprolol
  - 50–200 mg PO b.i.d
- Atenolol
  - Start at 50 mg PO every day and increase after 10–14 days to a maximum of 100 mg every day
- Propranolol
  - Only to be used after adequate α blockade has been instituted
  - Start 40 mg PO b.i.d. and increase every 3–7 days to a maximum of 480 mg daily in divided doses (b.i.d.)

Fluid management

Surgical management

- Timing depends on
  - Medical control
  - Tumor size
  - Risk of malignancy
  - Stage of pregnancy (Best in second trimester)
  - laparoscopy vs. laparotomy
- Third trimester
  - C/S after confirmation of lung maturity with adrenalectomy OR
  - vaginal delivery and laparoscopic removal of tumor postpartum

which persist after complete α-blockade and volume repletion. β-blockade without prior α-blockade is contraindicated because the unopposed α-adrenergic activity may lead to vasoconstriction and hypertensive crisis. Propranolol has been successfully used after appropriate α-blockade in pregnancy. β blockers may be associated with fetal bradycardia and intrauterine fetal growth restriction when used early in pregnancy. All of these potential fetal risks are small compared to the risk of fetal wastage from unblocked high maternal levels of catecholamines. Hypertensive emergencies should be treated with phentolamine or nitroprusside. The definitive treatment of pheochromocytoma is surgical removal of the tumor(s) and this should ideally be accomplished before 24 weeks of gestation, and only after achieving adequate α-blockade. Successful laparoscopic excision of a pheochromocytoma has been described in the second trimester of pregnancy. After 24 weeks of gestation, uterine size makes abdominal exploration and access to the tumor difficult and it is generally recommended that surgery be delayed until fetal maturity is reached. To that end, steroid therapy may be used to hasten fetal lung maturity. Once delivery is entertained, adequate α-blockade should be instituted and elective cesarean delivery may be performed, followed immediately by adrenal exploration. Cesarean section is recommended for delivery based on the work of Schenker and Granat who reported higher maternal mortality rates with vaginal delivery (31 percent) compared to cesarean delivery (19 percent). Labor may result in uncontrolled release of catecholamines secondary to pain and uterine contractions. Severe maternal hypertension may lead to placental ischemia and fetal hypoxia. However, in the well-blocked patient, vaginal delivery may be possible if cesarean section is not possible, as long as there is intensive pain management with epidural anesthesia, avoidance of mechanical compression, passive descent, and instrumental delivery.

There is no available information regarding the impact of maternal use of phenoxybenzamine on the nursing neonate. Malignant pheochromocytoma may recur in pregnancy. Life-long monitoring is necessary in all patients, with extra caution in those who are pregnant.

PRIMARY HYPERALDOSTERONISM

Primary hyperaldosteronism is a rare cause of hypertension in pregnancy. Occasionally this hypertension can be severe, and can be confused with preeclampsia. In addition, the degree of hypertension can be variable and can significantly worsen in the first six weeks of the postpartum period.

Patients with classic hyperaldosteronism present with hypertension, hypokalemia, and elevated urine potassium levels. Before biochemical diagnosis, hypokalemia should be corrected because low potassium levels may suppress aldosterone. When making the diagnosis, potassium replacement should be initiated, all diuretics should be discontinued for at least two weeks, and high doses of β-blockers should be reduced because they reduce renin production. Calcium channel blockers should not be used for at least 2 to 3 hours before testing.

It must be remembered that the measurement of plasma aldosterone levels may not be useful in the diagnosis of hyperaldosteronism in pregnant women because of the physiological increase in aldosterone levels in pregnancy. The levels measured during normal pregnancy are often within the primary hyperaldosteronism range. Pregnant women may have less urinary potassium wasting than patients with primary hyperaldosteronism because of the antagonizing effects of progesterone. Another factor that may complicate the diagnosis during pregnancy is the increase in plasma renin levels in normal pregnancy. In primary hyperaldosteronism, plasma renin levels are usually decreased, and in pregnancy the decrease may be attenuated. Outside of pregnancy salt-loading studies are desirable to confirm the autonomous secretion of aldosterone, but during pregnancy there are concerns about volume overload, worsening of hypokalemia, and the lack of specific reference ranges for pregnancy. One test that can be used in pregnancy involves prolonged positioning of the patient in an upright posture. This usually causes a modest increase in plasma renin activity. However, if there is primary hyperaldosteronism, the renin activity remains suppressed.

Ultrasonography and MRI are the preferred imaging methods in pregnant women for localizing the tumor, but if necessary, any appropriate imaging modality should be used to confirm the presence of a tumor.

If an adrenal adenoma is detected, the preferred treatment is unilateral adrenalectomy. Cases of successful adrenalectomy in the second trimester have been reported. Early delivery may need to be considered in the third trimester since spironolactone and angiotensin-converting enzyme inhibitors are generally avoided in pregnancy. The goals of therapy are to reduce blood pressure and replace potassium and while α-methyl dopa, β blockers, and calcium channel blockers can be used, they have variable success rates.

DIABETES INSIPIDUS

Diabetes insipidus in pregnancy is caused by either an abnormality of vasopressin secretion, an abnormality of vasopressin action or vasopressin degradation. The presenting features are polydipsia, polyuria, and dehydration. Three types of diabetes insipidus can be found in pregnancy: central, nephrogenic, and transient vasopressin resistant (Table 10-15).

Central Diabetes Insipidus

Central diabetes insipidus is caused by decreased production of vasopressin by the paraventricular nuclei of the hypothalamus. It complicates 1 in 15,000 deliveries. The most common presentation is that of a woman who has central

TABLE 10-15 Causes of Diabetes Insipidus in Pregnancy

Type of DI	Cause
Central	• Pregnancy worsening of prior DI • CNS tumor, e.g., prolactinoma • Granuloma, e.g., sarcoid • Histiocytosis x • Aneurysm • Lymphocytic hypophysitis • Sheehan syndrome
Nephrogenic	• x-linked abnormality of vasopressin V2 receptor
Transient vasopressin resistant	• Increased vasopressinase activity due to decreased vasopressinase degradation due to hepatic disease (e.g., acute fatty liver, HELLP syndrome, or Hepatitis)

diabetes insipidus before conception, arising from a pituitary tumor or another invasive disease such as histiocytosis X. Central diabetes insipidus often worsens during pregnancy due to an increase in the clearance of endogenous vasopressin by placental vasopressinase. Vasopressinase concentration increases during pregnancy in proportion to the placental weight. It is metabolized by the liver, thus its activity is increased in liver disease. Subclinical central diabetes insipidus may be unmasked for the first time during pregnancy, because the need for vasopressin release, low serum osmolality and because of increased clearance of vasopressinase. During pregnancy 60 percent of established cases of central diabetes insipidus worsen, but 25 percent improve, and 15 percent remain the same.

The diagnosis of central diabetes insipidus during pregnancy has been seen following development of Sheehan syndrome and as a result of the enlargement of a prolactinoma, histiocytosis X, and lymphocytic hypophysitis. It has also been reported as a complication of ventriculoperitoneal shunt during pregnancy.

The diagnosis of central diabetes insipidus that occurs for the first time during pregnancy requires modification of the standard water deprivation test. Nonpregnant patients normally need to lose up to 5 percent of their total body weight before the induced dehydration adequately stimulates vasopressin release. Such dehydration can be dangerous in pregnancy and should not be used. The use of DDAVP as a test of urinary concentrating ability has been described and is currently the preferred method. Maximum urine osmolality over the 11 hours after administration of DDAVP is assessed. Any value greater than 700 mosmol/kg is considered normal.

The treatment of central diabetes insipidus in pregnancy is with DDAVP, 2 to 20 μg intranasally twice daily. This treatment can be given parenterally after cesarean section, but intravenous dosing is 5 to 20 fold more potent than the intranasal spray and the dose should be adjusted accordingly. DDAVP is not degraded by vasopressinase and no further adjustment is needed in patients with increased vasopressinase activity. Transfer of DDAVP to breast milk is minimal, and breastfeeding is not contraindicated. Treatment of central maternal diabetes insipidus with DDAVP throughout pregnancy does not pose a risk to the infant.

Labor proceeds normally in women with central diabetes insipidus, and surges of oxytocin can be detected during labor and the puerperium. This suggests that women with central diabetes insipidus, although they are vasopressin deficient, still secrete oxytocin normally. Lactation is not impaired.

Nephrogenic Diabetes Insipidus

Nephrogenic diabetes insipidus is a rare X-linked disorder. At least six mutations in this gene have been identified and direct mutation analysis can now be used for carrier detection and early prenatal diagnosis. Nonpregnant women with nephrogenic diabetes insipidus are usually treated with thiazide diuretics or chlorpropamide. Chlorpropamide stimulates vasopressin release and enhances its action on the renal tubule, but it may cause fetal hypoglycemia and neonatal diabetes insipidus, and therefore should not be used in pregnancy. Thiazide diuretics are the treatment of choice for nephrogenic diabetes insipidus during pregnancy.

Transient Vasopressin Resistant Diabetes Insipidus

Transient vasopressin-resistant diabetes insipidus is probably the most common form of diabetes insipidus seen in pregnancy. It is caused by increased vasopressinase activity due either to increased placental production of the enzyme or to decreased hepatic vasopressinase metabolism as a result of liver damage. Transient disturbances of liver function may be seen in acute fatty liver of pregnancy, preeclampsia, HELLP syndrome, and hepatitis.

The treatment of transient vasopressin-resistant diabetes insipidus in pregnancy requires DDAVP because DDAVP is not degraded by vasopressinase. Electrolyte and fluid balance should be closely monitored during the postpartum period. The symptoms of transient vasopressin-resistant diabetes insipidus resolve in a few days to a few weeks after delivery, when hepatic function returns to normal.

SHEEHAN SYNDROME

Severe hemorrhage, shock, or prolonged hypotension during or after delivery may lead to postpartum pituitary necrosis or the Sheehan syndrome. This condition is rare (1:10,000 deliveries) and its pathogenesis in still unclear. It is believed to be the result of spasm in the arterial supply to the anterior lobe of the pituitary gland leading to ischemia and edema and ultimate necrosis and thrombosis in the portal sinuses and capillaries. A second theory as to the etiology is based on the development of DIC and intrapituitary bleeding. Sheehan syndrome usually only involves anterior pituitary function because the posterior pituitary and hypothalamus are supplied by the inferior hypophyseal artery and the circle of Willis, which makes them less vulnerable to ischemic necrosis. In rare cases, however, some women with Sheehan syndrome may develop partial or overt diabetes insipidus due to reduced vasopressin (antid iuretic hormone; ADH) secretion. There is frequently poor correlation between the severity of the postpartum hemorrhage and the occurrence of Sheehan syndrome and patients suspected of this complication should be investigated regardless of the severity of their postpartum/intrapartum bleed.

The presentation of Sheehan syndrome is highly variable. It is estimated that 95 percent to 99 percent of the anterior pituitary gland needs to be destroyed before the characteristic postpartum failure of lactation, secondary amenorrhea, loss of axillary and pubic hair, genital and breast atrophy, increasing signs of secondary hypothyroidism, and adrenocortical insufficiency occur. The most specific early postpartum sign will be failure of lactation. Since mineralocorticoid secretion is not impaired, there are usually no electrolyte disturbances. However, hyponatremia has been reported in conjunction with Sheehan syndrome and appears to be on the basis of inappropriate ADH secretion (SIADH).

Less extensive pituitary destruction (50 to 95 percent) is associated with an atypical form of the disease with loss of one or more trophic hormones. Postpartum diagnosis of Sheehan syndrome requires dynamic provocative testing of both anterior and posterior lobes of the pituitary gland. The anterior pituitary gland function is best assessed with pituitary hormone response to standard stimulatory tests in conjunction with pituitary imaging with axial CT or MRI. Posterior pituitary function in Sheehan syndrome can be studied with plasma vasopressin response to either osmotic stimuli during 5 percent hypotonic saline infusion or following a water deprivation test. Spontaneous recovery from hypopituitarism due to postpartum hemorrhage has also been reported.

SUGGESTED READING

Aboul-Khair SA, Crooks J, Turnbull AC, et al.: The physiological changes in thyroid function during pregnancy. *Clin Sci* 1964;27:195.

Ahlawat SK, Jain S, Kumari S, et al.: Pheochromocytoma associated with pregnancy: case report and review of the literature. *Obstet Gynecol Surv* 1999;54(11):728–737.

Azizi F, Khoshniat M, Bahrainian M, et al.: Thyroid function and intellectual development of infants nursed by mothers taking methimazole. *J Clin Endocrinol Metab* 2000;85:3233–3238.

Azizi F: Effect of methimazole treatment of maternal thyrotoxicosis on thyroid function in breast-feeding infants. *J Pediatr* 1996;128:855.

Baron F, Sprauve ME, Hiddleston JF, et al.: Diagnosis and surgical treatment of primary hyperaldosteronism in pregnancy. *Obstet Gynecol* 1995;86:644.

Black JA: Neonatal goiter and mental deficiency: The role of iodides taken during pregnancy. *Arch Dis Child* 1963;38:526.

Burrow G: Thyroid function and hyperfunction during gestation. *Endocrinol Rev* 1993;14:194–202.

Burrow GN, Fisher DA, Larsen PR: Maternal and fetal thyroid function. *N Engl J Med* 1994;331:1074.

Cheong HI, Park HW, Ha IS, et al.: Six novel mutations in the vasopressin V2 receptor gene causing nephrogenic diabetes insipidus. *Nephron* 1997;75:431.

Davis L, Lucas M, Hankins G, et al.: Thyrotoxicosis complicating pregnancy. *Am J Obstet Gynecol* 1989;160:63.

Derksen RHWV, van der Wiel A, Poortman J, et al.: Plasma exchange in the treatment of severe thyrotoxicosis in pregnancy. *Eur J Obstet Gynecol Reprod Biol* 1984; 18:139.

Devoe LD, O'Dell BE, Castillo RA, et al.: Metastatic pheochromocytoma in pregnancy and fetal biophysical assessment after maternal administration of alpha-adrenergic, beta-adrenergic, and dopamine antagonists. *Obstet Gynecol* 1986; 68(Suppl 3):15S.

Durr JA, Hoggard JG, Hunt JM, et al.: Diabetes insipidus in pregnancy associated with abnormally high circulating vasopressinase activity. *N Engl J Med* 1982;316:1070.

Easterling T, Schmucker B, Carlson K, et al.: Maternal hemodynamics in pregnancies complicated by hyperthyroidism. *Obstet Gynecol* 1991;78:348.

Falterman CJ, Kreisberg R: Pheochromocytoma: Clinical diagnosis and management. *South Med J* 1982;75:321.

Finkenstedt G, Gasser RW, Hofle G, et al.: Pheochromocytoma and sub-clinical Cushing's syndrome during pregnancy: Diagnosis, medical pre-treatment and cure by laparoscopic unilateral adrenalectomy. *J Endocrinol Invest* 1999;22:551.

Freier DT, Eckhauser FE, Harrison TS: Pheochromocytoma. *Arch Surg* 1980;115:388.

Freier DT, Thompson NW: Pheochromocytoma and pregnancy: The epitome of high risk. *Surgery* 1993;114:1148.

Glinoer D, De Nayer P, Bourdoux P, et al.: Regulation of maternal thyroid during pregnancy. *J Clin Endocrinol Metab* 1990;71:276–287.

Glinoer D, Solo M, Bourdoux P, et al.: Pregnancy in patients with mild thyroid abnormalities: Maternal and neonatal repercussions. *J Clin Endocrinol Metab* 1991; 73:421–427.

Glinoer D: The regulation of thyroid function in pregnancy: pathways of endocrine adaptation from physiology to pathology. *Endocrine Rev* 1997;18:404–433.

Goodwin T, Montoro M, Mestman J, et al.: The role of chorionic gonadotropin in transient hyperthyroidism of hyperemesis gravidarum. *J Clin Endocrinol Metab* 1992;75:1333.

Gurlek A, Cobankara V, Bayraktar M: Liver tests in hyperthyroidism: Effect of antithyroid therapy. *J Clin Gastroenterol* 1997;24:180–183.

Haddow JE, Palomaki GE, Allan WC, et al.: Maternal thyroid deficiency during pregnancy and subsequent neuropsychological development of the child. *N Engl J Med* 1999;341:549–555.

Hall R, Richards C, Lazarus J: The thyroid and pregnancy. *Br J Obstet Gynaecol* 1993; 100:512.

Hammond TG, Buchanan JG, Scoggins BA, et al.: Primary hyperaldosteronism in pregnancy. *Aus NZ J Med* 1982;12:537.

Harper MA, Murnaghan GA, Kennedy L, et al.: Pheochromocytoma in pregnancy: Five cases and a review of the literature. *Br J Obstet Gynaecol* 1989;96:594.

Hime MC, Williams DJ: Osmoregulatory adaptation in pregnancy and its disorders. *J Endocrinol* 1992;132:7.

Huchon DJR, Van Zijl JAWM, et al.: Desmopressin as a test of urinary concentrating ability in pregnancy. *J Obstet Gynecol* 1982;2:206.

Ingbar SH: Management of emergencies, IX. Thyrotoxic storm. *N Engl J Med* 1966;274:1252.

Isely W, Dahl S, Gibbs H: Use of esmolol in managing a thyrotoxic patient needing emergency surgery. *Am J Med* 1990;89:122.

Jialal I, Desai RK, Rajput MC: An assessment of posterior pituitary function in patients with Sheehan syndrome. *Clin Endocrinol* 1987;27:91.

Jordan RM: Myxedema coma. Pathophysiology, therapy, and factors affecting prognosis. *Med Clin North Am* 1995;79(1):185–194.

Kageyama Y, Hirose S, Terashi K, et al.: A case of postpartum hypopituitarism associated with hyponatremia and congestive heart failure. *Jpn J Med* 1988;27:337.

Kalff V, Shapiro B, Lloyd R, et al.: The spectrum of pheochromocytoma in hypertensive patients with neurofibromatosis. *Arch Intern Med* 1982;142:2092.

Kallen BA, Carlsson SS, Bergen BK: Diabetes insipidus and the use of desmopressin during pregnancy. *Eur J Endocrinol* 1995;132:144–146.

Khunda S: Pregnancy and Addison's disease. *Obstet Gynecol* 1972;39:431.

Kothari A, Bethune M, Manwaring J, et al.: Massive bilateral pheochromocytomas in association with von Hippel Lindau syndrome in pregnancy. *Aust NZ J Obstet Gynaecol* 1999;39:381.

Lau P, Permezel M, Dawson P, et al.: Pheochromocytoma in pregnancy. *Aust N Z J Obstet Gynaecol* 1996;36:472.

Laurberg, et al.: *Eur J Endocrinol* 1998;139:584–586.

Laurel MT, Kabadi UM: Primary hyperaldosteronism. *Endocrine Practice* 1997;3:47.

Leung A, Millar L, Koonings P, et al.: Perinatal outcome in hypothyroid pregnancies. *Obstet Gynecol* 1993;81:349.

Levin N, McTighe A, Abdel Aziz MIE: Extra adrenal pheochromocytoma in pregnancy. *Maryland State Med J* 1983;32:377.

Liaw YF, Huang MJ, Fan KD, et al.: Hepatic injury during propylthiouracil therapy in patients with hyperthyroidism. *Ann Intern Med* 1993;118:424–428.

MacGillivray I: Acute suprarenal insufficiency in pregnancy. *BMJ* 1951;2:212.

Mandel SJ, Brent GA, Larsen PR: Review of antithyroid drug use during pregnancy and report of a case of aplasia cutis. *Thyroid* 1994;4:129.

Maragliano G, Zuppa AA, Florio MG, et al.: Efficacy of oral iodide therapy on neonatal hyperthyroidism caused by maternal Grave's disease. *Fetal Diagn Ther* 2000;15(2):122–126.

Mazzaferri EL: Evolution and management of common thyroid disorders in women. *Am J Obstet Gynecol* 1997;176:507.

Momotani N, Yamashita R, Yoshimoto M, et al.: Recovery from foetal hypothyroidism: Evidence for the safety of breast-feeding while taking propylthiouracil. *Clin Endocrinol* 1989;31:591.

Momotani, et al.: *J Clin Endocrinol Metab* 1997;82:3633–3636.

Monturo MN, Collea JA, Frasier SN, et al.: Successful outcome of pregnancy in women with hypothyroidism. *Ann Intern Med* 1981;94:31.

Moodley J, McFadyen ML, Dilraj A, et al.: Plasma noradrenaline and adrenaline levels in eclampsia. *S Afr Med J* 1991;80:191.

Ohyama T, Nagasaki A, Kakai A, et al.: Spontaneous recovery from hypopituitarism due to postpartum hemorrhage. *Horm Metab Res* 1989;21:320.

Oishi S, Sato T: Pheochromocytoma in pregnancy: a review of the Japanese literature. *Endocrine J* 1994;41:219.

Pederson EB, Rasmussen AB, Christensen NJ, et al.: Plasma noradrenaline and adrenaline in pre-eclampsia, essential hypertension in pregnancy and normotensive pregnant control subjects. *Acta Endocrinol (Copenh)* 99:594,1982.
Prihoda J, Davis L: Metabolic emergencies in obstetrics. *Obstet Gynecol Clin North Am* 1991;18:301.
Rubin PC: Beta-blockers in pregnancy. *N Engl J Med* 1983;18:73.
Saarikoski S: Fate of noradrenaline in the human fetoplacental unit. *Acta Physiol Scand* 1974;421 (Suppl): 1.
Safa AM, Schumacher OP, Rodriguez-Antunez A: Long-term follow-up results in children and adolescents treated with radioactive iodine (131I) for hypothyroidism. *N Engl J Med* 1975;292:167.
Sandstrom B: Antihypertensive treatment with the adrenergic beta-receptor blocker metoprolol during pregnancy. *Gynecol Invest* 1978;9:195.
Santeiro ML, Stromquist C, Wyble L: Phenoxybenzamine placental transfer during the third trimester. *Ann Pharmacother* 1996;30:1249.
Schenker JG, Granat M: Pheochromocytoma and pregnancy—an updated appraisal. *Aust NZ J Obstet Gynaecol* 1982;22:1.
Sheehan HL: Postpartum necrosis of the anterior pituitary. *J Path Bacteriol* 1937; 45:189.
Sheps SG, Jiang NS, Klee GC: Diagnostic evaluation of pheochromocytoma. *Endocrinol Metab Clin North Am* 1988;17:397.
Sitar D, Abu-Bakare A, Gardiner R: Propylthiouracil disposition in pregnant and postpartum women. *Pharmacology* 1982;25:57.
Soler NG, Nicholson H: Diabetes and thyroid disease during pregnancy. *Obstet Gynecol* 1979;54:318.
Solomon GC, Thiet M, Moore F, et al.: Primary hyperaldosteronism in pregnancy. *Obstet Gynecol* 1996;41:255.
Thorpe-Beeston J, Nicolaides K, Felton C, et al.: Maturation of the secretion of thyroid hormone and thyroid-stimulating hormone in the fetus. *N Engl J Med* 1991;324:531.
Uhrig JD, Hurley RM. Chlorpropamide in pregnancy and transient neonatal diabetes insipidus. *Can Med Assoc J* 1983;128:368.
Usta IM, Barton JR, Amon EA, et al.: Acute fatty liver of pregnancy: An experience in the diagnosis and management of fourteen cases. *Am J Obstet Gynecol* 1994; 171:1342.
Van Dijk, et al.: *Ann Intern Med* 1987;106:60–61.
Vaquero E, Lazzarin CD, Valensise H, et al.: Mild thyroid abnormalities and recurrent spontaneous abortion: Diagnostic and therapeutical approach. *Am J Reprod Immunol* 2000;43:204–208.
Vitug AC, Goldman JM: Hepatotoxicity from antithyroid drugs. *Hormone Res* 1985; 21:229–234.
Wartofsky L: Myxedema coma. In: Werner SC, Ingbar SH, Braverman LE, Utiger RD (eds), *Werner & Ingbar's the Thyroid: A Fundamental and Clinical Text,* 8th edn. Philadelphia, PA: Lipincott Williams & Wilkins, 2000; pp.843–847.
Wing DA, et al.: *Am J Obstet Gynecol* 1994;170:90–95.

11 Diabetic Ketoacidosis in Pregnancy

Michael R. Foley

INTRODUCTION

Despite recent advances in the evaluation and medical treatment of diabetes in pregnancy, diabetic ketoacidosis (DKA) remains a matter of significant concern. The fetal loss rate in most series has been estimated to range from 50 to 90 percent. Fortunately, since the advent and implementation of insulin therapy, the maternal mortality rate has declined to 1 percent or less. In order to favorably influence the outcome in these high-risk patients, it is imperative that the obstetrician/care giver be familiar with the basics of the pathophysiology, diagnosis, and treatment of diabetic ketoacidosis in pregnancy.

PATHOPHYSIOLOGY

Simply stated, DKA is characterized by hyperglycemia and accelerated ketogenesis. Both, a lack of insulin and an excess of glucagon and other counter-regulatory hormones significantly contribute to these problems and their resultant clinical manifestations. In a nutshell, glucose normally enters the cell secondary to the presence of insulin. The cell then may use glucose for nutrition and energy production. When insulin is lacking, glucose fails to enter the cell. The cell responds to this starvation by facilitating the release of counter-regulatory hormones including glucagon, catecholamines and cortisol. These counter-regulatory hormones are responsible for providing the cell with an alternative substrate for nutrition and energy production. By the process of gluconeogenesis, fatty acids from adipose tissue are broken down by hepatocytes to ketones (acetone, acetoacetate, and beta hydroxybutyrate = ketone bodies) which are then utilized by the cells of the body for nutrition and energy production (see Fig. 11-1). The lack of insulin also contributes to increased lipolysis and decreased reutilization of free fatty acids, thereby providing more substrate for hepatic ketogenesis. A basic review of the *Biochemistry of Diabetic Ketoacidosis* is presented in Fig. 11-1.

MATERNAL CONCERNS

Now that we have an understanding of how and why ketone bodies are produced during diabetic ketoacidosis, what are the maternal consequences resulting from excessive ketogenesis? In general, ketone bodies are considered to be moderately strong acids. In response to the fall in pH in most body fluids created by an accumulation of these acids, the body reacts physiologically to correct the resultant metabolic acidosis. The respiratory rate and depth increase (Kussmaul respirations) in an attempt to blow off carbon dioxide, initiating a corrective trend towards compensatory respiratory alkalosis. Serum bicarbonate levels decline and as a result the anion gap becomes abnormally elevated. In addition to increasing fatty acid production, poor glucose utilization results in severe hyperglycemia. Untreated hyperglycemia leads to marked glycosuria initiating a significant osmotic diuresis. As a result,

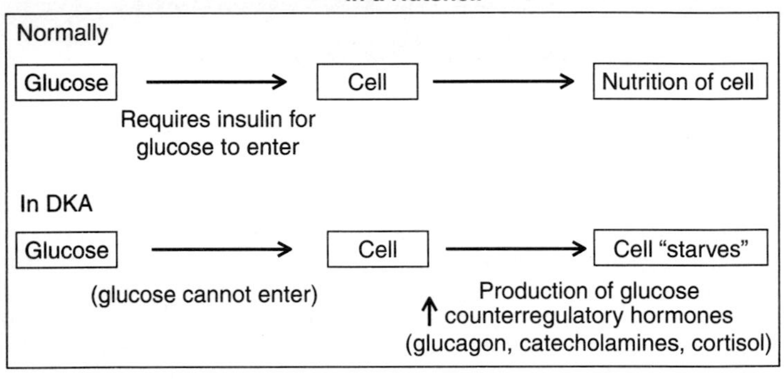

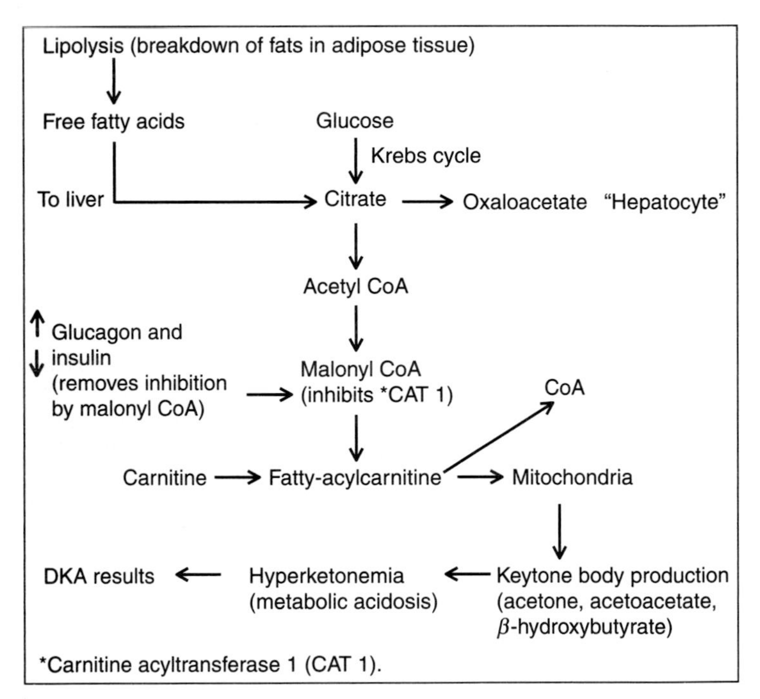

FIG. 11-1 Basic biochemistry of diabetic ketoacidosis. (*Adapted from Berkowitz RL (ed), Critical Care of the Obstetric Patient. New York: Churchill Livingstone, 1983; p. 416.*)

dehydration, electrolyte depletion, and if left untreated, cardiac failure and death may follow.

A vicious cycle is created by an increase in dehydration-mediated serum hyperosmolarity and catabolism, propagated by Kussmaul respiration, leading to a further production of glucose counter-regulatory hormones, lipolysis and subsequent hyperketonemia. An algorithm for this clinical pathophysiologic response is presented in Fig. 11-2.

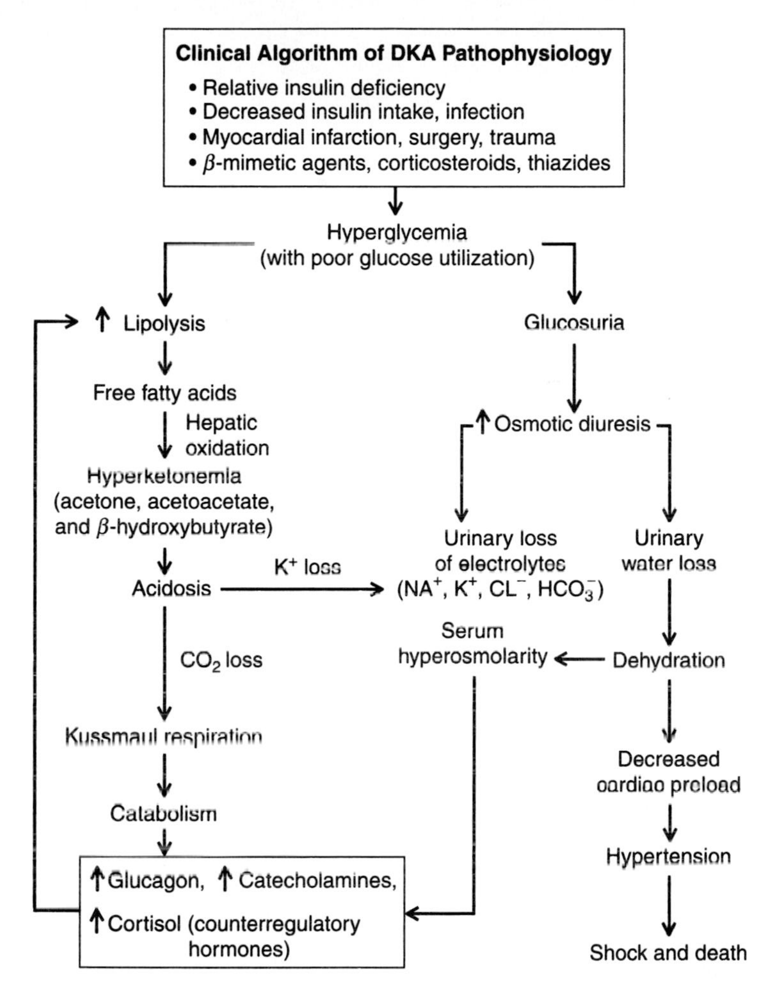

FIG. 11-2 Metabolic alterations in diabetic ketoacidosis. (*Modified from Hagay ZJ, Reece EA: Diabetes mellitus in pregnancy. In: Reece EA, Hubbins JC, Mahoney MJ, et al. (eds), Medicine of the Fetus and the Mother. Philadelphia: J.B. Lippincott, 1992; pp. 982–1020.*)

FETAL CONCERNS

The fetus appears to be at significant risk of sudden intrauterine death during an episode of maternal diabetic ketoacidosis. The mechanism for this sudden death is not completely understood; however, it appears to be related to a combination of factors. Alterations in fetal fluid and electrolyte balance, poor uterine perfusion resulting from maternal hypovolemia, and increased acid load in the form of fatty acids and lactate, all favor a reduction in fetal oxygenation and metabolic acid clearance. When caring for a patient in DKA who is carrying a potentially viable fetus, careful fetal monitoring should be

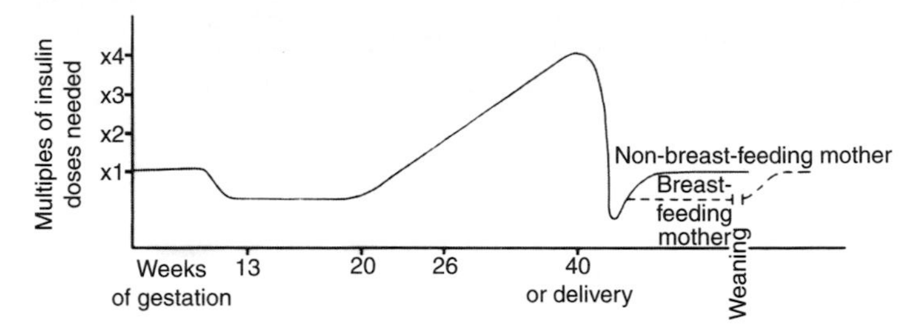

FIG. 11-3 Changing insulin needs during pregnancy caused by properties of placental hormones and enzyme (insulinase) and cortisol. (*Adapted from Bobak IM, Jensen MD, Zalar MK: Maternity and Gynecologic Care: The Nurse and the Family, 4th edn. St. Louis: C.V. Mosby, 1989; p. 783.*)

judiciously utilized. Often, signs of fetal stress become apparent reflecting the degree of maternal metabolic derangement. Delivery of a compromised baby should be prudently delayed until the mother is metabolically stable. Correction of maternal metabolic abnormalities generally results in a rapidly improved fetal condition. Therefore, efforts should be directed at improving maternal deficits reserving emergency operative intervention for unresponsive persistent fetal compromise.

MAKING THE DIAGNOSIS OF DKA

In pregnancy DKA may occur at a lower plasma glucose value as compared to the nonpregnant patient. DKA has been observed at plasma glucose levels as low as 180 mg/dL. It appears that a relative insulin resistance of pregnancy combined with a greater tendency toward ketosis reduces the threshold for DKA during pregnancy. The insulin resistance during pregnancy is related to an increased production of placental hormones, insulinase and cortisol (Fig. 11-3).

The maternal and fetal concerns resulting from DKA emphasize the importance of a rapid and reliable diagnosis. Following the axiom that laboratory tests should be utilized only to verify or nullify a clinical suspicion, the diagnosis of DKA should be based on clinical examination and supported by an evaluation of biochemical parameters. Table 11-1 summarizes the clinical presentation, the biochemical definition, and additional laboratory findings associated with diabetic ketoacidosis.

TREATMENT OF DKA

Diabetic ketoacidosis during pregnancy is a medical emergency. The patient should be admitted to an intensive care facility and consultations obtained from Maternal-Fetal Medicine, Endocrinology, and Neonatology. A detailed history and physical examination should be performed to search for underlying precipitatory factors for DKA such as noncompliance with insulin administration or infection (urine, skin, lungs, dental, and amniotic cavity). Fetal monitoring should be initiated if there is a potentially viable fetus (see Chap. 24). Intervention on behalf of the fetus should be withheld until the maternal metabolic condition is stabilized. Oxygen therapy and maternal position changes, however, should be initiated to help improve fetal perfusion while correcting maternal biochemical and plasma volume abnormalities (see Chap. 22). A detailed

TABLE 11-1 Diagnostic and Biochemical Parameters of DKA

Clinical features	
General	Neurologic
Malaise	Lethargy
Drowsiness	Coma
Weakness	Respiratory
Dehydration	Kussmaul respirations
Polyuria	Tachypnea
Polydipsia	Cardiovascular
Fruity breath	Tachycardia
Gastrointestinal	Hypotension
Nausea	
Vomiting	
Abdominal pain	
Ileus	
Biochemical definition (Memory AID)	
Diabetic → Glucose ≥100 mg%	
Keto → Serum acetone 1:2 or greater	
Acidosis → Arterial pH ≤ 7.3, HCO_3 ≤ 15, and anion gap $[Na^+ - (Cl^- + HCO_3^-)] > 12$	
Additional laboratory findings	
Glycosuria	Leukocytosis
Ketonuria	Elevated CPK
Metabolic acidosis	Elevated amylase
Hyperosmolality	Elevated transaminase
Hypokalemia	Elevated BUN
Hypomagnesemia	Elevated creatinine
Hypophosphatemia	

flow sheet including a comprehensive recording of serial laboratory values, at appropriate time intervals, should be started at bedside to facilitate patient assessment following therapy. The use of invasive hemodynamic monitoring should be reserved for the patient with severe renal compromise in an effort to properly guide rehydration while avoiding iatrogenic pulmonary edema. Other less invasive measures such as the initiation of an arterial line to follow serial arterial blood gases, a Foley catheter to monitor strict urinary output and continuous peripheral pulse oximetry should be initiated as an early adjunct to beginning therapy. The basic premise for the treatment of diabetic ketoacidosis in the pregnant patient is the simultaneous correction of fluid and electrolyte imbalance and treatment of hyperglycemia and acidosis (see Fig. 11-4).

TREATMENT OF HYPOVOLEMIA

Hypovolemia during diabetic ketoacidosis results primarily from hyperglycemia induced osmotic diuresis (see Fig. 11-2). Since the restoration of intravascular volume improves perfusion and augments systemic insulin delivery to peripheral tissues, repletion of the circulating intravascular volume is the number one treatment priority. The estimated total water deficit is calculated to be 100 mL/kg of actual body weight (4 to 10 L deficit). Once renal competence is established (urinary output of at least 0.5 cc/kg/h) fluid replacement may be initiated. Keeping in mind that many of the patients

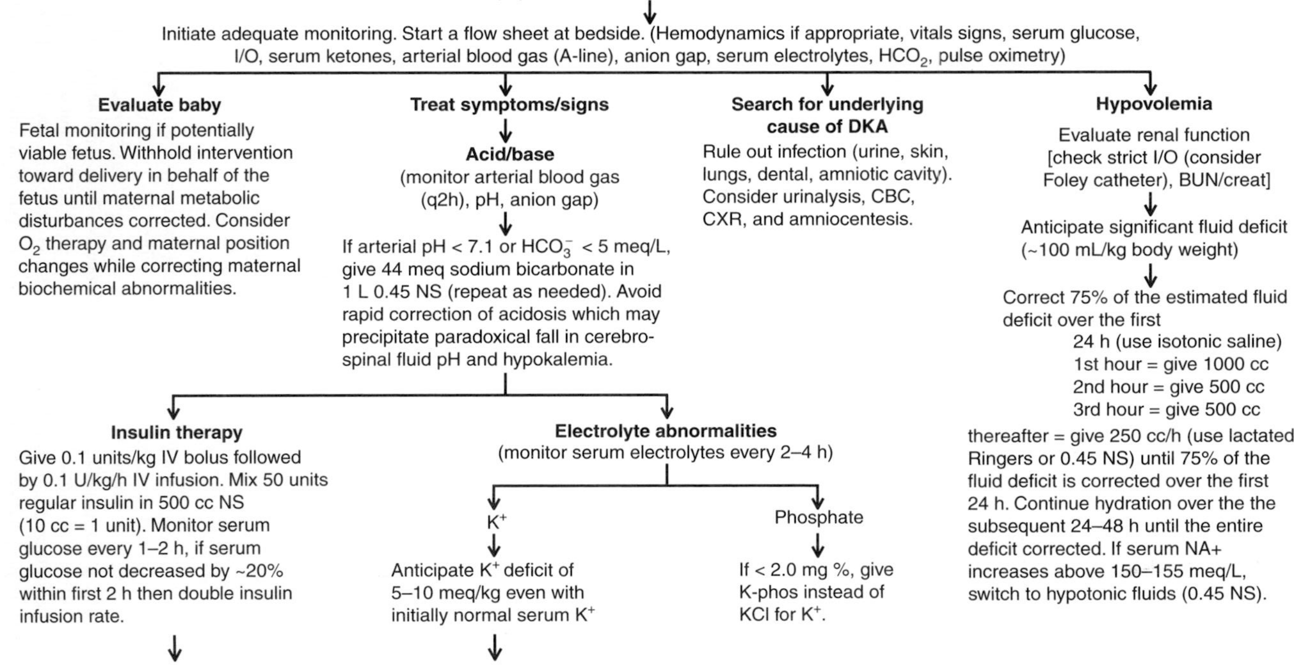
Admit to OB Intensive Care Unit or Equivalent
(Consult Maternal Fetal Medicine, Endocrinology, Neonatology, and Obstetric Anesthesiology)
Detailed physical exam, obtain IV access (two IV lines)
Initiate adequate monitoring. Start a flow sheet at bedside. (Hemodynamics if appropriate, vitals signs, serum glucose, I/O, serum ketones, arterial blood gas (A-line), anion gap, serum electrolytes, HCO2, pulse oximetry)
Evaluate baby
Fetal monitoring if potentially viable fetus. Withhold intervention toward delivery in behalf of the fetus until maternal metabolic disturbances corrected. Consider O2 therapy and maternal position changes while correcting maternal biochemical abnormalities.
Treat symptoms/signs
Acid/base
(monitor arterial blood gas (q2h), pH, anion gap)
If arterial pH < 7.1 or HCO3− < 5 meq/L, give 44 meq sodium bicarbonate in 1 L 0.45 NS (repeat as needed). Avoid rapid correction of acidosis which may precipitate paradoxical fall in cerebrospinal fluid pH and hypokalemia.
Search for underlying cause of DKA
Rule out infection (urine, skin, lungs, dental, amniotic cavity). Consider urinalysis, CBC, CXR, and amniocentesis.
Hypovolemia
Evaluate renal function [check strict I/O (consider Foley catheter), BUN/creat]
Anticipate significant fluid deficit (~100 mL/kg body weight)
Correct 75% of the estimated fluid deficit over the first
24 h (use isotonic saline)
1st hour = give 1000 cc
2nd hour = give 500 cc
3rd hour = give 500 cc
thereafter = give 250 cc/h (use lactated Ringers or 0.45 NS) until 75% of the fluid deficit is corrected over the first 24 h. Continue hydration over the the subsequent 24–48 h until the entire deficit corrected. If serum NA+ increases above 150–155 meq/L, switch to hypotonic fluids (0.45 NS).
Insulin therapy
Give 0.1 units/kg IV bolus followed by 0.1 U/kg/h IV infusion. Mix 50 units regular insulin in 500 cc NS (10 cc = 1 unit). Monitor serum glucose every 1–2 h, if serum glucose not decreased by ~20% within first 2 h then double insulin infusion rate.
Electrolyte abnormalities
(monitor serum electrolytes every 2–4 h)
K+
Anticipate K+ deficit of 5–10 meq/kg even with initially normal serum K+
Phosphate
If < 2.0 mg %, give K-phos instead of KCl for K+.

Glucose level should be decreased at a rate ≤ 60–75 mg % per hour to avoid rapid change in osmolarity which may precipitate cerebral edema: when the BG approaches 250 mg % add D5 to IV fluids and reduce insulin infusion by 1/2.

↓

Monitor serum ketones (every 2 h until stable) Be aware of the failure of the ketotest to measure β-hydroxybutyrate. The ketotest primarily measures acetone. Measured serum ketones may initially appear to increase after insulin therapy representing a shift of ketone production from β-hydroxybutyrate to acetone (oxidation) and acetoacetate.

↓

Continue IV insulin therapy until HCO_3^- and anion gap normalized HCO_3^- (18–31 meq/L), anion gap (<12).

↓

Give SQ insulin prior to discontinuing IV drip to prevent rebound hyperglycemia.

Establish and monitor for adequate urine output (at least 0.5 cc/kg/h) and wait for the serum K^+ to fall below 5 meq/L

↓

Replace K^+ with 40–60 meq of KCl/L IV normal saline. If plasma K is ≥ 4 meq/L, give 10–20 meq. If plasma K is < 4 meq/L give 30–40 meq. Maintain serum K^+ at 4.5–5.0 meq/L. (Initial replacement usually is initiated after the first 2–4 h of the patient's treatment.) Monitor serum K^+ every 2–4 h.

FIG. 11-4 Treatment algorithm for diabetic ketoacidosis.

TABLE 11-2 Common Intravenous Fluids

1 L	Glu (gm)	Na (meq)	Cl (meq)	K (meq)	Ca (meq)	Lactate (meq)	pH
5% Dextrose/water	50	0	0	0	0	0	3.5–6.5
0.9% NaCl normal saline	0	154	154	0	0	0	5.0
Lactated Ringer's	0	130	109	4	3	28	6.5

encountered with DKA during pregnancy may have preexisting renal compromise (class F DM), a baseline evaluation of serum BUN and creatinine would be prudent to avoid fluid overload in a patient with markedly reduced creatinine clearance. Most authorities recommend urinary isotonic normal saline as the intravenous fluid of choice for volume replacement instead of lactated Ringer's solution. The reason behind this recommendation is that the use of hypotonic solutions (0.45 NS or lactated Ringer's), as initial treatment, can lead to a rapid decline in plasma osmolarity which may lead to cellular swelling and resultant cerebral edema. Therefore, the recommended approach is to utilize isotonic normal saline and replace 75 percent of the total calculated fluid deficit within the first 24 hours of therapy. The remaining 25 percent of the deficit is replaced over the remainder of the patient's hospitalization. At our institution, 1 L of isotonic normal saline is given over the first hour, and 500 cc normal saline per hour is given over hours two and three. Isotonic normal saline, therefore, is used for the first three hours of therapy. Thereafter, however, lactated Ringer's or 0.45 normal saline is given at a rate of 250 cc/h until 75 percent of the total deficit is replaced over the first 24 hours. Lactated Ringer's solution is utilized to avoid further iatrogenic contributions to the fall in serum pH since the pH of lactated Ringer's is 6.5 compared to a pH of 5.0 for isotonic normal saline. In addition, the sodium load with isotonic saline may create hypernatremia fostering the recommendations to switch from isotonic saline to a more hypotonic solution (lactated Ringer's or 0.45 NS) when the patient's serum sodium increases above 150 to 155 meq/L (see Table 11-2).

INSULIN THERAPY

Intravenous insulin administration is the mainstay treatment for the pregnant patient in diabetic ketoacidosis. An initial intravenous loading dose of 0.1 units per kg followed by a constant infusion of 0.1 units/per kg per hour effectively inhibits lipolysis and ketogenesis leading to suppression of hepatic glucose output with resultant lower serum glucose levels. The insulin infusion is prepared by adding 50 units of regular insulin to 500 mL of normal saline (1 cc = 0.1 unit; 10 cc = 1 unit). General principles of an intravenous insulin infusion are listed in Table 11-3.

The intravenous insulin infusion should be titrated to reduce the serum glucose at a rate of less than or equal to 60 to 75 mg% per hour to avoid rapid changes in the serum osmolarity which may precipitate cerebral edema. A good rule of thumb is that if the plasma glucose does not decrease by 10 percent in the first hour or 20 percent by the second hour of therapy; repeat the intravenous loading dose or double the current continuous infusion rate. As the patient's blood glucose approaches 250 mg% add dextrose 5 percent to the IV infusion and reduce the hourly insulin infusion by one half. Be aware that

TABLE 11-3 General Principles of Intravenous Insulin Infusion

1. Use *regular* insulin when mixing the infusion
2. Pump monitor the infusion rate.
3. Clearly label the insulin infusion line with units of insulin per volume.
4. Intravenous insulin is compatible with both magnesium sulfate and pitocin.
5. To compensate for insulin binding to the plastic tubing gently mix the insulin in the bag and thoroughly flush the tubing with insulin before beginning administration.
6. Obtain blood samples from the patient's arm opposite the infusion.
7. Monitor the patient's blood glucose hourly during labor.
8. Have injectable dextrose 50% and dextrose 10% (500 mL) available at bedside for treatment of hypoglycemia.
9. Do not preload with glucose containing solutions before conduction anesthesia or as a bolus infusion to improve a nonreassuring fetal heart rate tracing.
10. Before discontinuing intravenous infusion give subcutaneous or intramuscular insulin to prevent rebound hyperglycemia.

Regular insulin half-lives

- Intravenous regular insulin: 5 minute half–life
- Intramuscular regular insulin: 2 hour half–life
- Subcutaneous regular insulin: 4 hour half–life

while monitoring serum ketones in response to insulin administration, a paradoxical increase in serum acetone should be anticipated. The ketotest primarily measures serum acetone. During insulin therapy while the overall production of ketones clearly diminishes, a shift of ketone production from hydroxybutyrate to acetone (oxidation) and acetoacetate is observed. This phenomenon results in the apparent paradoxical worsening of ketoacidemia at the onset of insulin therapy. The intravenous insulin infusion should be continued until the serum bicarbonate and anion gap normalize. Table 11-4 and Fig. 11-5 summarize the mechanics of changing from an intravenous insulin infusion to subcutaneous insulin or subcutaneous insulin pump, respectively. Table 11-5 provides additional helpful information regarding the insulin sensitivity factor.

POTASSIUM ADMINISTRATION

The anticipated potassium deficit in a pregnant patient with DKA is 5 to 10 meq/kg. Potassium replacement, however, is most often delayed for the first 2 to 4 hours of therapy since the initial serum potassium is usually normal to mildly elevated and adequate diuresis has yet to be established. Once fluid and insulin therapy have been instituted and corrections of the metabolic acidosis are underway, serum potassium may precipitously fall as a result of urinary loss and intracellular shift. When the patient's plasma potassium has fallen below 5 meq/L and an adequate diuresis has been established (at least 0.5 cc/kg/h) then potassium administration should be initiated. The usual method of potassium replacement is summarized as follows:

1. Mix 40 to 60 meq KCl/L NS
2. If plasma K+ is
   ≥4 meq/L, give 10 to 20 meq
   <4 meq/L, give 30 to 40 meq

TABLE 11-4 Managing the Conversion: Intravenous to Subcutaneous Insulin after Resolution of DKA

1. The patient should be tolerant of a full diet.
2. Calculate the total number of insulin units administered over 24 hours following stabilization.

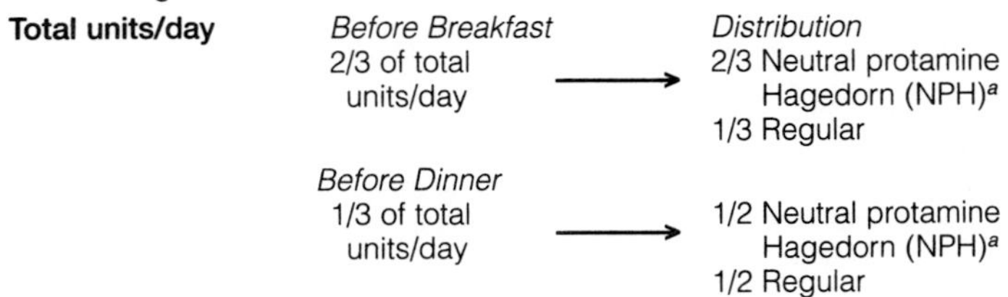

Total units/day		
Before Breakfast		*Distribution*
2/3 of total units/day	→	2/3 Neutral protamine Hagedorn (NPH)[a] 1/3 Regular
Before Dinner		
1/3 of total units/day	→	1/2 Neutral protamine Hagedorn (NPH)[a] 1/2 Regular

Example

Insulin infusion 2 units/hour × 24 hour (stabilized)
Total insulin/24 hour = 48 units

A.M. 2/3 × 48 = 32 → 2/3 as NPH = 21 units NPH
1/3 as regular = 11 units regular
P.M. 1/3 × 48 = 16 → 1/2 as NPH = 8 units NPH
as regular = 8 units regular

Insulin	Onset	Peak (maximum effect)	Duration
Regular	1 hour	2–3 hours	4–5 hours
NPH	2 hours	8 hours	24 hours

[a]NPH may be given at bedtime instead of at dinner if hypoglycemia occurs at 3 a.m.

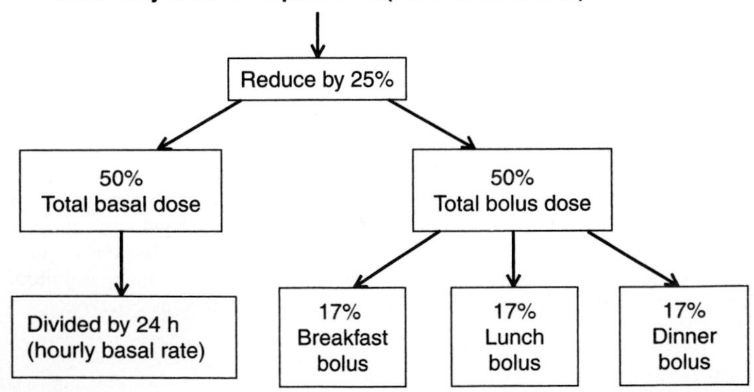

FIG. 11-5 Transition to subcutaneous insulin pump.

TABLE 11-5 Helpful Hints for the Insulin Pump

The insulin sensitivity factor
How much of a reduction in blood glucose should you expect for each 1.0 unit of insulin delivered to the patient?
The 1500 rule
$\text{Insulin sensitivity factor} = \dfrac{1500}{\text{Total daily insulin}}$
Example
If your patient receives a total daily insulin of 50 units
$\dfrac{1500}{50} = 30$ mg/dL blood glucose drop per 1.0 unit of insulin
To correct a patient's blood glucose to 100 mg/day:
$\dfrac{\text{Patient's blood glucose} - 100}{30} = \text{Supplemental units of insulin}$

3. Replace K+ cautiously, watching urinary output and serum K+ frequently
4. Replace entire K+ deficit over the span of the patient's entire hospitalization
5. Alternatively, in the face of DKA-induced maternal phosphate deficiency, K_2PO_4 (K-Phos) may be given as potassium replacement instead of KCL

BICARBONATE THERAPY

The use of sodium bicarbonate therapy in patients with DKA is usually reserved for those patients who have an arterial pH of <6.9–7.1 and/or a HCO_3 < 5 meq/L. Rapid undiluted correction of metabolic acidosis with sodium bicarbonate is unwarranted and may lead to severe hypokalemia, hypernatremia, impaired oxygen delivery, and a paradoxical fall in cerebrospinal fluid pH. One ampule (44 meq sodium bicarbonate) is diluted in 1000 mL of 0.45 normal saline. The total deficit of bicarbonate can be calculated (obtain base deficit on arterial blood gas):

$$\text{Bicarbonate (meq) regained to fully correct metabolic acidosis} = \frac{\text{Base deficit (meq/L)} \times \text{patient weight (kg)}}{4}$$

Since oxygen hemoglobin affinity is augmented in the presence of an alkalotic shift of the oxygen-hemoglobin disassociation curve to the left, it is prudent not to fully correct the patient's metabolic acidosis, ensuring better oxygen delivery to the fetus.

Please refer to Table 11-4 for an algorithmic summary of the treatment of diabetic ketoacidosis in pregnancy.

SUGGESTED READING

Coustan, Donald R, Diabetic ketoacidosis, in: Richard L Berkowitz (ed), *Critical Care of the Obstetric Patient*, Chap. 15. New York: Churchill Livingstone, 1983.

Diabetic ketoacidosis and nonketotic hyperosmolarity, in: Robert H Demling and Robert F Wilson (eds), *Decision Making in Surgical Critical Care.* Philadelphia: B.C. Kecker, 1988, p. 216.

Golde, Steven H, Diabetic ketoacidosis in pregnancy, in: Steven L Clark, David B Cotton, Gary DV Hankins, USAF, MC, and Jeffrey P. Phelan (eds), *Critical Care Obstetrics*, 2nd edn. Chap. 17. Boston: Blackwell Scientific Publications, 1991.

Hagay, Zion J: *Diabetic Ketoacidosis in Pregnancy: Etiology, Pathophysiology, and Management.* 1994;37:39–49.

Landon, Mark B, Diabetes mellitus and other endocrine diseases, in: Steven G Gabbe, Jennifer R Neibyl, and Joe Leigh Simpson (eds), *Obstetrics: Normal and Problem Pregnancies,* 2nd edn. New York: Churchill Livingstone, 1991.

Raff, Beverly S, RF, Faan and Ellen Fiore (eds): *Diabetes in Pregnancy—Series 2: Prenatal Care Module 10 by Barbara Plovie, ARNP, BSN, CDE-Sponsored by March of Dimes*, 1991.

Reece, Albert E (ed): *Clinical Obstetrics and Gynecology—Metabolic Disorders in Pregnancy.*

12 Respiratory Emergencies During Pregnancy

Alfredo F. Gei Victor R. Suarez

INTRODUCTION

Respiratory complications during pregnancy are not unusual and can be life threatening. A careful interview and physical examination, a chest x ray and an arterial blood analysis are the most useful interventions in the evaluation of these conditions.

Understanding of the cardiorespiratory changes during pregnancy is essential for the diagnosis and treatment of emergencies in normal pregnant women and in women with underlying cardiopulmonary diseases.

BASIC SCIENCE

Oxygen is the basis of every aerobic reaction in our organism. The procurement and delivery of oxygen is a vital process that the pregnant woman has to perform for herself and her unborn child. Nature has ensured satisfactory mechanisms of exchange of oxygen with air and delivery of it to her unborn child (and adapting body) through complex anatomic (Table 12-1) and physiologic changes (Table 12-2).

Respiration involves two different but interrelated phenomena: ventilation and oxygenation. The evaluation of these processes lies in the interpretation of arterial blood gases variables: PCO_2 and PO_2 (Figs. 12-1 and 12-2).

Respiration requires that O_2 be obtained from an extra-corporeal source (atmosphere or ventilator), then transferred across the alveolar-endothelial barrier, transported to the different organs in the periphery, and subsequently utilized in aerobic metabolism.

TABLE 12-1 Anatomic and Physiologic Respiratory Adaptations to Pregnancy

Upper airways	• Mucosal edema and friability • Capillary engorgement (A smaller-sized endotracheal tube may be required for intubation because of swelling of the arytenoid region of the vocal cords)
Chest wall	• Increases in chest wall circumference (6 cm) • Elevation of the diaphragm (5 cm) • Widening of the costal angles (from 70° to 104°) • Increase in diaphragmatic excursion (1.5 cm) (All these changes occur before significant increases in uterine size, maternal body weight, or intraabdominal pressure)
Respiratory musculature	• Respiratory muscle function is unchanged • Diaphragm and intercostals accessory muscles contribute equally to tidal volume during pregnancy • Maximum inspiratory and expiratory pressures are unchanged

TABLE 12-2 Changes in Respiratory Variables During Pregnancy

Parameter	Definition	Change in pregnancy
Respiratory Rate	Number of breaths per minute	• No change
Tidal Volume	Volume of air inspired and expired at each breath	• Increase up to 40% since early pregnancy remains essentially constant for the remainder of gestation (100–200 mL)
Minute Ventilation (RR × TV)	Total amount of air (gas) inspired and expired each minute Sum of the volume of air (gas) participating in gas exchange plus the one filling the airway's dead space (i.e., not participating in gas exchange)	• Increase up to 40% since early pregnancy and remains essentially constant for the remainder of gestation (100–200 mL)
Vital Capacity	Maximum volume of air that can be forcibly inspired after a maximum expiration	• Unchanged
Residual Volume	Volume of air remaining in the lungs after a maximum expiration	• Decreases by ~20% due to elevation of the diaphragm
Functional Residual Capacity (FRC)	Volume of air in lungs at resting expiratory level	• Decreases by ~20% due to elevation of the diaphragm
Inspiratory Capacity	Maximum volume of air that can be inspired from resting expiratory level	• Increases 100–300 mL (5–10%) as a result of the reduction in FRC

At term, there is a small (200–400 mL, 4%) decrease in total lung capacity. Vital capacity (VC) does not change significantly. Functional residual capacity (FRC) consistently decreases 300–500 mL (17–20%). Changing from a sitting to a supine position at term, causes a further decrease (25%) in FRC. This may increase closure of small airways, especially in obese patients in the supine or lithotomy position.

BASIC PHYSIOLOGIC OXYGENATION CONCEPTS

- **O_2 content.** The content of oxygen in arterial blood is the sum of that bound to hemoglobin (Hb) and that dissolved in plasma (normally about 1.5 percent). The main factor that determines the extent of O_2 binding to hemoglobin (saturation) is the PaO_2 (hemoglobin-oxygen dissociation curve). The shape of the curve indicates that unless the steep part of the curve is reached (a drop of PaO_2 to less than 60 mmHg) there will not be a significant deleterious effect on Hb saturation and O_2 arterial content.

- **O_2 affinity.** Several factors can change the affinity of Hb for O_2. Acidosis, fever, and increased 2,3-DPG shift the curve to the right. In the slightly acidic environment of peripheral tissues a right shift is important to unload O_2 to the cells. Alkalosis, hypothermia, and decreased 2,3-DPG shift the curve to the left. In the slightly alkalotic environment of the pulmonary capillary, a left shift is important to load O_2 to the red blood cells. Affinity is also shifted to the left in the fetal hemoglobin.
- **O_2 delivery.** Systemic O_2 delivery is the product of arterial O_2 content (mL/L of blood) and cardiac output (mL/min).
- **O_2 consumption.** In a normal adult at rest it is approximately 250 mL/min. During exercise it can rise to 3000 mL/min. When delivery cannot meet tissue demands, anaerobic metabolism occurs, leading to lactic acidosis.

RESPIRATORY PHYSIOLOGIC ADAPTATIONS OF PREGNANCY

Pregnancy increases O_2 consumption by 15 to 20 percent (Table 12-3). Half of this increase is associated with the requirements of the feto-placental unit, and the remaining half is secondary to the increased work by the maternal organs (heart, lungs, and kidneys). Increased cardiac output and minute ventilation explain how O_2 consumption increases despite no change in PaO_2 and a decrease in the arteriovenous O_2 difference (increase in oxygen delivery).

Despite the favorable effects of pregnancy (progesterone is a central stimulant) on ventilation, at least half of pregnant women complain of shortness of breath (dyspnea), fatigue, and decreased exercise tolerance during gestation.

OXYGENATION AND ACID-BASE HOMEOSTASIS

Pregnancy is characterized by a chronically compensated respiratory alkalosis due to the hyperventilation (rather than tachypnea) state of pregnancy. Pregnancy's increase in minute ventilation (progesterone-induced hyperventilation of pregnancy) results in a decrease in $PaCO_2$ to around 30 mmHg. Maternal pH reflects the chronic compensated mild respiratory alkalosis. Compensation is secondary to the decline in bicarbonate concentration (secondary to increased renal excretion). The net result of these changes is facilitation of CO_2 exchange from fetus to mother.

TABLE 12-3 Changes in Oxygenation Variables During Pregnancy

Parameter	Modification	Magnitude	Peak
Oxygen consumption (VO_2)	⇧	+20% + 40–60%	Term
Oxygen delivery (DO_2)	⇔ ⇧	700–400 mL/min	Term
Resistance of the pulmonary circulation	⇩	–34%	34 weeks

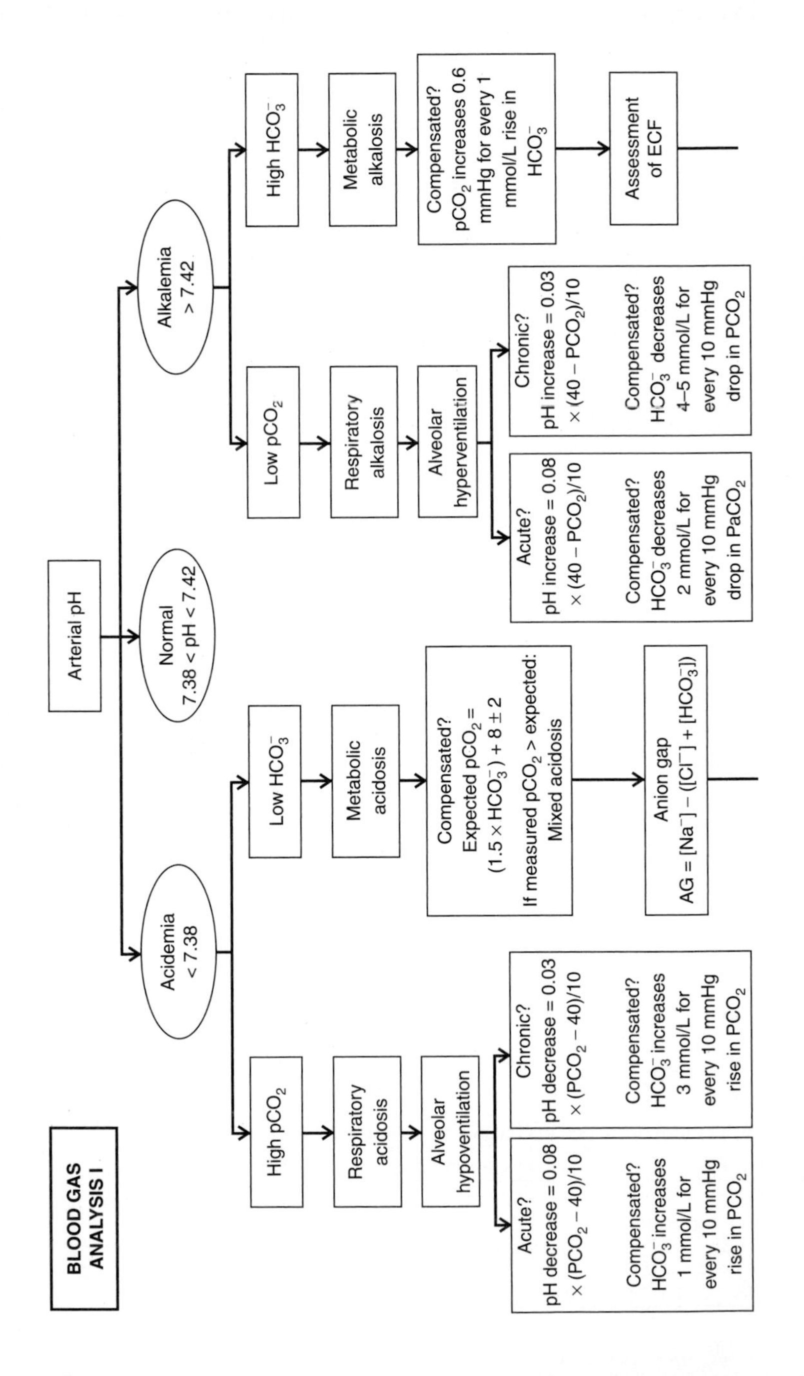

BLOOD GAS ANALYSIS I
Arterial pH
Acidemia < 7.38
Normal 7.38 < pH < 7.42
Alkalemia > 7.42
High pCO_2
Respiratory acidosis
Alveolar hypoventilation
Acute? pH decrease = 0.08 × (PCO_2 – 40)/10
Compensated? HCO_3^- increases 1 mmol/L for every 10 mmHg rise in PCO_2
Chronic? pH decrease = 0.03 × (PCO_2 – 40)/10
Compensated? HCO_3^- increases 3 mmol/L for every 10 mmHg rise in PCO_2
Low HCO_3^-
Metabolic acidosis
Compensated? Expected pCO_2 = (1.5 × HCO_3^-) + 8 ± 2
If measured pCO_2 > expected: Mixed acidosis
Anion gap
AG = [Na^+] – ([Cl^-] + [HCO_3^-])
Low pCO_2
Respiratory alkalosis
Alveolar hyperventilation
Acute? pH increase = 0.08 × (40 – PCO_2)/10
Compensated? HCO_3^- decreases 2 mmol/L for every 10 mmHg drop in $PaCO_2$
Chronic? pH increase = 0.03 × (40 – PCO_2)/10
Compensated? HCO_3^- decreases 4–5 mmol/L for every 10 mmHg drop in PCO_2
High HCO_3^-
Metabolic alkalosis
Compensated? pCO_2 increases 0.6 mmHg for every 1 mmol/L rise in HCO_3^-
Assessment of ECF

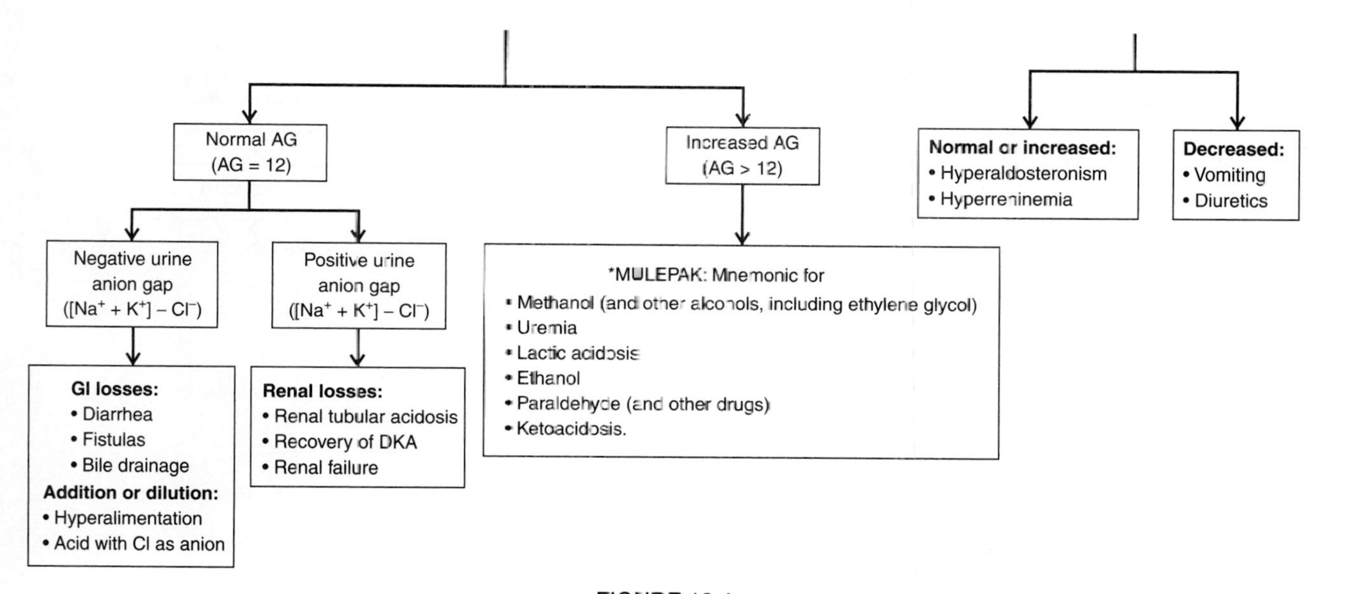
Normal AG
(AG = 12)
Increased AG
(AG > 12)
Normal or increased:
• Hyperaldosteronism
• Hyperreninemia
Decreased:
• Vomiting
• Diuretics
Negative urine
anion gap
([Na+ + K+] – Cl−)
Positive urine
anion gap
([Na+ + K+] – Cl−)
*MULEPAK: Mnemonic for
• Methanol (and other alcohols, including ethylene glycol)
• Uremia
• Lactic acidosis
• Ethanol
• Paraldehyde (and other drugs)
• Ketoacidosis.
GI losses:
• Diarrhea
• Fistulas
• Bile drainage
Addition or dilution:
• Hyperalimentation
• Acid with Cl as anion
Renal losses:
• Renal tubular acidosis
• Recovery of DKA
• Renal failure

FIGURE 12-1

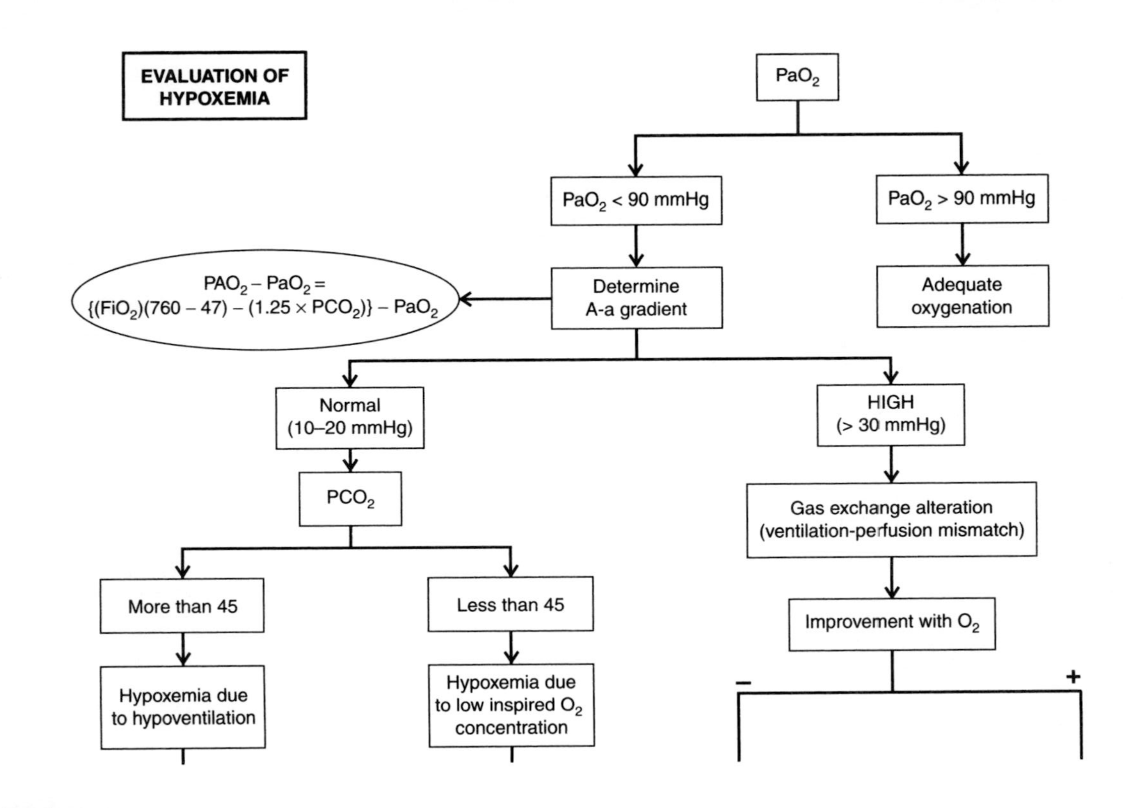
EVALUATION OF HYPOXEMIA
PaO2
PaO2 < 90 mmHg
PaO2 > 90 mmHg
Determine A-a gradient
Adequate oxygenation
PAO2 – PaO2 = {(FiO2)(760 – 47) – (1.25 × PCO2)} – PaO2
Normal (10–20 mmHg)
HIGH (> 30 mmHg)
PCO2
Gas exchange alteration (ventilation-perfusion mismatch)
More than 45
Less than 45
Improvement with O2
Hypoxemia due to hypoventilation
Hypoxemia due to low inspired O2 concentration
–
+

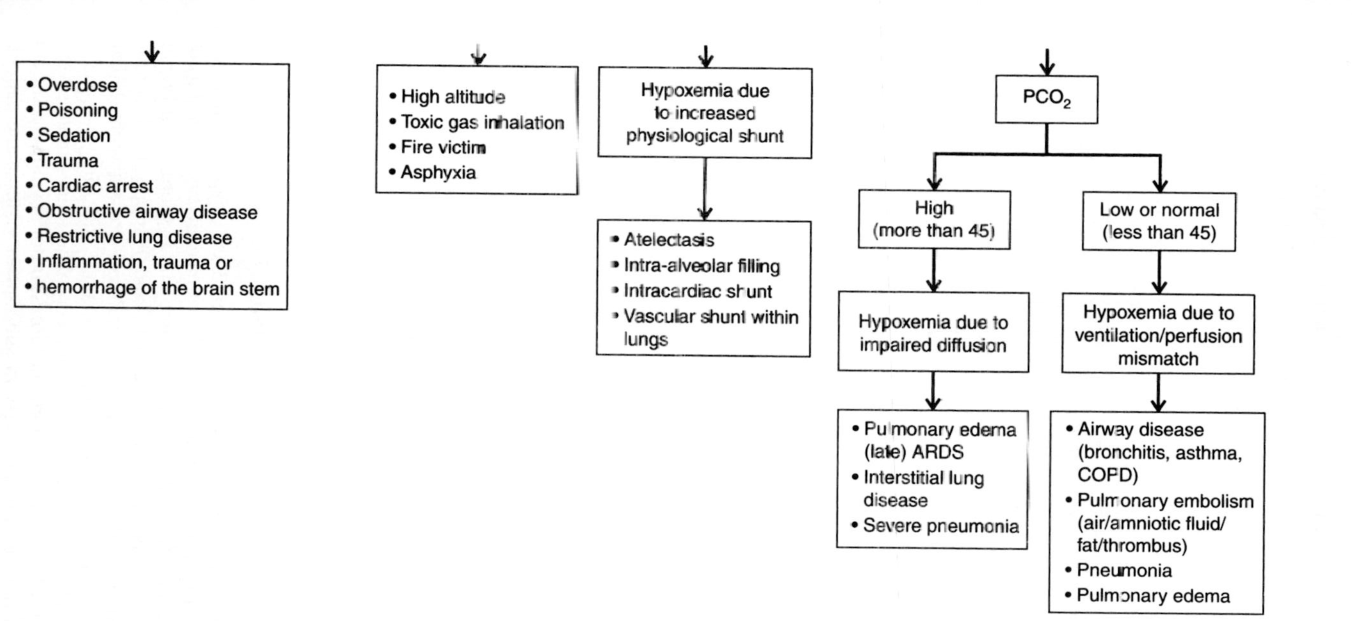
• Overdose
• Poisoning
• Sedation
• Trauma
• Cardiac arrest
• Obstructive airway disease
• Restrictive lung disease
• Inflammation, trauma or
• hemorrhage of the brain stem
• High altitude
• Toxic gas inhalation
• Fire victim
• Asphyxia
Hypoxemia due to increased physiological shunt
• Atelectasis
• Intra-alveolar filling
• Intracardiac shunt
• Vascular shunt within lungs
PCO2
High (more than 45)
Low or normal (less than 45)
Hypoxemia due to impaired diffusion
Hypoxemia due to ventilation/perfusion mismatch
• Pulmonary edema (late) ARDS
• Interstitial lung disease
• Severe pneumonia
• Airway disease (bronchitis, asthma, COPD)
• Pulmonary embolism (air/amniotic fluid/ fat/thrombus)
• Pneumonia
• Pulmonary edema

FIGURE 12-2

TABLE 12-4 Changes in Arterial Blood Gases During Pregnancy

ABG variable	Not pregnant adult	Pregnant
pH	7.35–7.43	7.40–7.47
PCO_2 (mmHg)	37–40	27–34 (there is a compensatory increase in renal bicarbonate excretion)
PO_2 (mmHg)	103	• 106–108 (sea level) • 101–104 (third trimester) • –13 (supine position and III trimester)
$P(A\text{-}a)O_2$ (mmHg)	14	• 20 • +6 (supine position and III trimester)
Bicarbonate (meq/L)	22–26	18–22
Base deficit (meq/L)	1	3

Oxygenation is affected in at least one fourth of pregnant women while in a supine position (lower PaO_2 and larger A-a gradient). These changes are reversed when the maternal position changes to the upright state (Table 12-4).

CLINICAL IMPLICATIONS

- It is not surprising that pregnant women complain of symptoms suggestive of pulmonary or cardiac disease. In most instances a careful interrogation and physical examination can establish whether these symptoms are physiologic or a possibility of a specific condition that needs to be addressed and evaluated (Fig. 3).
- Pregnant patients are prone to
  - hypoxemia (due to decreased FRC, increased alveolar ventilation, and increased O_2 consumption),
  - aspiration (slow gastric emptying, functional displacement of lower esophagus), and
  - anesthetic overdose (decreased minimal alveolar concentration of anesthetics, decreased functional residual capacity, and increased alveolar ventilation). Induction and emergence of and from general anesthesia occurs more rapidly in pregnant women.

RESPIRATORY EMERGENCIES DURING PREGNANCY

The anatomic and physiologic changes of the cardiac (Chap. 8) and respiratory systems explain why respiratory symptoms are common during pregnancy. The most frequent respiratory complaint is shortness of breath (dyspnea). Other symptoms include cough, and hemoptysis. Unfortunately both benign and life-threatening conditions present with similar complaints. A careful evaluation of these symptoms will allow the practitioner to discern between pregnancy-related complaints and a more severe condition. Even when deemed benign, cardiorespiratory symptoms should be noted and evaluated prospectively in subsequent visits of the patient.

TABLE 12-5 Changes in Chest x Ray During Pregnancy

Modifications
Apparent cardiomegaly (enlarged transverse diameter)
Enlarged left atrium (lateral views)
Increased vascular markings
Straightening of left heart border
Postpartum pleural effusion (right sided)

Some of the conditions that can be suggested by history or physical examination are included in the Fig. 12-3. Specific algorithms addressing the evaluation of dyspnea, cough, and hemoptysis (Figs. 12-4, 12-5, and 12-6) are suggested.

The two most helpful clinical adjuncts in the evaluation of respiratory conditions during pregnancy are:

- **Arterial blood gas interpretation.** The changes induced by the pregnant state are summarized in Table 12-4. Figures 12-1 and 12-2 illustrate the evaluation of ventilation and oxygenation through the laboratory analysis of an arterial blood sample.
- **Chest x ray interpretation.** Table 12-5 summarizes the changes described for pregnancy. Aside from heart enlargement secondary to hypervolemia and cardiac remodeling and some cephalad flow redistribution, all other criteria used to interpret chest radiograms remain the same as in the nonpregnant state. Figure 12-7 provides a guideline for evaluation of chest x rays and the most common pathologic processes encountered by the site of affliction. As was the case with the arterial blood gases, more than one process may coexist and affect the patient.

Several conditions specific to pregnancy and other intercurrent diseases in the pregnant woman may compromise the processes of oxygenation or ventilation. While the specific treatment of these conditions may differ, the recognition of the need for supportive respiratory therapy and the prompt institution of adequate ventilation and oxygenation support may be the dividing line between life and death. Clinical guidelines for the recognition of respiratory failure (Table 12-6), indications for endotracheal intubation

TABLE 12-6 Criteria for the Diagnosis of Respiratory Failure

Mnemonic: MOVE
1. Mechanical
a. Vital capacity <15 mL/kg
b. Maximal inspiratory force (MIF) < –25 cm H_2O
c. Respiratory rate >35/min
2. Oxygenation
a. PaO_2 < 70 mmHg with FIO_2 of 0.4
b. $P(A\text{-}a)O_2$: > 350 mmHg with FIO_2 of 1.0
3. Ventilation
a. $PaCO_2$ > 55 mmHg (if acute condition)
b. Dead space/tidal volume (Vd/Vt) > 0.6
4. End-inspiratory lung inflation inadequate for adequate gas exchange

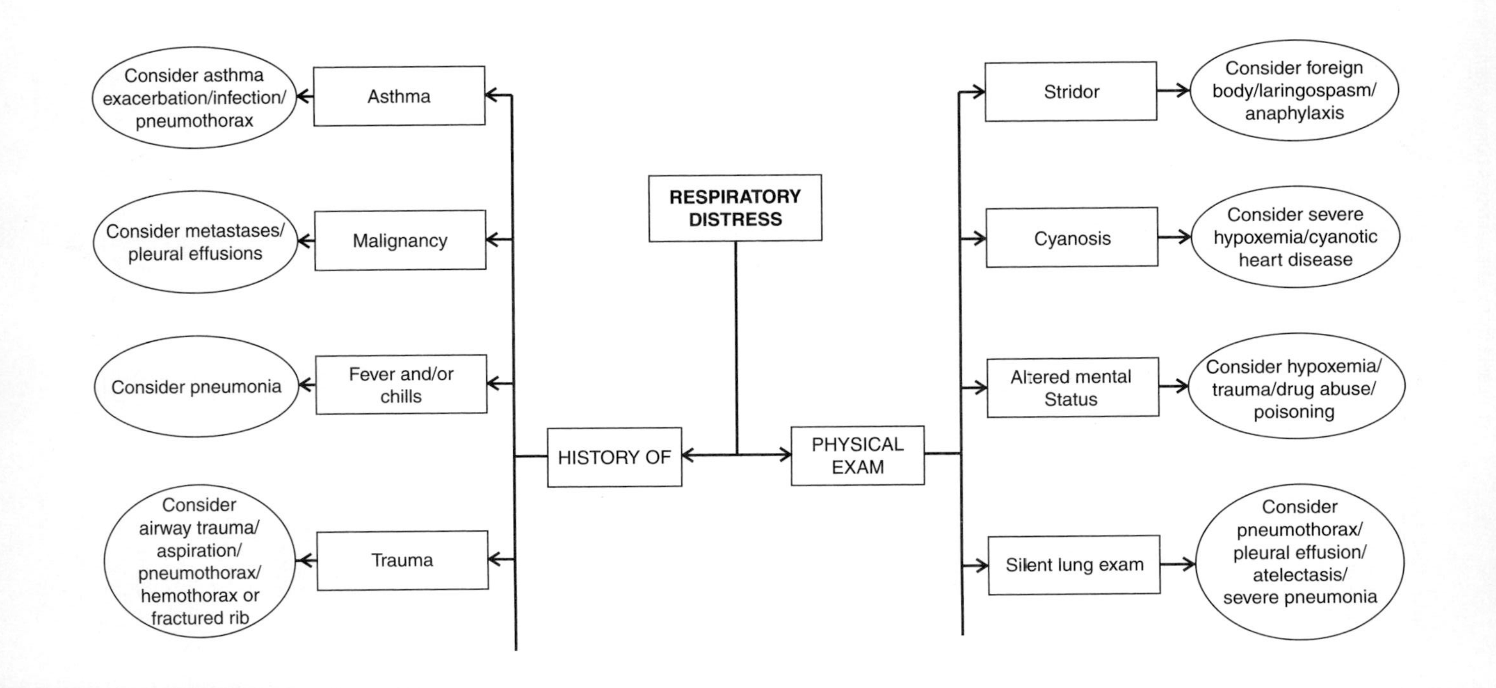
RESPIRATORY DISTRESS
HISTORY OF
Asthma
Consider asthma exacerbation/infection/ pneumothorax
Malignancy
Consider metastases/ pleural effusions
Fever and/or chills
Consider pneumonia
Trauma
Consider airway trauma/ aspiration/ pneumothorax/ hemothorax or fractured rib
PHYSICAL EXAM
Stridor
Consider foreign body/laringospasm/ anaphylaxis
Cyanosis
Consider severe hypoxemia/cyanotic heart disease
Altered mental Status
Consider hypoxemia/ trauma/drug abuse/ poisoning
Silent lung exam
Consider pneumothorax/ pleural effusion/ atelectasis/ severe pneumonia

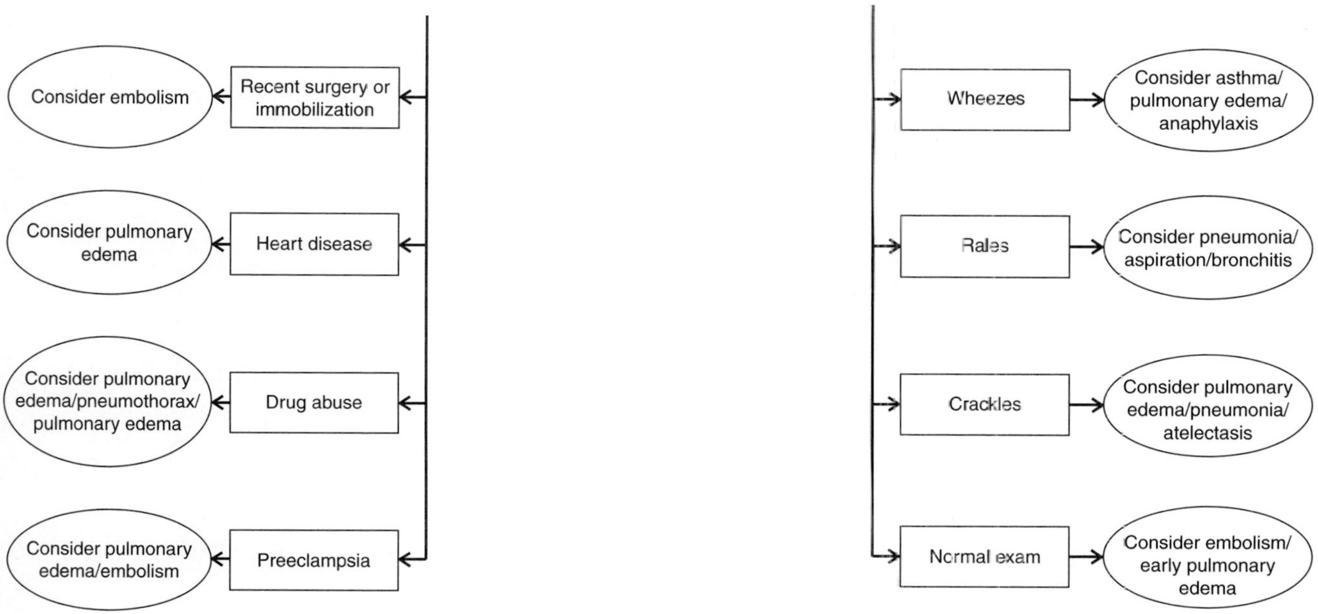

Recent surgery or immobilization → Consider embolism

Heart disease → Consider pulmonary edema

Drug abuse → Consider pulmonary edema/pneumothorax/ pulmonary edema

Preeclampsia → Consider pulmonary edema/embolism

Wheezes → Consider asthma/ pulmonary edema/ anaphylaxis

Rales → Consider pneumonia/ aspiration/bronchitis

Crackles → Consider pulmonary edema/pneumonia/ atelectasis

Normal exam → Consider embolism/ early pulmonary edema

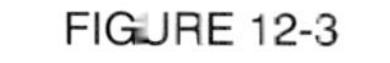

FIGURE 12-3

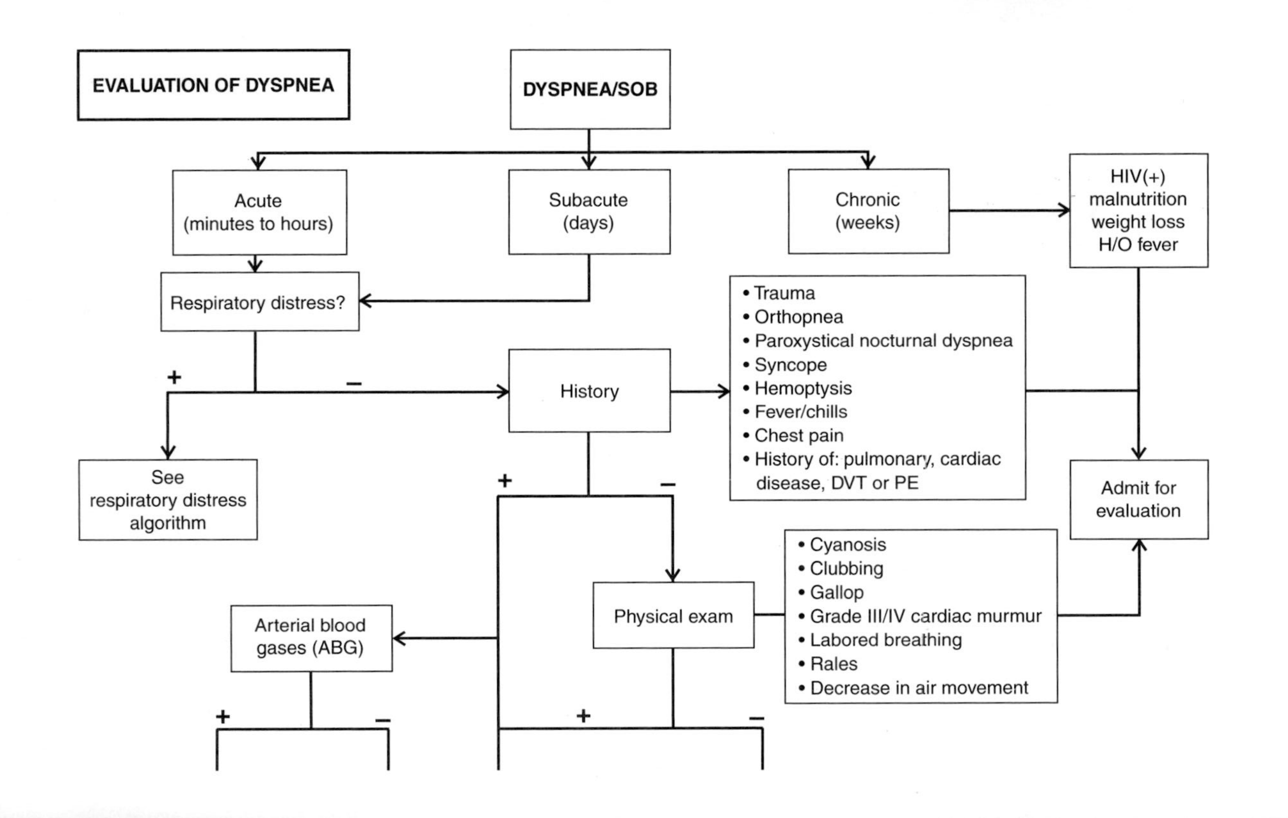
EVALUATION OF DYSPNEA
DYSPNEA/SOB
Acute
(minutes to hours)
Subacute
(days)
Chronic
(weeks)
HIV(+)
malnutrition
weight loss
H/O fever
Respiratory distress?
+
–
See
respiratory distress
algorithm
History
• Trauma
• Orthopnea
• Paroxystical nocturnal dyspnea
• Syncope
• Hemoptysis
• Fever/chills
• Chest pain
• History of: pulmonary, cardiac disease, DVT or PE
Admit for
evaluation
+
–
Physical exam
• Cyanosis
• Clubbing
• Gallop
• Grade III/IV cardiac murmur
• Labored breathing
• Rales
• Decrease in air movement
Arterial blood
gases (ABG)
+
–
+
–

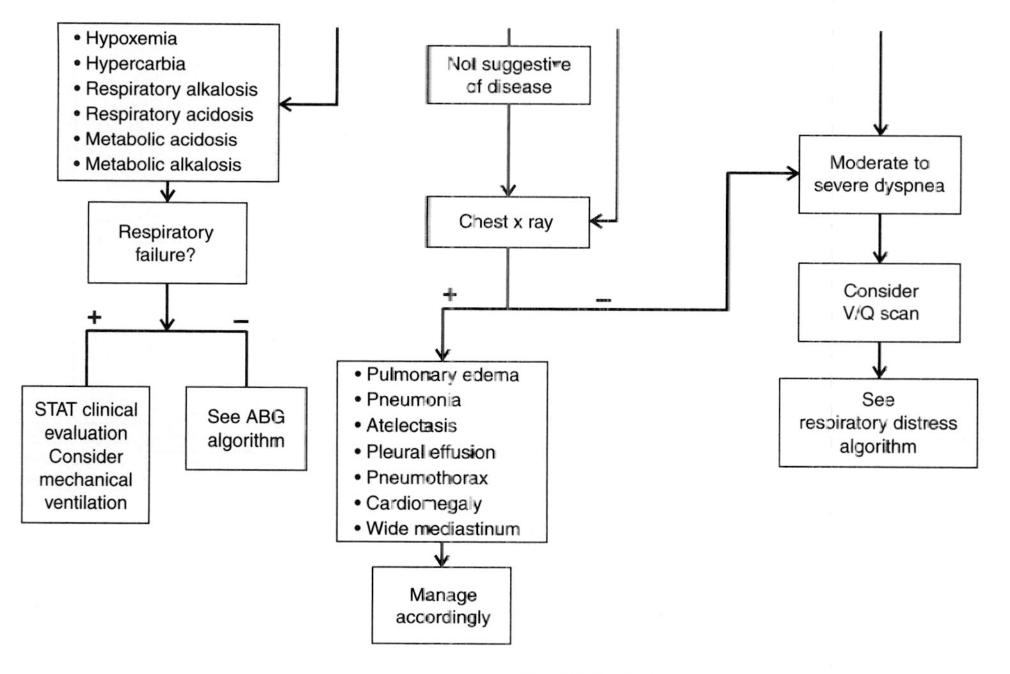
• Hypoxemia
• Hypercarbia
• Respiratory alkalosis
• Respiratory acidosis
• Metabolic acidosis
• Metabolic alkalosis
Respiratory failure?
+
–
STAT clinical evaluation Consider mechanical ventilation
See ABG algorithm
Not suggestive of disease
Chest x ray
+
–
• Pulmonary edema
• Pneumonia
• Atelectasis
• Pleural effusion
• Pneumothorax
• Cardiomegaly
• Wide mediastinum
Manage accordingly
Moderate to severe dyspnea
Consider V/Q scan
See respiratory distress algorithm

FIGURE 12-4

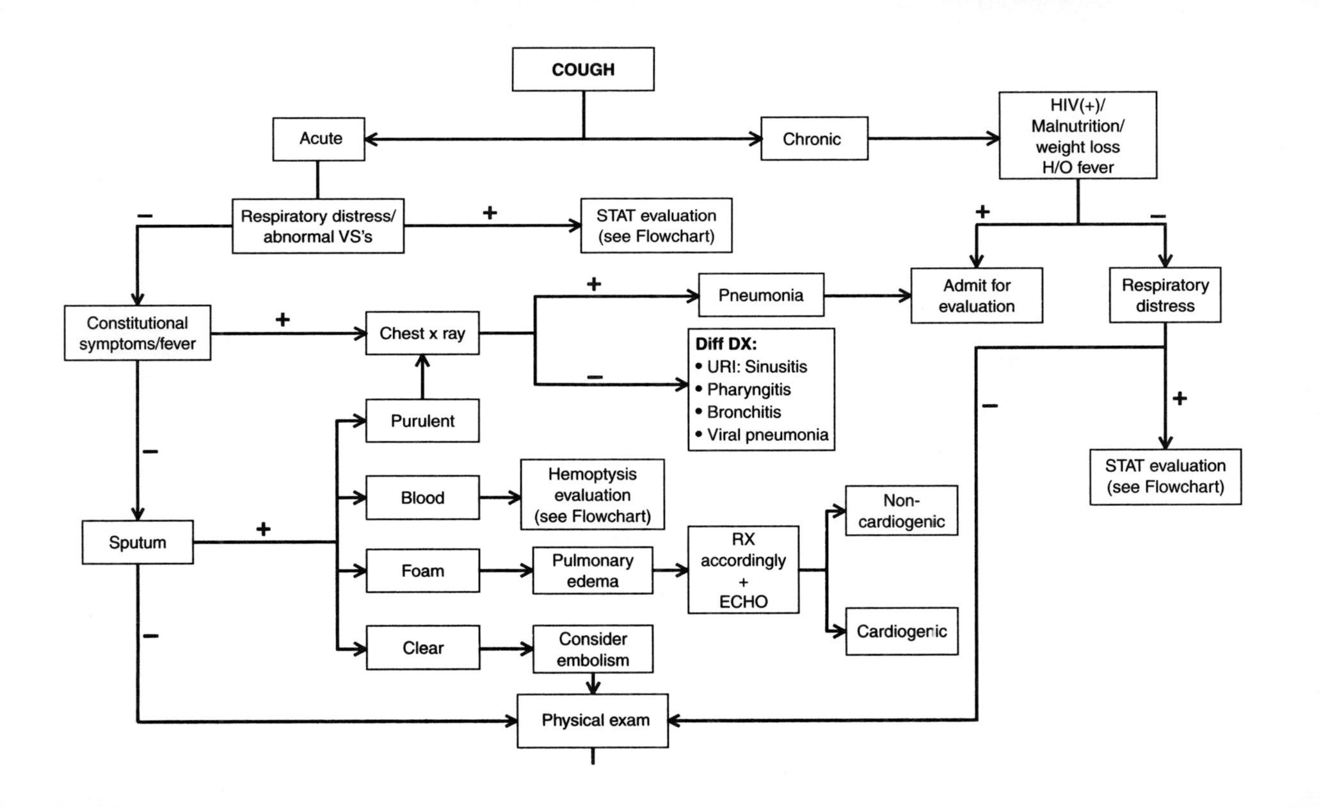

COUGH
Acute
Chronic
HIV(+)/
Malnutrition/
weight loss
H/O fever
Respiratory distress/
abnormal VS's
+
STAT evaluation
(see Flowchart)
−
+
−
Admit for
evaluation
Respiratory
distress
+
STAT evaluation
(see Flowchart)
−
Constitutional
symptoms/fever
+
Chest x ray
+
Pneumonia
−
Diff DX:
• URI: Sinusitis
• Pharyngitis
• Bronchitis
• Viral pneumonia
−
Sputum
+
Purulent
Blood
Hemoptysis
evaluation
(see Flowchart)
Foam
Pulmonary
edema
RX
accordingly
+
ECHO
Non-
cardiogenic
Cardiogenic
Clear
Consider
embolism
−
Physical exam

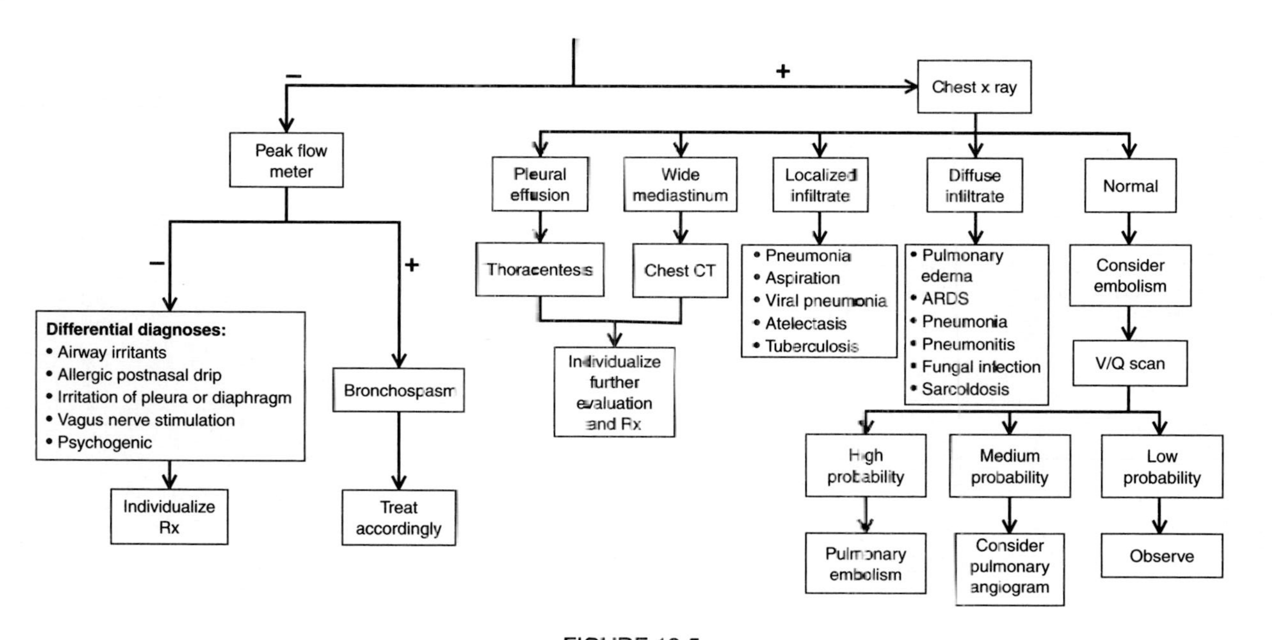

−
+
Chest x ray
Peak flow meter
Pleural effusion
Wide mediastinum
Localized infiltrate
Diffuse infiltrate
Normal
−
+
Thoracentesis
Chest CT
• Pneumonia
• Aspiration
• Viral pneumonia
• Atelectasis
• Tuberculosis
• Pulmonary edema
• ARDS
• Pneumonia
• Pneumonitis
• Fungal infection
• Sarcoidosis
Consider embolism
Differential diagnoses:
• Airway irritants
• Allergic postnasal drip
• Irritation of pleura or diaphragm
• Vagus nerve stimulation
• Psychogenic
Bronchospasm
Individualize further evaluation and Rx
V/Q scan
High probability
Medium probability
Low probability
Individualize Rx
Treat accordingly
Pulmonary embolism
Consider pulmonary angiogram
Observe

FIGURE 12-5

EVALUATION OF HEMOPTYSIS

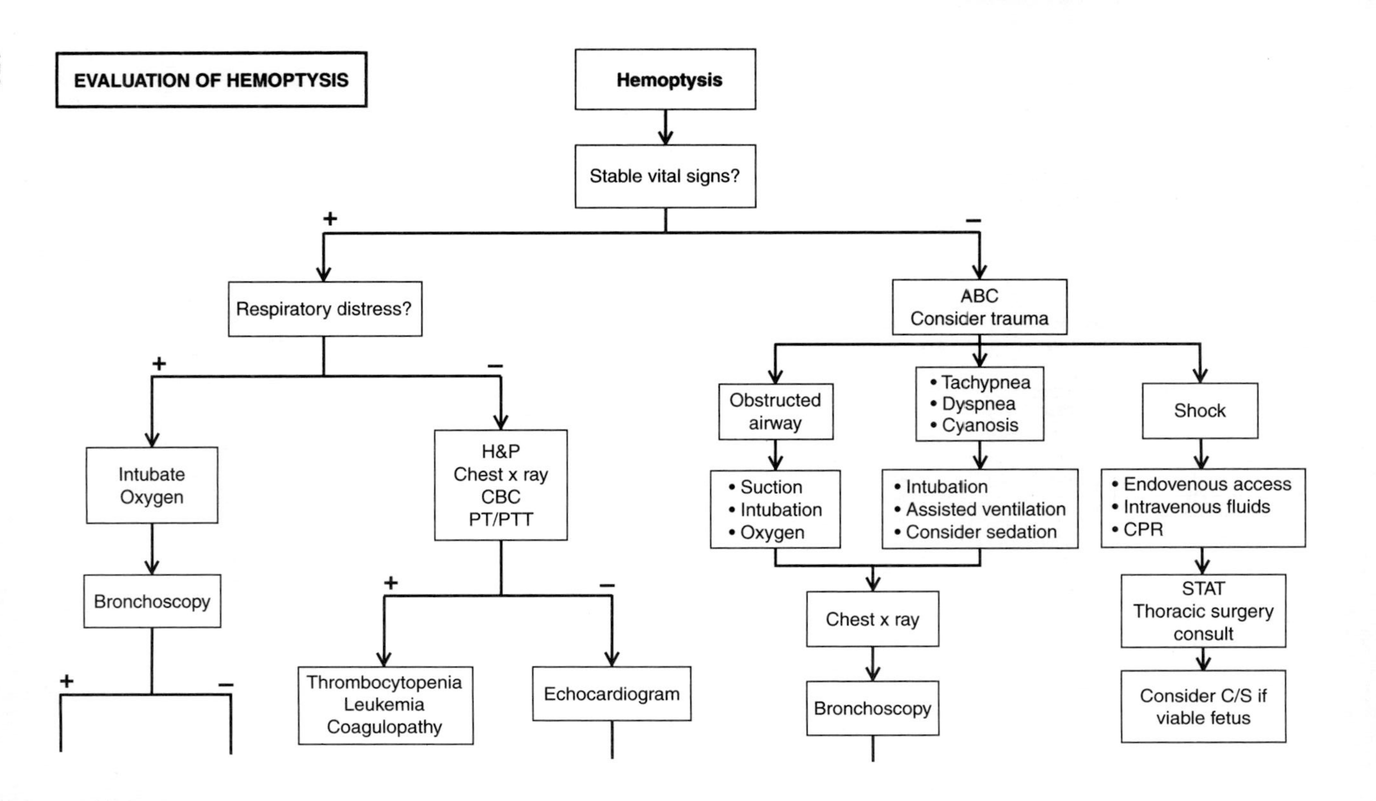

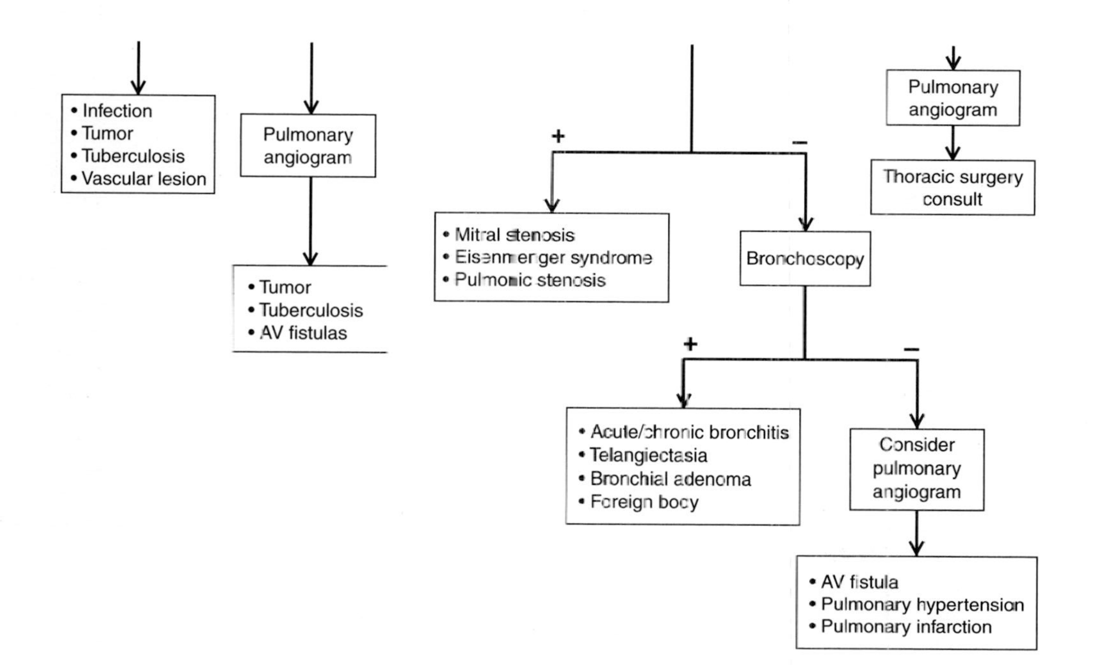
• Infection
• Tumor
• Tuberculosis
• Vascular lesion
Pulmonary angiogram
• Tumor
• Tuberculosis
• AV fistulas
+
–
• Mitral stenosis
• Eisenmenger syndrome
• Pulmonic stenosis
Bronchoscopy
+
–
• Acute/chronic bronchitis
• Telangiectasia
• Bronchial adenoma
• Foreign body
Consider pulmonary angiogram
• AV fistula
• Pulmonary hypertension
• Pulmonary infarction
Pulmonary angiogram
Thoracic surgery consult

FIGURE 12-6

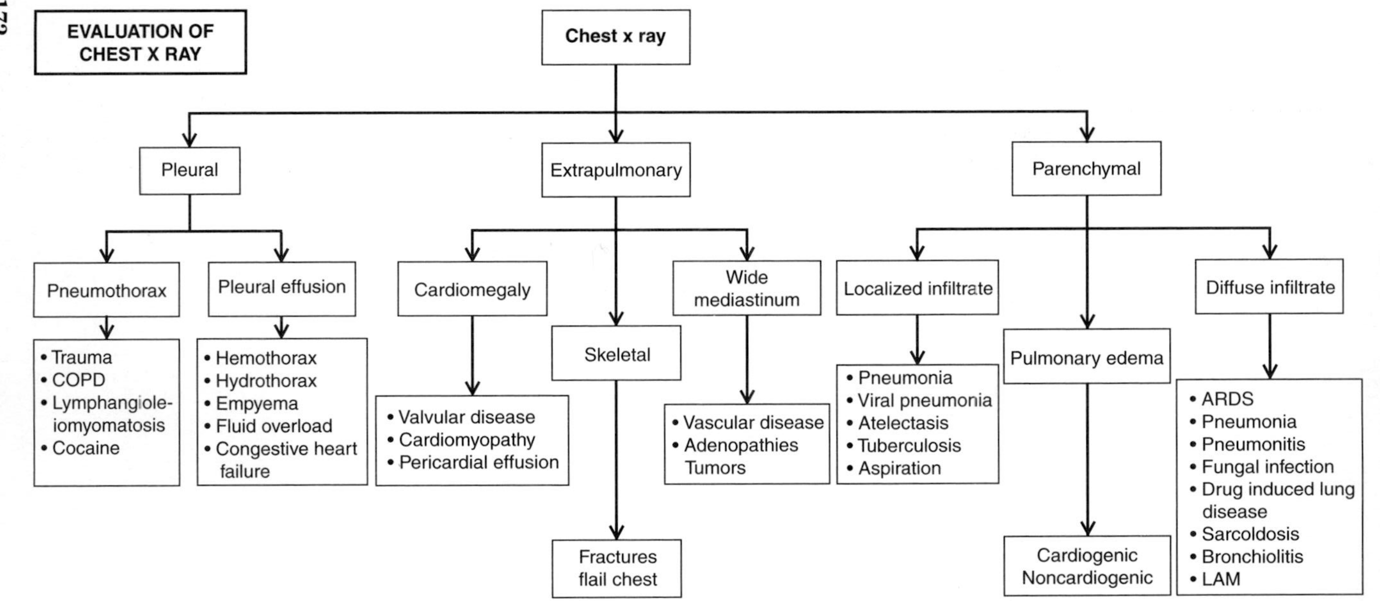
EVALUATION OF
CHEST X RAY
Chest x ray
Pleural
Extrapulmonary
Parenchymal
Pneumothorax
Pleural effusion
Cardiomegaly
Skeletal
Wide mediastinum
Localized infiltrate
Pulmonary edema
Diffuse infiltrate
• Trauma
• COPD
• Lymphangiole-iomyomatosis
• Cocaine
• Hemothorax
• Hydrothorax
• Empyema
• Fluid overload
• Congestive heart failure
• Valvular disease
• Cardiomyopathy
• Pericardial effusion
Fractures
flail chest
• Vascular disease
• Adenopathies
Tumors
• Pneumonia
• Viral pneumonia
• Atelectasis
• Tuberculosis
• Aspiration
Cardiogenic
Noncardiogenic
• ARDS
• Pneumonia
• Pneumonitis
• Fungal infection
• Drug induced lung disease
• Sarcoldosis
• Bronchiolitis
• LAM

FIGURE 12-7

TABLE 12-7 Indications for Endotracheal Intubation

Mnemonic: GARDD
1. Gastro-pulmonary reflux and aspiration
2. Airway obstruction (present or suspected)
3. Respiratory arrest (actual or impending)
4. Depressed mental status
5. Difficulty managing secretions

TABLE 12-8 Indications for Mechanical Ventilation (Invasive or Noninvasive)

A. Severe respiratory or combined respiratory and metabolic acidosis
B. Sustained respiratory rate of 40/min
C. Abnormal breathing pattern suggestive of increased respiratory workload and/or respiratory muscle fatigue
D. Depressed mental status
E. Severe hypoxemia

(Table 12-7), indications for mechanical ventilation (Table 12-8), means to provide noninvasive oxygen (Table 12-9), guidelines for the initiation (Table 12-10) and discontinuation of mechanical ventilation are provided (Table 12-11). In these situations, the processes of evaluation and treatment are frequently simultaneous (Figs. 12-4 and 12-8).

TABLE 12-9 Means to Provide Noninvasive Oxygen Therapy

Nasal cannulas
- Can provide 24–40% oxygen with flowrates up to 6 L/min
- Oxygen at flowrates of 4 L/min or less need not be humidified

Simple oxygen masks
- Can provide 35–50%, depending on fit, at flowrates from 5–10 L/min
- Flowrates need to be maintained at 5 L/min or higher to avoid rebreathing exhaled CO_2 that can be retained in the mask

Partial rebreathing mask (simple mask with a reservoir bag)
- Oxygen flow should be supplied to maintain the reservoir bag at least one-third to one-half full in inspiration
- At flow rates of 6–10 L/min the system can provide 40–70% oxygen

Nonrebreathing mask (similar to the partial rebreathing mask except it has a series of one-way valves; one valve is between the mask and the bag to prevent exhaled air from returning to the bag)
- The delivered FIO_2 of this system is 60–80%
- There should be a minimum flow of 10 L/min

Source: Modified from AARC Clinical Practice Guideline. *Respir Care* 2002;47(6):717.

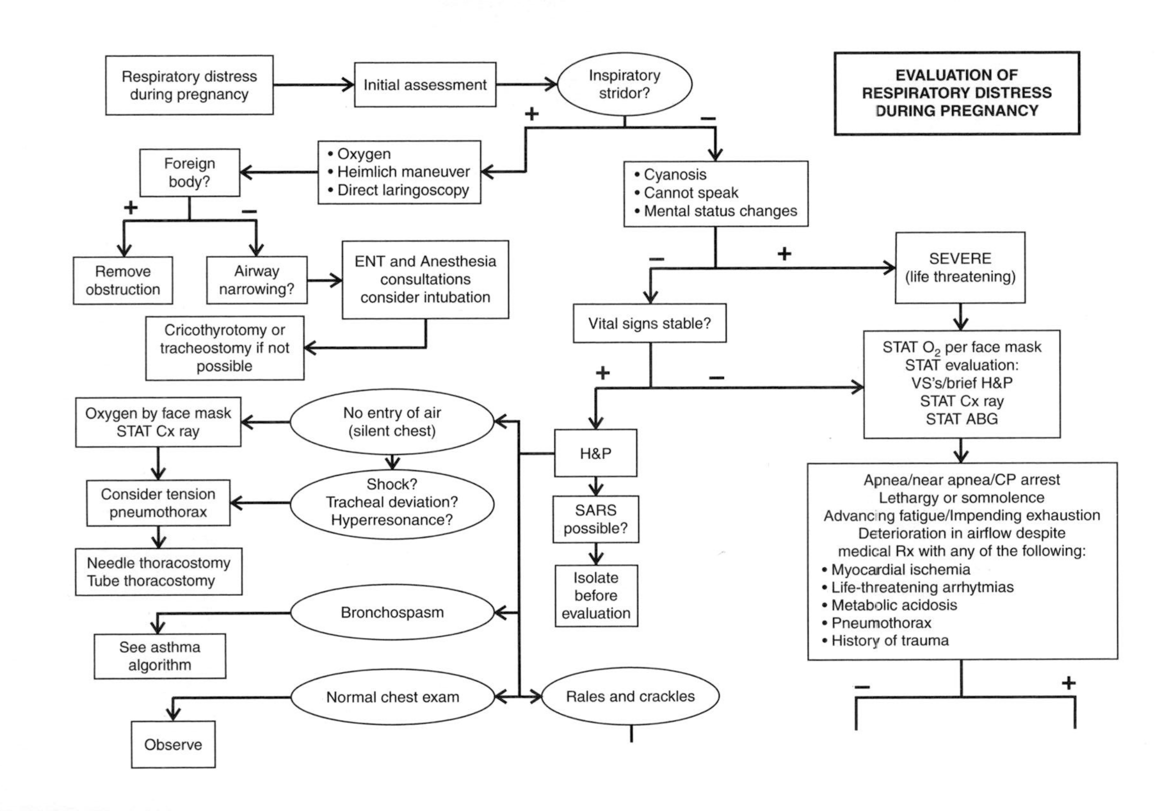
EVALUATION OF RESPIRATORY DISTRESS DURING PREGNANCY
Respiratory distress during pregnancy
Initial assessment
Inspiratory stridor?
+
−
• Oxygen
• Heimlich maneuver
• Direct laringoscopy
Foreign body?
+
−
Remove obstruction
Airway narrowing?
ENT and Anesthesia consultations consider intubation
Cricothyrotomy or tracheostomy if not possible
• Cyanosis
• Cannot speak
• Mental status changes
+
−
SEVERE (life threatening)
Vital signs stable?
+
−
STAT O_2 per face mask
STAT evaluation:
VS's/brief H&P
STAT Cx ray
STAT ABG
Apnea/near apnea/CP arrest
Lethargy or somnolence
Advancing fatigue/Impending exhaustion
Deterioration in airflow despite medical Rx with any of the following:
• Myocardial ischemia
• Life-threatening arrhytmias
• Metabolic acidosis
• Pneumothorax
• History of trauma
−
+
H&P
SARS possible?
Isolate before evaluation
No entry of air (silent chest)
Oxygen by face mask STAT Cx ray
Shock? Tracheal deviation? Hyperresonance?
Consider tension pneumothorax
Needle thoracostomy Tube thoracostomy
Bronchospasm
See asthma algorithm
Normal chest exam
Observe
Rales and crackles

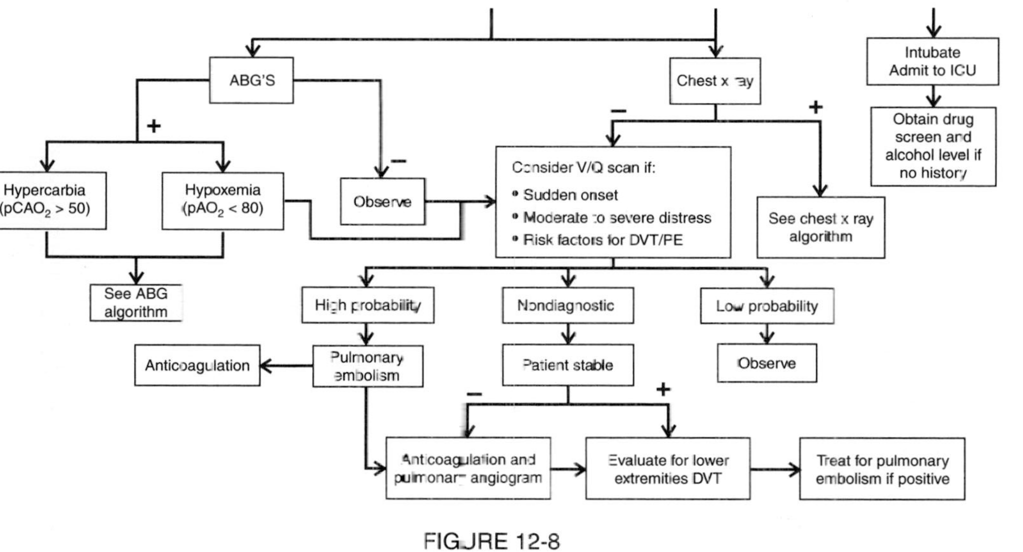
ABG'S
+
−
Hypercarbia ($pCAO_2 > 50$)
Hypoxemia ($pAO_2 < 80$)
See ABG algorithm
Observe
Chest x ray
−
+
Consider V/Q scan if:
• Sudden onset
• Moderate to severe distress
• Risk factors for DVT/PE
See chest x ray algorithm
Intubate Admit to ICU
Obtain drug screen and alcohol level if no history
High probability
Nondiagnostic
Low probability
Pulmonary embolism
Anticoagulation
Patient stable
Observe
−
+
Anticoagulation and pulmonary angiogram
Evaluate for lower extremities DVT
Treat for pulmonary embolism if positive

FIGURE 12-8

TABLE 12-10 Guidelines for the Initiation of Mechanical Ventilation

A. Primary goals of ventilatory support are
- Adequate oxygenation/ventilation
- Reduced work of breathing
- Synchrony between patient and ventilator
- Avoidance of high-end inspiration alveolar pressures

B. Five subsets of patients can be identified
- Normal lung mechanics and gas exchange (example: drug overdose)
  - Settings: ACV/PSV; FIO_2 of 0.5–1.0; TV: 8–15 mL/kg; RR: 8–12/min; inspiratory flow rate of 40–60 L/min; add sighs 6/h at 1.5 times Vt or PEEP of 5–7.5 cm H_2O to prevent atelectasis
- Severe airflow obstruction (example: drug overdose)
  - Settings: ACV/SIMV; FIO_2 of 0.5–1.0; TV: 5–7 mL/kg; RR: 12–15/min; inspiratory flow rate of 40–60 L/min; add PEEP if patient is triggering. Goals are to minimize alveolar overdistention (Pplat 15 < 30) and to minimize alveolar dynamic hyperinflation auto PEEP below 10 cm H_2O or end-expiratory lung volumes <20 mL/kg)
- Acute or chronic respiratory failure (example: status asthmaticus)
  - Settings: SIMV/ACV; FIO_2 of 0.4–0.6; TV: 5–7 mL/kg; RR: 24–28/min; inspiratory flow rate of 40–60 L/min
- Acute hypoxemic respiratory failure (example: ARDS)
  - Settings: ACV/PCV; FIO_2 of 1.0; TV: 5–7 mL/kg; RR: 24-28/min; minimal PEEP to keep SaO_2 of 90%. If volume is held constant, PEEP increases peak inspiratory airway pressure, a potentially undesirable effect in ARDS; PEEP levels > 15 cm H_2O are rarely necessary
- Restrictive lung or chest wall disease (example: sarcoidosis)
  - Settings: FIO_2 of 0.5–1.0; TV: 5–7 mL/kg; RR: 18–24/min

C. Other recommendations
- Avoid high inspiratory peak pressures (>30 cm H_2O)
- Target pH and not pCO_2 to make changes to respiratory rate and minute ventilation
- Use PEEP in diffuse lung injury to support oxygenation and reduce the FIO_2
- Set trigger sensitivity to allow a minimal patient effort to initiate the inspiration
- In patients at risk, avoid choosing ventilator settings that limit expiratory time and cause or worsen auto-PEEP
- When poor oxygenation, inadequate ventilation, or excessively high peak inspiratory pressures are thought to be related to patient intolerance of ventilator settings and are not corrected by ventilator adjustment, consider sedation, analgesia, and/or neuromuscular blockade

TABLE 12-11 Criteria for Determining Readiness for Extubation

- PaO_2 > 80 torr on FIO_2 of 0.6
- $PaCO_2$ < 45 torr
- Respiratory rate: < 35 breaths/min
- Tidal volume: > 5 mL/kg
- Vital capacity: > 10 mL/kg
- Minute ventilation: < 10 L/min
- Negative inspiratory force (NIF): < –20 cm H_2O
- Shallow breathing index (respiratory frequency/tidal volume): <80

TABLE 12-12 Risk Factors of Death From Asthma

- History of sudden severe exacerbations
- Prior intubations
- Prior admission to an ICU due to asthma
- >2 hospitalizations per year
- >3 ER visits for asthma
- Hospitalization or ER visit within last 30 days
- Use of >2 canisters of β_2 per month
- Current use of steroids or recent withdrawal from them
- Comorbidity (cardiovascular or COPD)
- Serious psychiatric illness
- Illicit drug use
- Poor perception of air flow or severity
- Low socioeconomic status
- Sensitivity to mold

In addition, an alogrithm for the evaluation and treatment of acute asthma is provided (Fig. 12-9) and a table with risk factors for asthma mortality included (Table12-12). Separate tables are provided covering the diagnosis of ARDS (Table 12-13) and SARS (Table 12-14) and general principles of management of pulmonary edema (Table 12-15), ARDS (Table 12-16), and the selection of antibiotic therapy for the treatment of community acquired pneumonia (Table 12-17).

TABLE 12-13 Consensus Criteria for the Diagnosis of ARDS

I. Acute onset
II. History compatible with specific risk factors
   - Trauma
   - Severe shock
   - Sepsis (septic abortion included)
   - Aspiration
   - Venous fluid, fat or amniotic fluid embolism
   - Pneumonia
   - Pancreatitis
   - Blood transfusion
   - Seizures (including eclampsia)
   - Overdose
   - Drug induced
   - Eclampsia
   - Abruptio placentae
   - Dead fetus syndrome or retained products of conception
   - Diabetic ketoacidosis
III. Clinical exclusion of cardiogenic pulmonary edema (or PCWP < 18 mmHg)
IV. Respiratory distress
V. Diffuse bilateral patchy opacities in chest x ray
VI. PaO_2/FIO_2 of < 200[a]

[a]Acute lung injury: Less severe form of ARDS with a PaO_2/FiO_2 between 201 and 300 mmHg.
Source: Modified from *Am J Respir Crit Care Med* 1994;149:818–824.

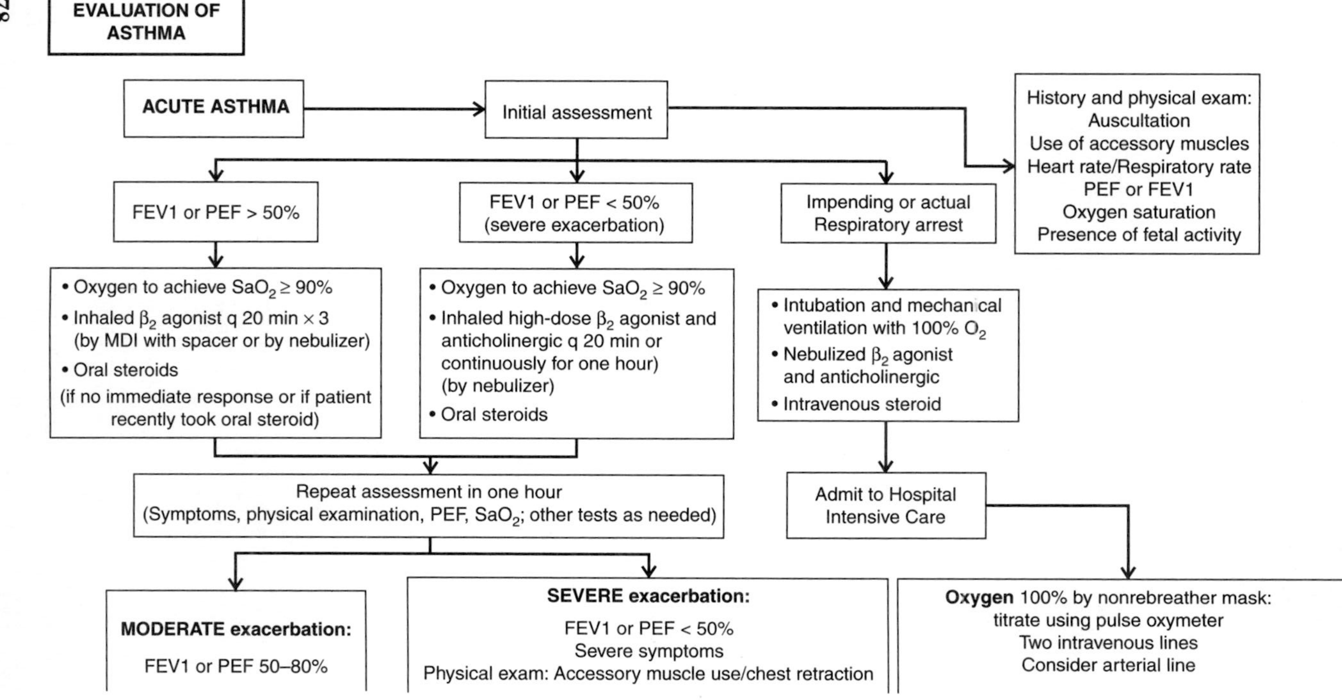
EVALUATION OF ASTHMA
ACUTE ASTHMA
Initial assessment
History and physical exam:
Auscultation
Use of accessory muscles
Heart rate/Respiratory rate
PEF or FEV1
Oxygen saturation
Presence of fetal activity
FEV1 or PEF > 50%
FEV1 or PEF < 50% (severe exacerbation)
Impending or actual Respiratory arrest
• Oxygen to achieve $SaO_2 \geq 90\%$
• Inhaled β_2 agonist q 20 min × 3 (by MDI with spacer or by nebulizer)
• Oral steroids
(if no immediate response or if patient recently took oral steroid)
• Oxygen to achieve $SaO_2 \geq 90\%$
• Inhaled high-dose β_2 agonist and anticholinergic q 20 min or continuously for one hour) (by nebulizer)
• Oral steroids
• Intubation and mechanical ventilation with 100% O_2
• Nebulized β_2 agonist and anticholinergic
• Intravenous steroid
Repeat assessment in one hour
(Symptoms, physical examination, PEF, SaO_2; other tests as needed)
Admit to Hospital Intensive Care
MODERATE exacerbation:
FEV1 or PEF 50–80%
SEVERE exacerbation:
FEV1 or PEF < 50%
Severe symptoms
Physical exam: Accessory muscle use/chest retraction
Oxygen 100% by nonrebreather mask:
titrate using pulse oxymeter
Two intravenous lines
Consider arterial line

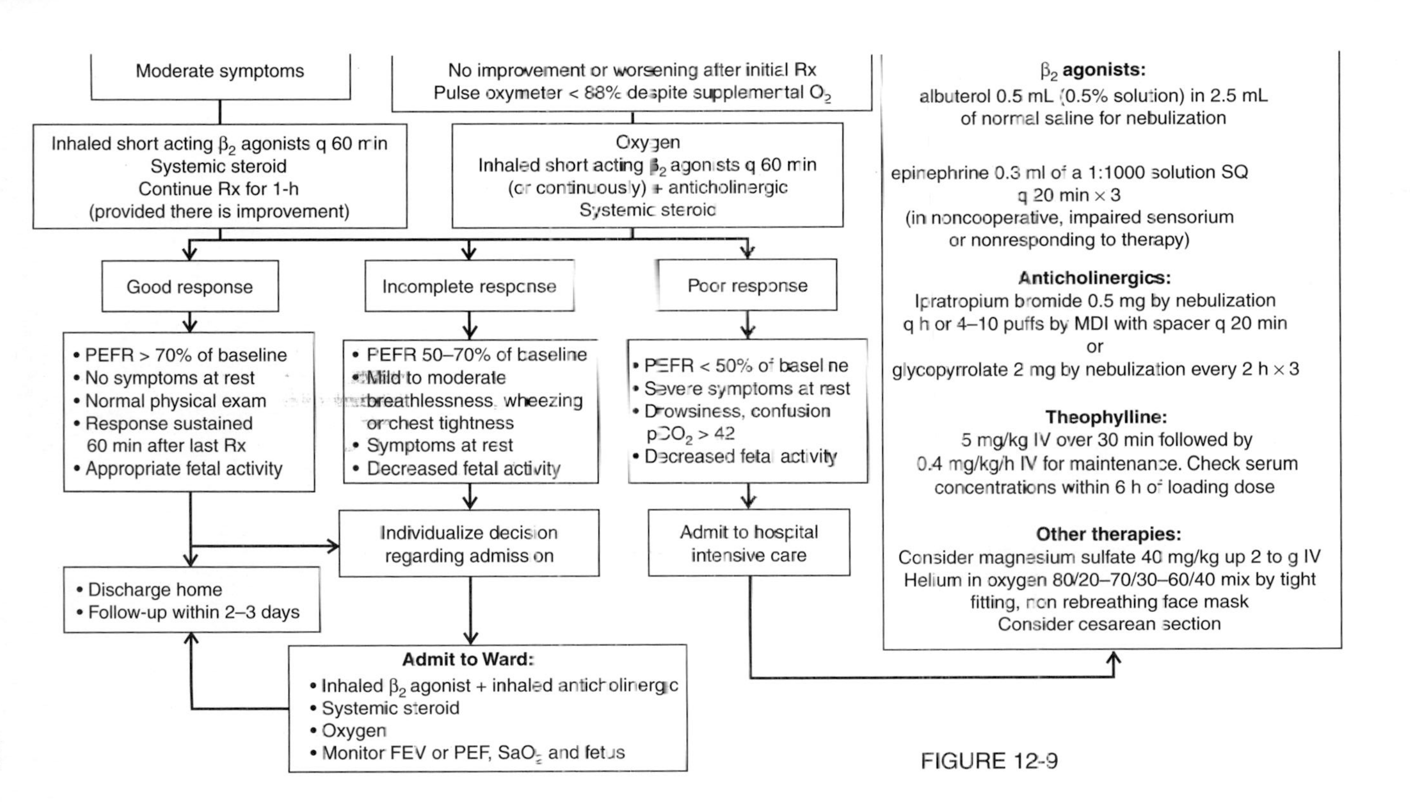
Moderate symptoms
No improvement or worsening after initial Rx
Pulse oxymeter < 88% despite supplemental O_2
Inhaled short acting β_2 agonists q 60 min
Systemic steroid
Continue Rx for 1-h
(provided there is improvement)
Oxygen
Inhaled short acting β_2 agonists q 60 min
(or continuously) + anticholinergic
Systemic steroid
Good response
Incomplete response
Poor response
• PEFR > 70% of baseline
• No symptoms at rest
• Normal physical exam
• Response sustained 60 min after last Rx
• Appropriate fetal activity
• PEFR 50–70% of baseline
• Mild to moderate breathlessness, wheezing or chest tightness
• Symptoms at rest
• Decreased fetal activity
• PEFR < 50% of baseline
• Severe symptoms at rest
• Drowsiness, confusion $pCO_2 > 42$
• Decreased fetal activity
Individualize decision regarding admission
Admit to hospital intensive care
• Discharge home
• Follow-up within 2–3 days
Admit to Ward:
• Inhaled β_2 agonist + inhaled anticholinergic
• Systemic steroid
• Oxygen
• Monitor FEV or PEF, SaO_2 and fetus
β_2 agonists:
albuterol 0.5 mL (0.5% solution) in 2.5 mL of normal saline for nebulization
epinephrine 0.3 ml of a 1:1000 solution SQ q 20 min × 3
(in noncooperative, impaired sensorium or nonresponding to therapy)
Anticholinergics:
Ipratropium bromide 0.5 mg by nebulization q h or 4–10 puffs by MDI with spacer q 20 min
or
glycopyrrolate 2 mg by nebulization every 2 h × 3
Theophylline:
5 mg/kg IV over 30 min followed by 0.4 mg/kg/h IV for maintenance. Check serum concentrations within 6 h of loading dose
Other therapies:
Consider magnesium sulfate 40 mg/kg up 2 to g IV
Helium in oxygen 80/20–70/30–60/40 mix by tight fitting, non rebreathing face mask
Consider cesarean section

FIGURE 12-9

TABLE 12-14 Case Definition of Severe Acute Respiratory Syndrome (SARS)

Case classification

- Suspect case: meets clinical criteria for moderate respiratory illness of unknown etiology, and epidemiologic criteria for exposure (laboratory criteria confirmed, negative, or undetermined)
- Probable case: meets clinical criteria for severe respiratory illness of unknown etiology and epidemiologic criteria for exposure (laboratory criteria confirmed, negative, or undetermined)

Clinical criteria

- Moderate respiratory illness
  - Temperature of >100.48°F (>38°C)*
  - One or more clinical findings of respiratory illness (e.g., cough, shortness of breath, difficulty breathing, or hypoxia)
- Severe respiratory illness
  - Temperature of >100.48°F (>38°C)*
  - One or more clinical findings of respiratory illness (e.g., cough, shortness of breath, difficulty breathing, or hypoxia), and
    - radiographic evidence of pneumonia, or
    - respiratory distress syndrome

Epidemiologic criteria

- Travel (including transit at an airport) within 10 days of onset of symptoms to an area with current or previously documented or suspected community transmission of SARS (mainland China, Hong Kong, Hanoi (Vietnam), Singapore, Toronto (Canada) or Taiwan), or
- Close contact within 10 days of onset of symptoms with a person known or suspected to have SARS

Exclusion criteria

A case may be excluded as a suspect or probable SARS case if

- An alternative diagnosis can fully explain the illness
- The case was reported on the basis of contact with an index case that was subsequently excluded as a case of SARS (e.g., another etiology fully explains the illness) provided other possible epidemiologic exposure criteria are not present

Source: Modified from Updated Interim U.S. Case Definition of Severe Acute Respiratory Syndrome (SARS). *CDC*. 5/23/2003.

TABLE 12-15 Principles of Management of Pulmonary Edema

Diagnosis
- Progressive (not sudden) shortness of breath
- Desaturation
- Tachypnea
- Occasionally hypertension
- Bilateral crackles
- S3/Gallop (not always)

Predisposing factors
- Fluid overload
- Preeclampsia
- Tocolytic treatment
- Uncontrolled hypertension

Management
- Semi-Fowler position: Elevate head and chest to improve ventilation
- Oxygen: Administer at 10 L/min via nonrebreather face mask or with CPAP (intubation may be required)
- Continuous pulse oxymetry and cardiac monitoring
- Establish IV access; limit intravenous fluid infusion (30–50 mL/h)
- Identify and control predisposing factor(s)

Pharmacologic therapy
- Morphine sulfate: 3–5 mg IV may be given; (avoid in the presence of altered consciousness, increased intracranial pressure or severe COPD)
- Furosemide: 20–40 mg IV; repeat as necessary (do not use more than 120 mg/h and give slowly to prevent ototoxicity)
- Nitroglycerin: 2 in of paste to chest or 1 pill (1/150) until IV access is secured or no other therapy available
- Hydralazine: 5–10 mg IV may be considered if severe hypertension is mediating the pulmonary edema

Monitor
- Input and output
- Blood pressure and fetal heart rate monitoring if appropriate according to GA

TABLE 12-16 Principles of Treatment of ARDS

Therapeutic goals
- Adequate oxygenation
- Avoidance of barotraumas with treatment
- Avoidance of cardiovascular compromise

Management
- Semi-Fowler position: Elevate head and chest to improve ventilation
- Oxygen: Administer at 10 L/min via nonrebreather face mask or with CPAP (Intubation may be required)
- Continuous pulse oxymetry and cardiac monitoring
- Establish IV access. Consider placement of arterial line and a central line
- Identify and control predisposing factor(s)

Pharmacologic therapy: None specific available. In severe cases consult pulmonary services for consideration of nitric oxide, pulmonary vasodilatation, corticosteroids, exogenous surfactant administration, prone ventilation, or extracellular membrane oxygenation (ECMO)

Monitor
- Input and output
- Blood pressure and fetal heart rate monitoring if appropriate according to GA

TABLE 12-17 Empirical Selection of Antibiotics for Patients with Community-Acquired Pneumonia

Specific therapy is desirable within 8 h of onset of empirical therapy to narrow the spectrum and direct the treatment

Hospitalized patients

I. General medical ward
   - Generally preferred are an extended spectrum cephalosporin combined with a macrolide or a fluoroquinolone (alone) OR
   - β-lactam/β-lactamase inhibitor combined with either a macrolide or a fluoroquinolone

II. Intensive care unit
   - Generally preferred are an extended-spectrum cephalosporin or β-lactam/β-lactamase inhibitor plus a macrolide
     - If structural lung disease: antipseudomonal agents (piperacillin, piperacillin-tazobactam, carbapenem, or cefepime) plus a fluoroquinolone (including high-dose ciprofloxacin)
     - If β-lactam allergy: fluoroquinolone ± clindamycin
     - If suspected aspiration: fluoroquinolone with or without clindamycin, metronidazole, or a β-lactam/β-lactamase inhibitor

Outpatients

- Generally preferred are (not in any particular order): doxycycline, a macrolide or a fluoroquinolone.
  - Penicillin-resistant pneumococci may be resistant to macrolides and/or doxycycline. Selection should be influenced by regional antibiotic susceptibility patterns for *S. pneumoniae* and the presence of other risk factors for drug-resistant *S. pneumoniae*

Note

- *β-Lactam/β-lactamase inhibitor:* ampicillin-sulbactam or piperacillin-tazobactam
- *Extended-spectrum cephalosporin:* cefotaxime or ceftriaxone
- *Fluoroquinolone:* gatifloxacin, levofloxacin, moxifloxacin, or other fluoroquinolone with enhanced activity against *S. pneumoniae*
- *Macrolide:* azithromycin, clarithromycin, or erythromycin

Source: From *Clin Infect Diseases* 2000;31:347–382.

Abbreviations Used

BP	Blood pressure
Hb	Hemoglobin
ICU	Intensive care unit
O_2	Oxygen
PaO_2	Arterial oxygen's partial pressure
$PaCO_2$	Arterial carbon dioxide's partial pressure
$P(A\text{-}a)O_2$	Alveolar-arterial oxygen difference
PEEP	Positive end expiratory pressure
SOB	Shortness of breath
Vd	Dead space
Vt	Tidal volume
Wga	Weeks of gestational age
ECF	Extracellular fluid
AG	Anion gap

SUGGESTED READING

AARC Clinical Practice Guideline: Oxygen therapy for adults in the acute care facility-2002 revision and update. *Respir Care* 2002;47:717.

American College of Emergency Physicians: Clinical policy for the initial approach to adults presenting with the chief complaint of chest pain, with no history of trauma. *Ann Emerg Med* 1995;25:274.

American Thoracic Society: The diagnostic approach to acute venous thromboembolism. *Am J Respir Care Med* 1999;160:1043.

Bartlett JG, Dowell SF, Mandell LA, et al.: Guidelines from the Infectious Diseases Society of America. Practice Guidelines for the Management of Community-Acquired Pneumonia in Adults. *CID* 2000;31:347.

Crapo RO: Normal cardiopulmonary physiology during pregnancy. *Clin Obstet Gynecol* 1999;39:3.

Deblieux PM, Summer WR: Acute respiratory failure in pregnancy. *Clin Obstet Gynecol* 1996;39:143.

Gei AF, Vadhera RB, Hankins GDV: Embolism during pregnancy: thrombus, air and amniotic fluid. *Anesthesiology Clin N Am* 2003;21:165.

George RB, Light RW, Mathay MA, et al.: Chest Medicine. *Essentials of Pulmonary and Critical Care Medicine,* 4th edn. Philadelphia, PA: Lippincott Williams and Wilkins, 2000.

Goodrum LA: Pneumonia in pregnancy. *Semin Perinatol* 1997;21:276.

Ie S, Rubio ER, Alper B, et al.: Respiratory complications of pregnancy. *Obstet Gynecol Survey* 2001;57:39.

King TE: Restrictive lung disease in pregnancy. *Clin Chest Med* 1992;13:607.

Lee RW: Pulmonary embolism. *Chest Surg Clin N Am* 2002;12:417.

National Asthma Education Program: National Institute of Health. *Practical Guide for the Diagnosis and Management of Asthma.* NIH Publication A97-4053, 1997.

O'Day M: Cardiorespiratory physiological adaptation of pregnancy. *Semin Perinatol* 1997;21:268.

Rodgers L, Dangel-Palmer MC, Berner N: Acute circulatory and respiratory collapse in obstetrical patients: A case report and review of the literature. *AANA J* 1985;68:444.

Rowe TF: Acute gastric aspiration: prevention and treatment. *Semin Perinatol* 1997;21:313.

Saade GR: Human immunodeficiency virus (HIV)-related pulmonary complications in pregnancy. *Semin Perinatol* 1997;21:336.

Van Hook JW: Acute respiratory distress syndrome in pregnancy. *Semin Perinatol* 1997;21:320.

Witlin AG: Asthma in pregnancy. *Semin Perinatol* 1997;21:284.

Zimmerman JL: *Fundamental critical care support*, 3rd edn., Society of Critical Care Medicine. Des Plaines IL, 2001.

Zlatnik MG: Pulmonary edema: etiology and treatment. *Semin Perinatol* 1997;21:298.

13 Acute Renal Failure in Pregnancy

Tamerou Asrat   Michael P. Nageotte

INTRODUCTION

Acute renal failure can occur in patients with multiple complications but is predominantly observed in hospitalized patients. This is not a rare medical condition since as many as five percent of all hospitalized patients have some degree of acute renal failure. With respect to the obstetrical patient, however, acute renal failure has become an uncommon complication of pregnancy in developed countries. It is estimated that the current incidence of acute renal failure (ARF) complicating pregnancy approximates 1 per 10,000 pregnant women. In three successive periods of 10 years between 1958 and 1987, Stratta and colleagues have reported a continued decrease in ARF requiring emergency renal dialysis from a rate of 1 in 3000 in 1958 to 1 in 15,000 pregnancies in 1987. They documented 81 cases of ARF in pregnancy of which 11.6 percent experienced irreversible renal damage. A majority of these cases of ARF resulted from complications of either severe preeclampsia or eclampsia. Possible explanations for this dramatic trend in this subset of patients include ready availability of prenatal care and the legalization of medical abortions, as main factors responsible for this reduction in the incidence of ARF requiring dialytic support. However, in the underdeveloped countries of the world, ARF remains a frequent complication of pregnancy and has an attendant maternal mortality surpassing 50 percent. In these countries, ARF has a bimodal distribution with peaks in the first and third trimester, presumably reflective of the continued practice of illegal abortions, the lack of access to quality prenatal care and the occurrence of preeclampsia or eclampsia. Whatever the explanation, acute renal failure in pregnancy can be the result of any of the disorders which lead to severe renal dysfunction in nonpregnant patients or may result from disorders that are unique to the pregnant condition.

RENAL ANATOMY AND FUNCTION DURING PREGNANCY

An understanding of the dramatic changes, which occur normally in renal architecture, function, and blood flow, is essential for the correct diagnosis and management of renal disease in the pregnant patient (Table 13-1).

Anatomic Changes

There is a marked increase in kidney size during pregnancy. This increase in size is primarily due to the increase in renal vascular volume and in the capacity of the collecting system. Hormonal influence is the most likely cause of the dilatation of the urinary collecting system. In addition, increased production of prostaglandin E_2 (PGE_2), which inhibits urethral peristalsis, and mechanical obstruction by the enlarging uterus and distended iliac vessels (particularly on the right side) contributes to these changes, which are evident as early as the first trimester and may continue for as long as 12 weeks postpartum.

TABLE 13-1 Renal Changes in Normal Pregnancy

Alteration	Change	Clinical relevance
Increased renal size	Renal length about 1 cm greater on x rays	Postpartum decrease in size should not be mistaken for parenchymal loss
Dilation of pelves, calyces, and ureters	Resembles hydronephrosis on ultrasound or IVP	Not to be mistaken for obstructive uropathy, increased rates of upper tract infections
Increased renal hemodynamics	Increased GFR and renal plasma flow	Decreased serum creatinine and BUN, increased excretion of amino acids, protein, and glucose
Changes in acid base metabolism	Renal bicarbonate threshold decreases	Serum bicarbonate are 4–5 meq/L
Renal water handling	Osmoregulation altered with decreased osmotic thresholds for AVP release, and thirst	Serum osmolality decreases 10 mOsm/L during normal gestation

Changes in Renal Blood Flow, Glomerular Filtration Rate and Renal Tubular Function

Substantial increases in renal blood flow occur beginning early in the first trimester. This increase in renal blood flow is caused by both an increase in cardiac output and a decrease in renal vascular resistance. Renal vasodilatation is believed to be the most important mechanism for the dramatic rise in renal blood flow. Estimates of renal vascular resistance reveal a 50 percent decrease in renal vascular resistance by the end of the first trimester. The underlying physiologic processes and causes of this pregnancy related renal-vasodilatation are not clearly understood. The large increases in the concentration of PGE_2 and prostacyclin (PGI_2) are believed to contribute to this effect, but do not appear to be the only mechanism. Prolactin may be a hormonal mediator of renal vasodilatation in pregnancy. Estimation of renal plasma flow from *p*-aminohippuric acid clearance studies indicates an effective renal plasma flow of 809 mL/mm in the first trimester, 695 mL/mm in the last 10 weeks of pregnancy, and 482 mL/mm during the postpartum period. The most important consequence of this increase in renal blood flow during pregnancy is a dramatic rise in glomerular filtration rate (GFR). An increase in GFR of about 45 percent is seen as early as at the end of the first trimester, and unlike renal plasma flow, this increase in GFR is maintained until term.

Despite this marked increase in GFR, the renal tubules are not only able to preserve normal sodium (Na+) balance, but are also able to achieve a cumulative Na+ retention of 500 to 900 meq during the course of a normal pregnancy. Further, pregnant women maintain a normal sodium balance in settings when sodium intake is either increased or decreased. Pregnant women also maintain normal water balance and retain the ability to produce appropriately concentrated or dilute urine despite a significant alteration in the thirst and argenine vasopressin (AVP) release thresholds during normal pregnancy.

Similarly potassium (K^+) metabolism in pregnancy is unchanged. There is a physiologic requirement for the retention of approximately 350 meq of potassium for the developing fetal-placental unit along with a significant expansion of maternal red cell volume. This increase in potassium retention occurs despite the dramatically elevated levels of aldosterone in the plasma of pregnant patients.

Pregnancy results in a respiratory alkalosis with a decrease of about 10 mmHg in the arterial Pco_2. The slight respiratory alkalosis is compensated by an increased excretion of bicarbonate by the kidneys resulting in a decrease in the plasma bicarbonate level to 18 to 20 meq/L.

These physiologic anatomic and functional changes seen in the renal systems of pregnant patients have practical consequences. For example, dilated collecting systems make the diagnosis of an obstructive uropathy challenging. The increased GFR and tubular functions result in changes of the normal laboratory values for the commonly employed serum tests of renal function. Examples include normal blood urea nitrogen values in pregnancy average 8.7 ± 1.5 mg/dL and serum creatinine levels average 0.46 ± 0.13 mg/dL. Glucosuria is also a common finding during normal pregnancy.

Acute Renal Failure in Pregnancy

Acute renal failure (ARF) is a syndrome characterized by the rapid (hours to weeks) decline in renal function resulting in the retention of nitrogenous waste products such as BUN and creatinine along with the inability to maintain normal fluid and electrolyte balances. Nonpregnant patients with acute renal failure are often asymptomatic but, when seen in pregnancy, ARF is rarely encountered in the absence of significant clinical findings or events complicating the gestation. ARF may complicate a host of diseases that, for purposes of diagnoses and management, are conveniently divided into three categories (Table 13-2):

1. Diseases characterized by renal hypoperfusion in which the integrity of renal parenchymal tissue is preserved (prerenal azotemia, prerenal ARF). This is the most common form of ARF, and has the best prognosis.
2. Diseases involving renal parenchymal tissue (intrarenal azotemia, or intrinsic renal ARF).
3. Diseases associated with an acute obstruction of the urinary tract (postrenal azotemia, postrenal ARF).

Most acute intrinsic renal azotemia is caused by ischemia or nephrotoxins and is classically associated with acute tubular necrosis (ATN). Thus, in clinical practice the term ATN is commonly used to denote ischemic or nephrotoxic ARF.

In prerenal ARF, impaired renal perfusion is the problem and this may be secondary to true intravascular volume depletion, decreased effective circulating volume to the kidneys secondary to impaired cardiac output or due to agents which alter renal perfusion. Prerenal ARF may be rarely seen in the first trimester of pregnancy as a complication of severe hyperemesis gravidarum. In the second and third trimesters, severe blood loss as a complication of uterine hemorrhage in the antepartum, intrapartum or postpartum periods is an important and not an uncommon cause of hypovolemia and subsequent ARF. It is important to remember that maternal bleeding may be concealed behind the placenta in some patients with serious placental abruption and this

TABLE 13-2 Acute Renal Failure in Pregnancy

Differential diagnosis
Prerenal azotemia
• Hyperemesis gravidarum
• Hemorrhage from any cause
Intrarenal azotemia or acute tubular necrosis
• Preeclampsia
• HELLP syndrome
• Acute fatty liver of pregnancy
• Postpartum renal failure
• Bilateral renal cortical necrosis
• Pyelonephritis
• Acute interstitial nephritis
• Acute glomerulonephritis
Obstructive
• Post renal azotemia

condition may also be accompanied by varying degrees of a consumptive coagulopathy which can further complicate the degree of renal dysfunction.

Pregnancy is associated with a higher incidence of both bladder infections and pyelonephritis. This increased incidence of both upper and lower urinary tract infections, estimated to complicate approximately 2 percent of all pregnancies, is believed to result from both hormonal and mechanical changes, which result in stasis within the urinary collecting system. Unlike their nonpregnant counterparts, pregnant women with pyelonephritis can manifest a substantial decrease in creatinine clearance and rarely may experience some degree of transient ARF. Patients with pyelonephritis in pregnancy complicated by ARF often have evidence of chronic renal parenchymal infection and recovery following appropriate antimicrobial therapy may be incomplete.

Severe preeclampsia and eclampsia account for a majority of the ARF cases unique to pregnancy. Renal failure is unusual even with severe diseases, unless there has also been significant blood loss with hemodynamic instablility or severe disseminated intravascular coagulopathy. Usually the clinical picture of ARF seen in such patients is that of ATN and typically resolves spontaneously within the first two weeks postpartum. While in the short term, some of these patients with preeclampsia/eclampsia induced ATN may require dialytic support, in general even these more seriously affected patients experience complete recovery and have an excellent long term prognosis. In the patients with ATN secondary to preeclampsia, in whom the disease persists and long term dialysis is necessary, frequently, it appears that pregnancy and/or preeclampsia have unmasked a chronic renal disorder or there has been some degree of renal cortical necrosis. When ARF develops in patients with severe preeclampsia or eclampsia, consideration should be given to effecting delivery as safely and as expeditiously as possible since the maternal condition will frequently improve drametically, postpartum.

Preeclamptic/eclamptic patients, patients who develop placental abruption with or without coagulopathy, pregnancies in which there is a prolonged intrauterine fetal demise complicated with DIC, or women experiencing an amniotic fluid embolism are at an increased risk of developing renal cortical necrosis. Renal cortical necrosis, a pathologic process which destroys the renal cortex partially or completely while sparing the medulla, is heralded by the abrupt onset of oliguria or anuria which may be accompanied by flank pain, gross hematuria, and hypotension. This triad of anuria, gross hematuria, and flank pain is unusual in the other causes of renal failure in pregnancy. Renal cortical necrosis is not unique to pregnancy. However, pregnancy related cases account for up to 70 percent of all cases. This entity is diagnosed based upon the clinical presentation and can usually be established with ultrasonography or CT scanning of the kidneys. The characteristic findings are hypoechoic or hypodense areas in the renal cortex. There is no specific therapy that has been shown to be effective for patients with renal cortical necrosis with many women requiring chronic hemodialysis. Approximately 30 to 40 percent of patients experience at least partial recovery and have markedly compromised creatinine clearances.

Other clinical entities more commonly associated with pregnancy and acute renal failure, with varying degrees of proteinuria, are seen in patients with hemolysis, elevated liver function tests and low platelets (HELLP syndrome), acute fatty liver of pregnancy, postpartum renal failure due to adult hemolytic uremic syndrome (HUS) and thrombotic thrombocytopenic purpura (TTP). Some investigators group these disease processes and preeclampsia under the same rubric of microangiopathic hemolytic processes of pregnancy, because they share a common histologic feature of anemia with evidence of red cell destruction on peripheral smears. The clinical manifestation and the nomenclature of the disease reflect the primary target organ. However, it is believed that there may be a unifying pathophysiologic process of profound vasoconstriction of arterioles resulting from an, as yet, unidentified toxin or mechanism likely to involve the vascular endothelium. Consequently, in acute fatty liver of pregnancy, although this rare complication of pregnancy is associated with ARF in up to 60 percent of the cases, the target organ is primarily the liver, with accompanying alterations of normal laboratory values such as transaminases, bilirubin, glucose metabolism, and various clotting factors (e.g., antithrombin III, fibrinogen). Similarly, in postpartum renal failure resulting from HUS, the kidneys appear to be the target organs with resultant alterations in normal renal function assays and, in comparison to renal dysfunction associated with HELLP syndrome or acute fatty liver of pregnancy, protracted acute renal failure may result. While HUS is generally a postpartum disease and HELLP syndrome is a form of severe preeclampsia usually confined to the late second or third trimesters, TTP almost always occurs antepartum and, although it may occur in the third trimester, many cases appear before 24 weeks of gestation. TTP is characterized by the pentad of microangiopathic hemolytic anemia, thrombocytopenia, renal insufficiency, fever, and neurologic abnormalities. The severity of renal dysfunction is usually mild, particularly in comparison with the more striking neurological involvement, fever, and thrombocytopenia.

Diagnosis of ARF

Regardless of the underlying cause of ARF the diagnosis usually hinges on serial analysis of BUN, creatinine, urinalysis, and urinary sediment analysis. It must be emphasized, however, that measurements of BUN and creatinine are relatively insensitive indices of glomerular function. For instance, the GFR may fall by 50 percent before the serum creatinine values rise. Conversely a relatively large increment in the serum creatinine value reflects

TABLE 13-3 Clinical Approach to the Diagnosis of ARF

History and physical: including drug history, previous records, and detailed review of the hospital chart
Urinalysis: specific gravity, microscopic, dipstick, and staining for eosinophils
Flow charts: daily weights, serial blood pressures, serial BUN and creatinine, and major clinical events and interventions
Routine blood chemistry and hematology tests: BUN, creatinine, electrolytes and red and white cell counts
Selected special investigations: Urine chemistry, eosinophils, and/or immunoelectrophoresis
Serologic tests: antiglomerular basement membrane antibodies, ANA, cryoglobulins, antistreptolysin O antibodies, and anti-DNase titers
Radiologic evaluations: plain abdominal films, renal ultrasonography, intravenous pyelography, and renal angiography
Renal biopsy: rarely used

relatively small decrement in GFR in patients with preexisting chronic renal disease (Tables 13-3, 13-4, and 13-5).

The clinical approach to the diagnosis of acute renal failure involves a detailed history and physical, urinalysis, flow charts of serial blood pressures, daily weights, urine output and intake, routine laboratory assessments, and special diagnostic procedures (Table 13-2).

The clinical course of ATN can be divided into three phases, irrespective of the underlying disease process: the initiation phase, the maintenance phase, and the recovery phase. In the initiation phase, patients have been exposed to the insult, either ischemia, or toxins, and while the picture is evolving, renal parenchymal injury is not yet established. The initiation phase is followed by the maintenance phase, in which the renal parenchymal injury is established and GFR stabilizes at a value of 5 to 10 mL/min. Urine output is usually lowest during this period. This phase typically lasts one to two weeks, but

TABLE 13-4 Urine Indices Used in the Differential Diagnosis of Prerenal and Ischemic Intrinsic Renal Azotemia

Diagnositc index	Prerenal azotemia	Ischemic intrinsic azotemia
Fractional excretion of Na^+ (%) $\frac{U_{Na} \times P_{cr}}{P_{Na} \times U_{Na}} \times 100$	<1	>1
Urinary Na^+ concentration (meq/L)	<10	>10
Urinary creatinine/plasma creatinine ratio	>40	<20
Urinary urea nitrogen/plasma urea nitrogen, ratio	>8	<3
Urine specific gravity	>1.018	<1.012
Urine osmolality (mOsm/kg H_2O)	>500	<250
Plasma BUN/cretinine ratio	>20	<10–15
Renal failure index $U_{Na}/U_{cr}/P_{cr}$	<1	>1
Urine sediment	Hyaline casts	Muddy brown granular casts

TABLE 13-5 Urine Sediment in the Differential Diagnosis of Acute Renal Failure

Normal or few red blood cells or white blood cells
Prerenal azotemia
Arterial thrombosis or embolism
Preglomerular vasculitis
HUS or TTP
Scleroderma crisis
  Post renal azotemia

Granular casts
ATN (muddy brown)
Glomerulonephritis or vasculitis
  Interstitial nephritis

Red blood cell casts
Glomerulonephritis or vasculitis
Malignant hypertension
Rarely interstitial nephritis

White blood cell casts
Acute interstitial nephritis or exudative glomerulonephritis
  Severe pyelonephritis
  Marked leukemic or lymphomatous infiltration
Eosinophiluria (>5%)
  Allergic interstitial nephritis (antibiotics> NSAIDS)
  Atheroembolic disease
Crsytalluria
  Acute urate nephropathy
  Calcium oxalate (ethylene glycol toxicity)
  Acyclovir
  Sulfonamides
  Radiocontrast agents

may be prolonged for 1 to 11 months depending upon the etiology before recovery, if any. Uremic complications usually arise during this phase. The recovery phase is heralded by a gradual restoration of the urine output and a decline in the serum BUN and creatinine. The recovery phase is frequently accompanied by a marked diuresis which results in profound electrolyte disturbances unless correctly monitored and corrected.

Management of Acute Renal Failure

The initial therapy for acute renal failure should be focused on correction of the specific etiology of the renal dysfunction, reestablishing normal fluid and electrolyte abnormalities, being cognizant of potential complications, and maintaining appropriate nutritional and medical requirements (Tables 13-6, 13-7, and 13-8). Prerenal azotemia is rapidly reversible upon restoration of renal perfusion. The source of the loss of fluid determines the composition of the replacement fluid. Hypovolemia, caused by hemorrhage, is ideally corrected with packed red blood cells. Isotonic saline is usually an appropriate replacement for plasma losses. Urinary or gastrointestinal fluids are generally hypotonic. Accordingly, initial replacement can be achieved with hypotonic solutions (e.g., 0.45% saline) and subsequent replacement should be based on laboratory values. Serum potassium and acid base status

TABLE 13-6 Common Complications of ARF

Metabolic	Hematologic
Hyperkalemia	Anemia
Metabolic acidosis	• Bleeding
Hyponatremia	**Neurologic**
Hypocalcemia	Neuromuscular irritability
• Hyperphosphotemia	Asterixis
• Hypermagnesemia	Seizures
Hyperurecemia	Mental status changes
Cardiovascular	• Somnolence
Pulmonary edema	• Coma
• Arrhythmias	**Infectious**
• Pericarditis	Pneumonia
• Pericardial effusion	• Wound infections
• Hypertension	• Intravenous line infections
• Myocardial infarction	• Septicemia
• Pulmonary embolus	• Urinary tract infection
• Pneumonitis	**Other**
Gastrointestinal	Hiccups
Nausea	• Decreased insulin catabolism
• Vomiting	• Mild insulin resistance
• Malnutrition	• Elevated parathyroid hormone
• Gastritis	• Reduced 1,25-dihydroxy and 25-vitamin D
• Gastrointestinal ulcers	• hydroxyvitamin
• Gastrointestinal bleeding	Low total T_3 and T_4
Stomatitis or gingivitis	Normal free T_4
Parotitis or pancreatitis	

TABLE 13-7 Supportive Management of Intrinsic ARF

Intravascular volume overload
Restriction of salt (1–2 g/day and water usually <1 L/day)
Diuretics (usually loop blockers ± thiazides)
Ultrafiltration or dialysis

Hyponatremia
Restriction of free water intake (oral and dextrose containing solutions)

Hyperkalemia
Restriction of dietary potassium intake (Eliminate K^+ supplements and K^+ sparing diuretics)
K^+ binding ion exchange resins
Glucose (50 mL of 50% dextrose) and insulin (10 U regular)
Sodium bicarbonate (usually 50–100 meq)
Calcium gluconate (10 mL of 10% solution over 5 min)
Dialysis

Metabolic acidosis
Restriction of dietary protein
Sodium bicarbonate (maintain serum HCO_3^- > 15 meq/L)
Dialysis

TABLE 13-8 Supportive Management of Intrinsic ARF

Hyperphosphatemia
Restriction of dietary phosphate intake. Use PO_4^{3-} binding agents (calcium carbonate, aluminum hydroxide)
Hypocalcemia
Calcium carbonate (if symptomatic or if sodium bicarbonate is to be administered)
Calcium gluconate (10–20 mL of 10% solution)
Hypermagnesemia
Discontinue Mg^{++} containing antacids
Hyperuricemia
Treatment usually not necessary (if <15 mg/dL)
Nutrition
Restriction of dietary protein (~0.5 g/kg/day)
Carbohydrate (~100 g/day)
Enteral or parenteral nutrition (if recovery is prolonged)
Drug dosage
Adjust dosage for degree of renal impairment

should be monitored in all patients. In certain instances, use of insulin and glucose replacement may be necessary to lower the plasma potassium levels. Alternative therapies include sodium polystyrene sulfonate (Kayexalate) orally or as an enema or consideration of dialysis.

Fluid management is particularly difficult in patients with ARF, resulting from underlying severe preeclampsia, since they are not necessarily volume depleted and are at increased risk for developing pulmonary edema. Liberal use of invasive monitoring with a pulmonary artery catheter has been recommended. In patients with ARF, due to severe preelampsia, there may be a poor correlation between the central venous pressure (CVP) value and the pulmonary capillary wedge pressure (PCWP). Therefore, it is preferable to use a pulmonary artery catheter, which can measure the PCWP, in order to be able to correctly determine the optimal fluid and pharmacologic management of such patients. Similarly, measurements of urinary indices may not accurately reflect the volume status of the patient and allow the clinician to differentiate between prerenal azotemia and intrinsic renal disease. Patients who do not respond to initial fluid boluses of 500 to 1000 cc should have a pulmonary artery catheter inserted to assist with further management decisions. If the pulmonary capillary wedge pressures indicate euvolemia or hypervolemia and the cause of the renal failure is not prerenal, then efforts should be directed towards medical therapy with diuretics and to selectively dilate the renal vascular bed such as with the use of renal doses of dopamine. Furosemide (Lasix) administration intravenously is the initial treatment for volume-overloaded patients with ARF. If the initial response is inadequate, the administered dosage is doubled or a continuous furosemide drip is initiated until adequate urine output results (0.5 µ/kg/h). As an additional point, all medications should be carefully reviewed and dosages adjusted to maintain appropriate serum levels.

The single most important factor in the appropriate management of intrinsic renal azotemia is the optimization of both cardiovascular function and intravascular volume. The clinician must have an appreciation for the potential complications seen in patients with intrinsic renal azotemia and adopt an aggressive preventative management protocol in order to attempt prevention of significant worsening of acute renal failure. Pregnancy represents a unique challenge in such patients, as there are both maternal and fetal concerns. Regardless of the underlying etiology of ARF, there are general guidelines and principles governing its management in pregnancy. As discussed, most cases of ARF complicating pregnancy develop in the postpartum period, thus obviating concerns about fetal well-being. However, in cases of severe preeclampsia/eclampsia or any of the microangiopathic thrombotic processes complicated by ARF, expeditious delivery of the fetus should be carefully considered with appropriate and judicious use of blood product replacement. Oliguria in the pregnant patient is frequently mismanaged. Fluid replacement must be carefully monitored. Indeed, worsening of the medical condition resulting from efforts to reestablish urine production is a common complication of ARF in pregnancy. As with aggressive but inappropriate fluid replacement, the use of potent diuretics, such as furosemide, may increase urine output transiently without correcting the underlying pathology and, in certain instances, such therapy may exacerbate the disease and worsen the clinical condition. One example of this is the oliguric phase of severe preeclampsia, which is managed most appropriately with support and minimal fluid replacement rather than aggressively giving fluid and/or diuretics with the intent to simply establish a greater amount of urine production.

The available data support an early and aggressive use of hemodialysis in ARF which does not respond to fluid replacement and diuretics. This is also applicable to the pregnant patient although the use of acute hemodialysis during pregnancy is quite rare. However, following delivery, it may indeed be necessary to employ this important clinical modality, particularly for patients experiencing protracted renal failure, such as may be seen with hemolytic uremic syndrome or acute cortical necrosis complicating pregnancy. Dialysis has been shown to decrease maternal mortality and accelerate recovery of renal function. Typically, initiation of dialysis should be considered when the BUN reaches 50 to 70 mg/dL or when the serum creatinine is greater than 6 to 7 mg/dL. These are levels lower than those for the nonpregnant patient (Table 13-9).

For women requiring dialysis for renal failure, the reported pregnancy outcomes have been generally poor. In 1980, the European Dialysis and Transplant Association (EDTA) reported a 23 percent successful pregnancy outcome in women conceiving after starting dialysis. Subsequently, there have been reports of a possible improvement with peritoneal dialysis in pregnant women requiring dialysis when compared to the EDTA report. The question of continuing a pregnancy in patients either already dialysis-dependent or who have moderate renal insufficiency at conception, but experience a rapid deterioration of renal function during pregnancy leading to chronic dialysis, is critically important in counseling women with end-stage renal disease. Pregnancy termination with the hopes of improving renal function does not appear to be a

TABLE 13-9 Indications for Dialysis in Pregnancy

1. Clinical evidence of uremia
2. Intractable intravascular volume overload
3. Hyperkalemia or severe acidosis resistant to conservative measures
4. Prophylactic dialysis when BUN > 50–70 mg/dL, or creatinine >6–7 mg/dL

good option. In a recent series of 82 pregnancies in women with chronic renal insufficiency, Jones and Hayslett reported that only 15 percent of the women had a return to baseline renal function at six months postpartum. More recently, in a review of 2300 dialysis units in the United States, Okundaye and colleagues report that over a four-year period, two percent of the female dialysis patients of childbearing age became pregnant. Of the hemodialysis women, 2.4 percent conceived, while 1.1 percent of the peritoneal dialysis women conceived. Of 184 pregnancies occurring in women who conceived after starting dialysis, the infant survival rate was 40.2 percent. Comparatively, the infant survival rate for the 57 pregnancies in women starting dialysis after conception was 73.6 percent. There was no difference in outcome between women receiving hemodialysis versus peritoneal dialysis and these investigators do not recommend switching from one modality to another during pregnancy. However, they do report a possible association between improved outcome and increased time and frequency of dialysis. The major complication remains premature birth resulting in both significant mortality as well as morbidity in the surviving infants.

The role of renal biopsy in pregnancies complicated with ARF is not without controversy. Although such a procedure is valuable in many nonpregnant patients and plays a critical role in establishing the specific renal pathology, renal biopsy has potentially significant complications which may be of more concern in the pregnant patient. Consequently, renal biopsy should rarely, if ever, be performed in a patient with ARF while pregnant.

SUGGESTED READING

Baylis C, Reckelhoff JF: Renal hemodynamics in normal and hypertensive pregnancy: Lessons from micropuncture. *Am J Kidney Dis* 1991;17:98.

Brady HR, Brenner BM, Lieberthal W: Acute Renal Failure. In: Brenner BM (ed), *The Kidney*, 5th edn., Philadelphia: W.B. Saunders, 1996; pp.1200–1252.

Christensen T, Klebe JG, Bertelsen V, et al.: Changes in renal volume during normal pregnancy. *Acta Obstet Gynecol Scand* 1989;68:541.

Davidson J: Changes in renal function and other aspects of homeostasis in early pregnancy. *J Obstet Gynaecol Br Commonw* 1974;81:1003.

Davison J: Renal disease. In: deSwiet M (ed), *Medical Disorders in Obstetric Practice.* Oxford: Blackwell, 1984; p. 236.

Davison JM, Dunlop W: Renal hemodynamics and tubular function in normal human pregnancy. *Kidney Int* 1980;18:152.

DeAlvarez RR: Renal glomerulotubular mechanisms during normal pregnancy: I. Glomerular filtration rate, renal plasma flow and creatinine clearance. *Am J Obstet Gynecol* 1958;75:931.

Donohue JF. Acute bilateral cortical necrosis. In: Brenner BM, Lazarus J (eds), *Acute renal failure*, 1st edn., Philadelphia: WB Saunders, 1983; pp. 252–269.

Dunlop W, Davison JM: The effect of normal pregnancy upon the renal handling of uric acid. *Br J Obstet Gynaecol* 1977;84:13.

Dunlop W: Renal physiology in pregnancy. *Postgrad med J* 1979;55:329.

Grunfeld JP, Ganeval D, Bournerias F: Acute renal failure in pregnancy. *Kidney Int* 1980;18:179–191.

Grunfeld JP, Pertuiset N: Acute renal failure in pregnancy. *Am J Kidney Dis* 1987;9:359–362.

Hankins GDV, Cunningham FG: Severe preeclampsia and eclampsia: Controversies in management. *Williams Obstetrics*, 18th edn. (Suppl 12), Norwalk, CT: Appleton & Lange, 1991.

Hankins GDV, Wendel GW, Jr, Cunningham FG, et al.: Longitudinal evaluation of hemodynamic changes in eclampsia. *Am J Obstet Gynecol* 1984;150:506.

Hayslett JP: Postpartum renal failure. *N Engl J Med* 1985;312:1556–1559.

Krane NK: Acute renal failure in pregnancy. *Arch Intern Med* 1988;148:2347–2357.

Lee W, Gonik B, Cotton DB: Urinary diagnostic indices in preeclampsia-associated oliguria: Correlation with invasive hemodynamic monitoring. *Am J Obstet Gynecol* 1987;156:100.

Lindheimer M, Grunfeld JP, Davison JM: Renal disorders. In: Barron WM, Lindheimer M (eds), *Medical Disorders During Pregnancy.* St. Louis: CV Mosby, 2000; p. 39.

Lindheimer MD, Barron WM, Davison JM: Osmotic and volume control of vasopressin release in pregnancy. *Am J Kidney Dis* 1991;17:105.

Lindheimer MD, Katz AI, Ganeval D, et al.: Acute renal failure in pregnancy. In: Brenner BN, Lazarus JM (eds), *Acute Renal Failure.* New York: Churchill Livingstone, 1988; pp. 597–620.

Lindheimer MD, Richardson DA, Ehrlich EN, et al.: Potassium homeostasis in pregnancy. *J Reprod Med* 1987;32:517.

Lindheimer MD, Weston PV: Effect of hypotonic expansion on sodium, water and urea excretion in late pregnancy: The influence of posture on these results. *J Clin Invest* 1969;48:947.

Martin JN, Blake PG, Perry KG, et al.: The natural history of HELLP syndrome:patterns of disease; progression and regression. *Am J Obstet Gyencol* 1991;164:1500–1513.

Pertuiser N, Grunfeld JP: Acute renal failure in pregnancy. *Baillieres Clin Obstet Gynaecol* 1987;1:873.

Pertuiset N, Ganeval D, Grunfeld JP: Acute renal failure in pregnancy: an update. *Semin Nephrol* 1984;3:232–239.

Stratta P, Canavese C, Colla L, et al.: Acute renal failure in preeclampsia eclampsia. *Gynecol Obstet Invest* 1987;27:225.

Stratta P, Canavese C, Dogliani M, et al.: Pregnancy related acute renal failure. *Clin nephrol* 1989;32:14.

Usta IM, Barton JR, Amon EA, et al.: Acute fatty liver of pregnancy: an experience in the diagnosis and management of fourteen cases. *Am J Obstet Gynecol* 1994;171:142–147.

Weiner CP: Thrombotic microangiopathy in pregnancy and the postpartum period. *Semin Hematol* 1987;24:119–129.

Whalley PJ, Cunningham FG, Martin FG: Transient renal dysfunction associated with acute pyelonephritis of pregnancy. *Obstet Gynecol* 1975;46:174–177.

14 Amniotic Fluid Embolism

Steven L. Clark *Gary A. Dildy*

INTRODUCTION

Amniotic fluid embolism (AFE) is a rare obstetric disorder with a maternal mortality rate of 60 to 80 percent. This condition is a leading cause of maternal mortality in developed countries. In its most classic form, AFE is characterized by hypoxia, hemodynamic collapse, and disseminated intravascular coagulation (DIC). Despite numerous attempts to develop an animal model, AFE remains incompletely understood. Nevertheless, during the past decade, there have been several significant advances in our understanding of this condition. A recent survey of over one million deliveries in California during 1994 to 1995 suggested an incidence of one in 20,000; many patients given this diagnosis lacked more serious features of the classic syndrome. Fortunately, patients developing the complete AFE syndrome appear to be less common.

HISTORIC CONSIDERATIONS

The earliest description of AFE was by Meyer in 1926, however, this condition was not widely recognized until the report of Steiner and Luschbaugh in 1941. These investigators described autopsy findings in eight pregnant women with sudden shock and pulmonary edema during labor. In all cases, squamous cells or mucin, presumably of fetal origin, were found in the pulmonary vasculature. In another report in 1969 by Liban and Raz, cellular debris was also observed in organs such as the kidneys, liver, spleen, pancreas, and brain of several such patients. Squamous cells also were identified in the uterine veins of several control patients in this series, a finding confirmed in the report of Thompson and Budd in a patient without clinical AFE. It should be noted, however, that in the initial description of Steiner and Luschbaugh (1941), seven of the eight patients carried clinical diagnoses other than AFE (including sepsis and unrecognized uterine rupture) which could have accounted for their deaths. Only one of the eight patients in the classic AFE group died of *obstetric shock* without an additional clinical diagnosis. Thus, the relevance of this original report to patients presently dying of AFE, after the exclusion of other diagnoses, is uncertain.

Since the initial descriptions of AFE, more than 300 case reports have appeared in published literature. Although most cases were reported during labor, sudden death in pregnancy has been attributed to AFE under many widely varying circumstances, including amniocentesis and early abortion. In 1948, Eastman stated, "Let us be careful not to make [the diagnosis of AFE] a waste basket for cases of unexplained death in labor." Fortunately, increased understanding of the syndrome of AFE makes such errors less likely today.

CLINICAL PRESENTATION

Diagnostic criteria for AFE as proposed in the National Registry are summarized in Table 14-1. Clinical signs and symptoms of AFE from this series are presented in Table 14-2. In a typical case, a patient laboring, having just undergone cesarean delivery or immediately following vaginal delivery or pregnancy termination, suffers the acute onset of profound hypoxia and

TABLE 14-1 Diagnostic Criteria of AFE

1. Acute hypotension or cardiac arrest.
2. Acute hypoxia, defined as dyspnea, cyanosis, or respiratory arrest.
3. Coagulopathy, defined as laboratory evidence of intravascular consumption, fibrinolysis or severe clinical hemorrhage in the absence of other explanations.
4. Onset of the above during labor, cesarean section, dilatation and evacuation, or within 30 min postpartum.
5. Absence of any other significant confounding condition or potential explanation for the signs and symptoms observed.

Source: As suggested by Clark et al. Amniotic fluid embolism: analysis of the National Registry. *Am J Obstet Gynecol* 1995;172:1158–1169.

hypotension followed by cardiopulmonary arrest. If the fetus is in utero at the time of this event, a fetal heart rate pattern suggesting fetal hypoxia is virtually always seen, and often precedes actual signs of maternal collapse. The initial episode often is complicated by the development of a consumptive coagulopathy, which may lead to exsanguination, even if attempts to restore hemodynamic and respiratory function have been successful. It must be emphasized, however, that in any individual patient, any of the three principal phases (hypoxia, hypotension, or coagulopathy) may either dominate or be entirely absent. Clinical variations in this syndrome may be related to variations in either the nature of the antigenic exposure or maternal response. Initial laboratory investigation is summarized in Table 14-3. As with any pathologic condition, a differential diagnosis should be considered (Table 14-4).

Maternal outcome is dismal in patients with AFE syndrome. The overall maternal mortality rate appears to be 60 to 80 percent and only 15 percent of patients survive neurologically intact. In a number of cases, following successful hemodynamic resuscitation and reversal of DIC, life-support systems were withdrawn because of brain death resulting from the initial

TABLE 14-2 Signs and Symptoms Noted in Patients with AFE

Sign or symptom	*N*	%
Hypotension	43	100
Fetal distress	30	100
Pulmonary edema or ARDS	28	93
Cardiopulmonary arrest	40	87
Cyanosis	38	83
Coagulopathy	38	83
Dyspnea	22	49
Seizure	22	48
Atony	11	23
Bronchospasm	7	15
Transient hypertension	5	11
Cough	3	7
Headache	3	7
Chest pain	1	2

Source: Reproduced by permission from Clark SL, Hankins GD, Dudley DA, et al.: Amniotic fluid embolism: analysis of a national registry. *Am J Obstet Gynecol* 1995;172:1158–1169.

TABLE 14-3 Evaluation of Suspected AFE

1. Arterial blood gas
2. CBC & platelets
3. PT & PTT
4. Fibrinogen & fibrin split products
5. Blood type & crossmatch
6. Chest x ray
7. 12 lead electrocardiogram

profound hypoxia. In patients progressing to cardiac arrest, only 8 percent survive neurologically intact. In the National Registry data, no form of therapy appeared to be consistently associated with improved outcome. A more recent series of patients in whom the diagnosis of AFE was obtained from the discharge summary reported a 26 percent mortality rate. Notably, however, many patients in this series lacked one or more potentially lethal clinical manifestations of the disease classically considered mandatory for diagnosis, thus casting doubt upon the accuracy of the diagnosis. However, if one assumes that the discharge diagnosis of these patients was accurate, this data suggests improved outcome for those women with milder forms of the disease.

Neonatal outcome is also poor. If the event occurs prior to delivery, the neonatal survival rate is approximately 80 percent with half of these fetuses suffering hypoxic brain injury during the maternal collapse prior to delivery. Fetuses surviving to delivery generally demonstrate profound respiratory acidemia. Although at the present time no form of therapy appears to be associated with improved maternal outcome, there is a clear relationship between neonatal outcome and event-to-delivery interval in those women suffering cardiac arrest (Table 14-5). Similar findings were reported by Katz et al. for patients suffering cardiac arrest in a number of different clinical situations.

HEMODYNAMIC ALTERATIONS

In humans, an initial, transient phase of hemodynamic change involving both systemic and pulmonary vasospasm (Table 14-6) leads to a more often recognized secondary phase involving hypotension and depressed ventricular function. These events may occur simultaneously and manifest as sudden cardiorespiratory arrest. The mechanism of left ventricular dysfunction or failure is uncertain. Work in the rat model by Richards and co-workers suggested the presence of possible coronary artery spasm and myocardial ischemia. On the other hand, the global hypoxia commonly seen in patients with AFE could also account for depressed ventricular function. The in vitro observation of decreased myometrial contractility in the presence of amniotic fluid also

TABLE 14-4 Differential Diagnosis of AFE

1. Septic shock
2. Acute myocardial infarction
3. Aspiration pneumonia
4. Pulmonary thromboembolism
5. Placental abruption
6. Anesthetic accident

TABLE 14-5 Cardiac Arrest-to-Delivery Interval and Neonatal Outcome

Interval (min)	Survival	Intact survival
<5	3/3	2/3 (67%)
5–15	3/3	2/3 (67%)
16–25	2/5	2/5 (40%)
26–35	3/4	1/4 (25%)
36–54	0/1	0/1 (0%)

Source: Reproduced by permission from Clark SL, Hankins GD, Dudley DA, et al.: Amniotic fluid embolism: analysis of the National Registry. *Am J Obstet Gynecol* 1995;172:1158–1169.

suggests the possibility of a direct depressant effect of amniotic fluid on myocardium.

PULMONARY MANIFESTATIONS

Patients suffering from AFE typically develop rapid and often profound hypoxia, which may result in permanent neurologic impairment in the survivors of this condition. We have been impressed at the manner in which even brief periods of cardiac standstill and respiratory arrest with subsequent resuscitation may result in maternal neurologic impairment, implying a potential-specific effect of this syndrome on cerebral vasculature or perfusion. The initial systemic hypoxia is likely due to a combination of initial pulmonary vasospasm and ventricular dysfunction. A case report of transesophageal echocardiography findings during the hyper-acute stage of AFE revealed acute right ventricular failure and suprasystemic right sided pressures. In both animal models and human experience, however, this initial hypoxia is often transient. Table 14-7 details arterial blood gas findings in a group of patients with AFE for whom paired data are available, demonstrating initial profound shunting followed by rapid recovery of oxygenation. In survivors, primary lung injury often leads to acute respiratory distress syndrome.

TABLE 14-6 Hemodynamic Indices (mean ± SD) in Nonpregnant Women, Normal Women in the Third Trimester, and Women with AFE

	MPAP (mmHg)	PCWP (mmHg)	PVR (dyn s cm^{-5})	LVSWI (gm m M^{-2})
Nonpregnant (*n* = 10)	11.9 ± 2.0[b]	6.3 ± 2.1[a]	119 ± 47[a]	41 ± 8[a]
Normal third trimester (*n* = 10)	12.5 ± 2.0[b]	7.5 ± 1.8[a]	78 ± 22[a]	48 ± 6[a]
AFE (*n* = 15)	26.2 ± 15.7[c]	18.9 ± 9.2[c]	176 ± 72[c]	26 ± 19[c]

Note: MPAP, mean pulmonary artery pressure; PCWP, pulmonary capillary wedge pressure; PVR, pulmonary vascular resistance; LVSWI, left ventricular stroke work index.

[a]Clark et al. *Am J Obstet Gynecol* 1989;161:1439–1442.

[b]Clark et al. (unpublished data).

[c]Clark et al. *Am J Obstet Gynecol* 1988;158:1124–1126 and unpublished data from the National AFE Registry.

TABLE 14-7 Resolution of Hypoxia After AFE

Patient No.	Initial pO_2 (mmHg)	Time from AFE (min)	Next pO_2 (mmHg)	Time from AFE (min)
2	34	11	242	62
4	19	20	587	40
12	98	21	388	45
22	24	60	128	75
25	12	37	484	96

Source: Reproduced by permission from Clark SL, Hankins GD, Dudley DA, et al.: Amniotic fluid embolism: analysis of the National Registry. *Am J Obstet Gynecol* 1995;172:1158–1169.

COAGULOPATHY

Patients surviving the initial hemodynamic insult may later die of uncontrollable bleeding due to DIC. The exact incidence of the coagulopathy is unknown. Coagulopathy was an entry criterion for inclusion in the initial analysis of the National AFE Registry; however, several patients submitted to the registry for potential analysis, who clearly had AFE, did not have clinical evidence of coagulopathy. In a similar manner, several patients have been observed who developed an acute obstetric coagulopathy alone in the absence of placental abruption and suffered fatal exsanguination without any evidence of primary hemodynamic or pulmonary insult.

As with experimental investigations into hemodynamic alterations associated with AFE, investigations of the nature of the DIC have yielded contradictory results. Amniotic fluid has been shown in vitro to shorten whole blood clotting time, to have a thromboplastin-like effect, to induce platelet aggregation and release of platelet factor III, and to activate the complement cascade. In addition, Courtney and Allington showed that amniotic fluid contains a direct factor X activating factor. Although confirming the factor X activating properties of amniotic fluid, Phillips and Davidson concluded that the amount of procoagulant in clear amniotic fluid is insufficient to cause clinically significant intravascular coagulation, a finding disputed by studies of Lockwood and colleagues (1991) and Phillips et al. (1972).

In the experimental animal models discussed previously, DIC has likewise been an inconsistent finding. Thus, the exact nature of the consumptive coagulopathy demonstrated in humans with AFE is yet to be satisfactorily explained. The powerful thromboplastin effects of trophoblast are well established. The coagulopathy associated with severe placental abruption and that seen with AFE are probably similar in origin; both represent an activation of the coagulation cascade following exposure of the maternal circulation to fetal antigens with varying thromboplastin-like effects.

PATHOPHYSIOLOGY

In an analysis of the National AFE Registry, a marked similarity was noted between many of the clinical, hemodynamic, and hematologic manifestations of AFE and both septic and anaphylactic shock. The clinical manifestations of these conditions are not identical; fever is unique to septic shock and cutaneous manifestations are more common in anaphylaxis. Nevertheless, the marked clinical similarities of these conditions suggest similar pathophysiologic mechanisms.

Septic shock and anaphylactic shock involve the entrance of a foreign substance (bacterial endotoxin or specific antigens) into the circulation, which then results in the release of various primary and secondary endogenous mediators. Similar pathophysiology has also been demonstrated in nonpregnant patients with pulmonary fat embolism. It is the release of these mediators that results in the principal physiologic derangements characterizing these various syndromes. Such abnormalities include profound myocardial depression and decreased cardiac output, described in both animals and humans; pulmonary hypertension, demonstrated in lower primate models of anaphylaxis and DIC, described in both human anaphylactic reactions and septic shock. Further, the temporal sequence of hemodynamic decompensation and recovery seen in experimental AFE is virtually identical to that described in canine anaphylaxis. It is also intriguing that upon admission to the hospital, 41 percent of patients in the AFE registry gave a history of either drug allergy or atopy.

Earlier anecdotal reports suggested a relationship between hypertonic uterine contractions or oxytocin use and AFE. Although disputed on statistical grounds by Morgan in 1979, this misconception persisted in some writings until recently. The historic anecdotal association between hypertonic uterine contractions and the onset of symptoms in AFE was made clear by the analysis of the National Registry. These data demonstrated that the hypertonic contractions commonly seen in association with AFE appear to be a result of the release of catecholamines into the circulation as part of the initial human hemodynamic response to any massive physiologic insult. Under these circumstances, norepinephrine, in particular, acts as a potent uterotonic agent. Thus, while the association of hypertonic contractions and AFE appears to be valid, this contraction pattern is a sign of AFE rather than the cause. There is a complete cessation of uterine blood flow in the presence of uterine contractions exceeding 35 to 40 mmHg. Thus, a tetanic contraction is the least likely time during the labor process for any exchange between the maternal and fetal compartments. Oxytocin is not used with increased frequency in patients suffering AFE compared with the general population, nor does oxytocin-induced hyperstimulation commonly precede this condition (Clark, 1995). Thus, several authorities, including the American College of Obstetricians and Gynecologists, have concluded that oxytocin use has no causative relationship to the occurrence of AFE.

The syndrome of AFE appears to be initiated after maternal intravascular exposure to various types of fetal tissue and antigens. Such exposure may occur during the course of normal labor and delivery; after potentially minor traumatic events, such as uneventful intrauterine pressure catheter placement; or during cesarean section. Because fetal-to-maternal tissue transfer is virtually universal at some point during the delivery process, actions by health-care providers, such as intrauterine manipulation or cesarean delivery may affect the timing of the exposure, however no evidence exists to suggest that exposure itself can be avoided by altering clinical management. Simple exposure of the maternal circulatory system to even small amounts of fetal tissue may, under the right circumstances, initiate the syndrome of AFE. This understanding explains the well-documented occurrence of fatal AFE during early pregnancy termination at a time when neither the volume of fluid nor positive intrauterine pressure could be contributing factors. Whereas much has been written about the importance to the fetus of an immunologic barrier between the mother and the antigenically different products of conception, little attention has been paid to the potential importance of this barrier to maternal health. The observations of the National Registry as well as cumulative data for the past several decades suggest that breaches of this barrier may, in susceptible maternal-fetal pairs, be of tremendous significance to the mother as well.

Previous experimental evidence in animals and humans unequivocally demonstrates that the intravenous administration of even large amounts of amniotic fluid per se is innocuous. Further, the clinical findings described in classic cases of AFE are not consistent with an embolic event as commonly understood. Thus, the term *amniotic fluid embolism* itself appears to be somewhat of a misnomer. In the National Registry analysis, the authors suggested that the term *amniotic fluid embolism* be discarded and the syndrome of acute peripartum hypoxia, hemodynamic collapse, and coagulopathy might more accurately be designated in a more descriptive manner, as *anaphylactoid syndrome of pregnancy*.

DIAGNOSIS

In the past, histologic confirmation of the clinical syndrome of AFE was often sought by the detection of cellular or amorphous debris of presumed fetal origin either in the distal port of a pulmonary artery catheter or at the autopsy. Several studies conducted during the past decade, however, suggest that such findings are commonly encountered, even in normal pregnant women. In the analysis of the National AFE Registry, fetal elements were found in 50 percent of cases in which the pulmonary artery catheter aspirate was analyzed and in 75 percent of patients undergoing autopsy. The frequency with which such findings are encountered varies with the number of histologic sections obtained. In addition, multiple special stains often are required to document such debris. Thus, AFE remains a clinical diagnosis; histologic findings are neither sensitive nor specific. It is interesting to note that similar conclusions have been drawn regarding the diagnostic significance of histologic findings in patients with pulmonary fat embolism.

TREATMENT

For the mother with the classic form of this syndrome, maternal death is the rule. In the National Registry, we noted no difference in survival among patients suffering initial cardiac arrest in small rural hospitals attended by family practitioners when compared with those suffering identical clinical signs and symptoms in tertiary-level centers attended by board-certified anesthesiologists, cardiologists, and maternal-fetal medicine specialists. Nevertheless, several generalizations can be drawn and management is summarized in Fig. 14-1.

1. The initial treatment for AFE is supportive. Cardiopulmonary resuscitation is performed if the patient is suffering from a lethal dysrhythmia. Oxygen should be provided at high concentrations.
2. In the patient who survives the initial cardiopulmonary insult, it should be remembered that left ventricular failure is commonly seen. Thus, volume expansion to optimize ventricular preload is performed, and if the patient remains significantly hypotensive, the addition of an inotropic agent seems most appropriate (Table14-8). In patients who remain unstable following the

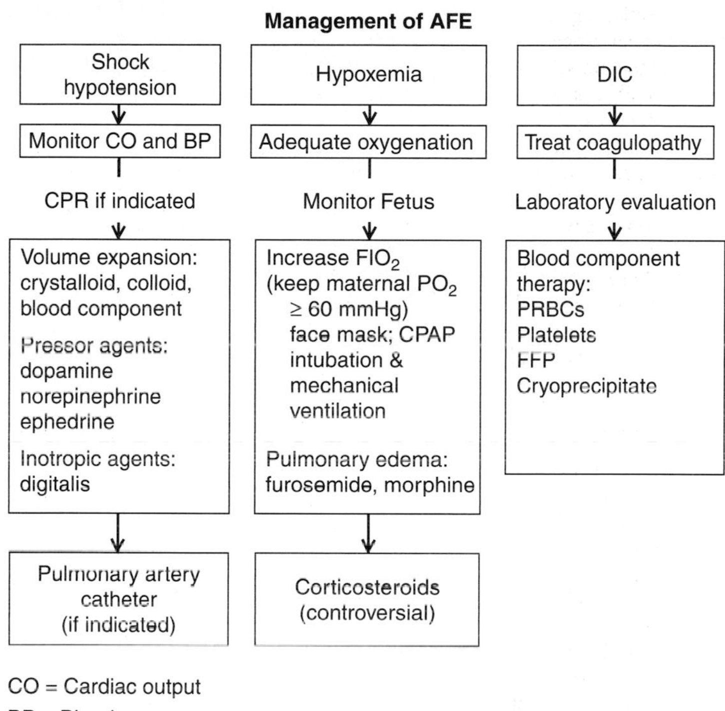

CO = Cardiac output
BP = Blood pressure
CPR = Cardiopulmonary resuscitation
FIO_2 = Inspired oxygen concentration
ET = Endotracheal
DIC = Disseminated intravascular coagulation
PRBCs = Packed red blood cells
FFP = Fresh frozen plasma
CPAP = Continuous positive airway pressure

FIG. 14-1 Management of AFE.

initial resuscitative efforts, pulmonary artery catheterization may be of benefit to guide hemodynamic manipulation.

3. In antepartum cases of AFE, careful attention must be paid to the fetal condition. In a mother who is hemodynamically unstable but has not yet undergone cardiac arrest, maternal considerations must be weighed carefully against those of the fetus. The decision to subject such an unstable mother to a major abdominal operation (cesarean section) is a difficult one, and each case must be individualized. However, it is axiomatic in these situations that where a choice must be made, maternal well-being must take precedence over that of the fetus.

TABLE 14-8 Pharmocologic Agents Used to Treat AFE

Agent	Mechanism of action	Dosage	Comments
Dopamine	Dopaminergic (0.5–5.0 μg/kg/min) vasodilation of renal and mesenteric vasculature β_1-Adrenergic (5.0–10.0 μg/kg/min) increased myocardial contractility, SV, CO α-Adrenergic (15–20 μg/kg/min) increased general vasoconstriction	2–5 μg/kg/min and titrate to BP & CO	Protect from light. Do not use if injection is discolored.
Norepinephrine	α-Adrenergic—peripheral vasoconstriction β-Adrenergic—inotropic stimulator of the heart and dilator of coronary arteries	Initial dose 8–12 μg/min and titrate to blood pressure	Contraindicated in hypovolemic hypotension .
Ephedrine	α and β sympathominetic effects increase blood pressure	25–50 mg SQ or IM 5–25 mg slow IVP, repeat in 5–10 min if necessary	Peripheral actions partly secondary to release of norepinephrine.
Digoxin	Improved contractility of myocardium	0.5 mg IV push and 0.25 mg q 4 h × 2, then 0.25–0.37 mg/day	Narrow toxic-to-therapeutic ratio, especially with potassium depletion.
Hydrocortisone Sodium Succinate	Naturally occurring glucocorticoid, modifies immune system response to diverse stimuli	500 mg IV every 6 h until condition stabilizes	Sodium retention and hypernatremia may occur if administered beyond 48–72 h.

Note: Refer to package insert for further information regarding preparation, contraindications, dosage, etc.

4. In mothers who have progressed to frank cardiac arrest, the situation is different. Under these circumstances, maternal survival is highly unlikely, regardless of the therapy rendered. In such women, it is unlikely that the performance of cesarean section would significantly alter the maternal outcome. Even properly performed cardiopulmonary resuscitation, difficult at best in a pregnant woman, provides only a maximum of 30 percent of normal cardiac output. Under these circumstances, it is fair to assume that the proportion of blood directed to the uterus and other splanchnic beds is minimal. Thus, the fetus will be profoundly hypoxic at all times following maternal cardiac arrest, even during ideal performance of cardiopulmonary resuscitation. Because the interval from maternal arrest to delivery is directly correlated with newborn outcome, perimortum cesarean section should be initiated immediately on the diagnosis of maternal cardiac arrest in patients with AFE, assuming that sufficient personnel are available to continue to provide care to the mother and deliver the baby. For the pregnant patient, the standard ABCs of cardiopulmonary resuscitation should be modified to include a fourth category, D: delivery.

There are limited data on the risk of recurrence in a subsequent pregnancy for women who experience AFE; at present, fewer than 10 cases are reported in published literature. New modalities for the treatment of AFE, such as extracorporeal membrane oxygenation with intraaortic balloon counterpulsation and continuous hemodiafiltration have been reported in survivors. However, such techniques are of unproven benefit and remain investigational.

Despite many advances in the understanding of this condition, AFE or anaphylactoid syndrome of pregnancy remains enigmatic and in most cases is associated with dismal maternal and fetal outcomes, regardless of the quality of care rendered. Thus, AFE remains unpredictable, unpreventable, and, for the most part, untreatable. It is anticipated that new insight into the pathophysiology of AFE suggested by the U.S. Registry Data may allow future advances in the treatment of this condition. Recently, a new AFE Registry has been initiated in the United Kingdom, which may provide further understanding of this condition.

SUGGESTED READING

Clark SL, Montz FJ, Phelan JP: Hemodynamic alterations in amniotic fluid embolism: a reappraisal. *Am J Obstet Gynecol* 1985;151:617.

Clark SL, Pavlova Z, Horenstein J, et al.: Squamous cells in the maternal pulmonary circulation. *Am J Obstet Gynecol* 1986;154:104–106.

Clark SL, Cotton DB, Gonik B, et al.: Central hemodynamic alterations in amniotic fluid embolism. *Am J Obstet Gynecol* 1988;158:1124–1126.

Clark SL. New concepts of amniotic fluid embolism: a review. *Obstet Gynecol Surv* 1990;45:360–368.

Clark SL. Successful pregnancy outcomes after amniotic fluid embolism. *Am J Obstet Gynecol* 1992;167:511–512.

Clark SL, Hankins GDV, Dudley DA, et al.: Amniotic fluid embolism: analysis of a National Registry. *Am J Obstet Gynecol* 1995;172:1158–1169.

De Swiet M. Maternal mortality: confidential enquiries into maternal deaths in the United Kingdom. *Am J Obstet Gynecol* 2000;182:760–766.

Gilbert WM, Danielsen B: Amniotic fluid embolism: decreased mortality in a population-based study. *Obstet Gynecol* 1999;93:973–977.

Grimes DA: The morbidity and mortality of pregnancy: still a risky business. *Am J Obstet Gynecol* 1994;170:1489.

Katz VJ, Dotters DJ, Droegemueller W: Perimortem cesarean delivery. *Obstet Gynecol* 1986;68:571–576.

Lockwood CJ, Bach R, Guha A, et al.: Amniotic fluid contains tissue factor, a potent initiator of coagulation. *Am J Obstet Gynecol* 1991;165:1335–1341.

Parrillo JE: Pathogenic mechanisms of septic shock. *N Engl J Med* 1993; 328:1471–1477.

Phillips LL, Davidson EC: Procoagulant properties of amniotic fluid. *Am J Obstet Gynecol* 1972;113:911.

Plauche WC: Amniotic fluid embolism. *Am J Obstet Gynecol* 1983;147:982–983.

Shechtman M, Ziser A, Markovits R, et al.: Amniotic fluid embolism: early findings of transesophageal echocardiography. *Anesth Analg* 1999;89:1456–1458.

Stiller RJ, Siddiqui D, Laifer SA, et al.: Successful pregnancy after suspected anaphylactoid syndrome of pregnancy (amniotic fluid embolus). A case report. *J Reprod Med* 2000;45:1007–1009.

Tuffnell DJ, Johnson H. Amniotic fluid embolism: the UK register. *Hosp Med* 2000;61:532–534.

15 Acute Fatty Liver of Pregnancy

Jennifer McNulty

ACUTE FATTY LIVER OF PREGNANCY

Acute fatty liver of pregnancy (AFLP) is an uncommon but potentially fatal complication of pregnancy, which results in microvesicular fat deposition in the liver, resulting in severe liver dysfunction. Hallmarks of the disease include jaundice, coagulopathy, and encephalopathy. Although most commonly a disorder of the late third trimester, rare cases have been reported as early as 23 and 26 weeks. The incidence of AFLP appears to have increased over the past thirty years (from 1:15,900 to 1:6692 deliveries) possibly as more widespread recognition of the disease and identification of milder cases occurs. Prior to the 1970s, maternal and fetal mortality rates were reported to be as high as 75 and 85 percent, respectively. However, recent reports suggest markedly improved maternal mortality, ranging from 0 to 10 percent and fetal mortality from 8 to 25 percent. Deaths have been attributed to bleeding complications, aspiration, renal failure, and sepsis. Survivors of AFLP generally recover without sequelae.

Pathophysiology

The precise etiology of AFLP remains unknown. However, research in the past decade has clearly linked an autosomal recessive fetal metabolic enzyme deficiency involved in the mitochondrial fatty acid oxidation pathway to the development of maternal AFLP in some cases. The largest study to date, of 27 women affected by AFLP, found that 19 percent of the offspring of these pregnancies had long-chain 3-hydroxyacyl coenzyme dehydrogenase (LCHAD) deficiency. In contrast, no newborns had LCHAD deficiency when 81 maternal HELLP syndrome cases were evaluated. It is postulated that toxic metabolites, such as free fatty acids from an impaired fetoplacental unit, result in maternal illness in these cases of AFLP. Importantly, LCHAD deficient infants are at subsequent risk for hepatic steatosis, hypoglycemia, coagulopathy, coma and death, all of which can be prevented with the use of a special diet and frequent regular feeding. Increasingly, it has been recommended that newborn infants of all women who were affected by AFLP should undergo molecular analysis for LCHAD gene mutations. Currently, there are also several states in the United States that include LCHAD enzyme testing as a part of routine newborn screening via tandem mass spectrometry and other states that include testing under a pilot program for expanded newborn screening. Abnormal LCHAD function could represent only one of a variety of metabolic disorders that might result in the clinical phenotype of AFLP.

The pathway of impaired mitochondrial oxidation has been implicated in other microvesicular liver disorders in nonpregnant individuals, that are remarkably similar to AFLP. Exogenous impairment of mitochondrial oxidation can occur with ingestion of aspirin, valproic acid, and tetracycline, and would, in susceptible individuals with latent oxidative enzyme deficiencies,

TABLE 15-1 Clinical Presenting Symptoms of Acute Fatty Liver of Pregnancy

Always
- Late second/early third trimester onset

Usual
- Jaundice
- Malaise
- Nausea and emesis

Common
- Abdominal pain (epigastric or right upper quadrant)
- Anorexia
- Clinical coagulopathy (GI bleeding, IV site bleeding, pelvic and postsurgical bleeding)
- CNS abnormalities (altered sensorium, lethargy, confusion, psychosis, restlessness, coma)
- Edema
- Hypertension with headache

result in liver dysfunction, such as is seen in Reyes disease, tetracycline toxicity, and valproic acid injury. Common histopathologic findings include the presence of fine fat droplets in swollen hepatocytes, due to the accumulation of triglycerides and particularly in AFLP, free fatty acids. Fat deposits are most prominent in pericentral and mid zones and spare the periportal cells. The microvesicular fat deposition can be missed if the tissue is fixed before examination, and Oil Red O or Sudan stains should be used on frozen tissue sections. Electron microscopy of the liver shows mitochondrial abnormalities. Intrahepatic cholestasis is usual and unlike in preeclampsia, cellular infiltration with lymphocytes is minimal. Although the diagnosis of AFLP can be made by liver biopsy, today the diagnosis is usually made clinically (Tables 15-1, 15-2, and 15-3).

Diagnostic Tests

Noninvasive radiologic techniques have been used in order to avoid liver biopsy and support a clinical diagnosis. Unfortunately, the reported sensitivities have not been high. Abnormalities in imaging studies in 19 patients with clinical AFLP were reported in 25 percent of ultrasounds, 50 percent of CT scans, and 0 percent of MRI studies. Imaging studies can be used to exclude biliary obstruction as a cause of jaundice, however.

Table 15-4 reviews the results of common liver assays in normal pregnancy and Table 15-5 presents the laboratory abnormalities encountered in AFLP. The laboratory hallmark of AFLP is hyperbilirubinemia, with values typically elevated to 3 to 10 mg/dL, with a reported range of 3 to 40 mg/dL. Alkaline phosphatase, normally elevated up to twofold in pregnancy, is commonly elevated up to 10-fold in AFLP. Due to decreased ammonia utilization by the urea cycle enzymes of the hepatocytes, serum ammonia is elevated, and associated with hepatic encephalopathy. Transaminase elevation is mild to moderate, usually less than 250 to 500 U/mL, but can be greater than 1000 U/mL. Transaminase elevation is not to the degree usually seen in acute hepatitis. Typically SGOT levels (aspartate) are greater than SGPT levels (alanine). Severe liver dysfunction also leads to coagulopathy. Production of vitamin K-dependent clotting factors by the liver is depressed, resulting in another hallmark of AFLP, an elevated prothrombin

TABLE 15-2 Physical Findings by System in Acute Fatty Liver of Pregnancy

Central nervous system
Asterixis
Fever, low grade
Mental status changes
Cardiovascular
Hypertensions
Tachycardia
Abdomen/gastrointestinal
Fluid wave or distension
Guaic positive stool or emesis
Pain (right upper quadrant or epigastric)
Small liver
Genitourinary
Hematuria
Oliguria
Polyuria (occasionally, due to diabetes insipidus)
Dermatologic
Edema
Icteric sclera, mucus membranes
Jaundiced skin
Mucus membrane (oropharynx, vagina)/IV site bleeding
Petechiae
Absent pruitis

time. With worsening liver failure, an elevated partial thromboplastin time results. Decreased fibrinogen production results with further liver dysfunction. A profound depression of antithrombin III (ATIII) activity is also reported in AFLP, to a far greater degree than in preeclampsia or HELLP syndrome. ATIII activity is not significantly affected by normal pregnancy, or pregnancy with chronic hypertension alone. The low levels in AFLP are probably due to derangement in liver production, but may also be associated with accelerated consumption and DIC. Despite the marked decrease in ATIII, which is a natural inhibitor of coagulation, clinical large vessel thrombosis does not occur, perhaps due to the proportional impairment of clotting activators.

Hypoglycemia is often present and is presumed to be due to the impairment of glycogenolysis within the liver, resulting from depression of glucose-6-phosphatase activity. Approximately 15 percent of patients with AFLP will

TABLE 15-3 Complications of Acute Fatty Liver of Pregnancy (PICKLE)

Pancreatitis
Infection (iatrogenic)
Coagulopathy
Anemia, GI bleeding, intraoperative hemorrhage, vaginal bleeding
Kidney failure
Oliguria, uremia, or diabetes insipidus occasionally
Liver failure
Acidosis, ascites, hepatic encephalopathy, hypoglycemia, hypovolemia
Edema
Pulmonary, hypoxia

TABLE 15-4 Liver Assays in Normal Pregnancy

Bilirubin	No change
Enzymes	
• Alkaline phosphatase	Increased twofold
• Amniotransferases	No change
• Gamma-glutamyl transpeptidase	No change
• LDH	No change
Hemostatic factors	
• Clotting factors VII, VIII, X	Elevated
• Clotting times (PT/PTT)	No change
• Fibrinogen	Elevated (by 50%)
Lipids	
• Triglycerides	Elevated
• Cholesterol	Increased twofold
Proteins	
• Albumin	Decreased (by 30% at term)
• Globulin	Slightly increased
• Hormone binding proteins	Increased
• Transferrin	Increased

have severe hypoglycemia and over 50 percent will require intravenous glucose supplementation with 10 percent dextrose to maintain adequate blood glucose.

Laboratory evaluation also reveals dysfunction of other organ systems. Renal insufficiency appears to be universal in AFLP, but generally not to a degree that would require dialysis. An elevated serum creatinine has been documented in some patients prior to development of liver failure, and renal insufficiency may not be due to hepatorenal syndrome as has been postulated. Instead, it may be due to inhibition of beta oxidation of fat in the kidneys, as in the liver, and thus might be a direct effect of the underlying mitochondrial dysfunction on the kidneys. Autopsy findings in patients with AFLP have shown microvesicular deposition of fat in the renal tubules. In addition, diabetes insipidus has been noted in up to 10 percent of patients with AFLP, resulting in polyuria and hypernatremia. The etiology is not yet clear. Pancreatitis, associated with microvesicular fat deposition in the pancreas, results in elevated amylase and lipase in some patients. Although hypoglycemia due to liver impairment is common in AFLP, hyperglycemia may be present if there is pancreatitis.

Differential Diagnosis

Table 15-6 outlines a comparison of liver diseases in pregnancy, which must be distinguished from AFLP, a task which in some cases may be very difficult. Atypical preeclampsia and HELLP syndrome (Hemolytic anemia, Elevated Liver function test, and Low Platelets) are probably the most common conditions the obstetrician will consider as alternate diagnoses to AFLP. Features in common to these entities include elevated transaminases, thrombocytopenia, and frequently an elevated serum creatinine. In addition, proteinuria and even hypertension are frequent in patients with AFLP, as is always seen in preeclampsia, and usually in HELLP syndrome. Importantly, in both AFLP and preeclampsia/HELLP, delivery is ultimately curative. Clinical jaundice, apparent when the bilirubin rises above 2 to 3 mg/dL, is a hallmark of AFLP,

TABLE 15-5 Laboratory Abnormalities in Acute Fatty Liver of Pregnancy by Affected System

Liver

Elevated
- Alkaline phosphatase
- Ammonia
- Bilirubin (usually 3–15 mg/dL)
- Transaminsases (usually <500 U/mL, unless cardiovascular collapse and liver hypoperfusion)

Decreased
- Antithrombin III activity (usually <20%)
- Fibrinogen
- Clotting factors
- Glucose

Renal

Elevated
- BUN
- Creatinine
- Proteinuria
- Sodium (if diabetes insipidus)
- Uric Acid
- Urobilinogen

Decreased
- Creatinine clearance
- Urine sodium

Hematologic

Elevated
- Smear morphology (schistocytes, normoblasts, giant platelets)
- Fibrin split products
- Prothrombin time, partial thromboplastin time
- WBCs (usually >15,000)

Decreased
- Antithrombin III activity
- Clotting factors
- Fibrinogen
- Hemoglobin/hematocrit

Pancreas

Elevated
- Amylase
- Lipase

but uncommon in preeclampsia/HELLP syndrome. While an elevated prothrombin time is a hallmark of AFLP, the prothrombin time and fibrinogen levels are usually normal in preeclampsia/HELLP, unless placental abruption or fetal death has occurred with associated DIC. Hypoglycemia, common in AFLP, is not expected in preeclampsia/HELLP.

Cholestasis of pregnancy is the most common liver disease in pregnant women. This entity can be associated with elevated transaminases and bilirubin, but usually to a lesser degree than in AFLP. Importantly, unlike in AFLP, cholestasis is associated with pruitis.

TABLE 15-6 Differential Diagnosis of Acute Fatty Liver in Pregnancy

	Fatty liver of pregnancy	Acute viral hepatitis	HELLP syndrome/preeclampsia/eclampsia
Onset (I/II/III trimester)	II/III, most >35 weeks, rare reports <30 weeks	Any	II/III (after 20 weeks)
Clinical findings	Malaise, nausea/emesis, jaundice, mental status changes, abdomen pain, ± hemorrhage, ± preeclampsia	Malaise, nausea/emesis, jaundice, abdomen pain	Malaise, hypertension, proteinuria, nausea, abdomen pain, rare jaundice, ± seizures, ± oliguria, ± coagulopathy
Laboratory			
Transaminases (U/mL)	↑ usually <500	↑ commonly >1000	Normal - ↑ 50x (> if liver hematoma)
Bilirubin (mg/dL)	↑ usually 3–10	↑	↑ occasionally (usually <2–3x)
Prothrombin time	↑	± ↑	Normal unless DIC/IUFD/abruption
Alkaline phosphatase	↑	± ↑	↑ occasionally
Other	↑ ammonia, very ↓ antithrombin III, ↓ platelets, ↓ fibrinogen, ↑ WBC, ↑ creatinine, proteinuria ↓ glucose	+ hepatitis serology, ↓ antithrombin III	Moderately ↓ antithrombin III, proteinuria, ↓ platelets, ↑ creatinine, ↑ uric acid
Liver histopathology	Centrilobular microvesicular fat, cholestasis	Marked inflammation and necrosis	Periportal fibrin deposits, hemorrhagic hepatocellular necrosis, inflammation
Treatment	Immediate delivery, supportive	Supportive	$MgSO_4$ seizure prophylaxis, delivery (delayed in very selected preterm cases), antihypertensive treatment

	Cholestasis of pregnancy	Hemolytic uremic syndrome (HUS)	Thrombotic thrombocytopenia purpura (TTP)
Onset (I/II/III trimester)	III, rare reports II	Any	Any, 60% <24 weeks
Clinical findings	Pruitis (worst in p.m., palms and soles), ± jaundice	Hypertension, acute renal failure, nausea/emesis, may have fever and neurologic findings, hallmarks microangiopathic anemia, severe thrombocytopenia	Often neurologic findings, fever and renal dysfunction, hallmarks microangiopathic anemia, severe thrombocytopenia
Laboratory			
Transaminases (U/mL)	↑ (usually <300)	Usually normal	Usually normal
Bilirubin (mg/dL)	Often ↑ (usually <5)	↑ (unconjugated)	↑ (uncongjugated)
Prothrombin time	Usually normal, may be ↑	Usually normal	Usually normal
Alkaline phosphatase	↑ (up to 4x normal)	Usually normal	Usually normal
Other	↑ serum bile acids	Normal antithrombin III, usually normal fibrinogen, ↑ WBC, ↓ platelets (often <20,000), significantly ↑ creatinine, ↑ uric acid, ± proteinuria	Normal antithrombin III, usually normal fibrinogen, ↑ WBC, ↓ platelets (often <20,000), normal – slightly ↑ creatinine, ± proteinuia
Liver histopathology	Centrolobular cholestasis, no inflammation	Unknown	Unknown
Treatment	Ursodeoxycholic acid, corticosteroids, cholestyramine all of reported benefit, vitamin K	For non diarrheal associated HUS probably plasma exchange, FFP infusion, hemodialysis, ?corticosteroids/antiplatelet agents	Plasma exchange, FFP infusion pending initiation of plasma exchange, ?corticosteroids/antiplatelet agents

The clinical presentation may be similar in both AFLP and viral hepatitis, including malaise, nausea, emesis, and a tender right upper quadrant. Fulminant acute viral hepatitis, is typically associated with much higher transaminase values than AFLP, usually >1000 U/L. In addition, unlike many patients with AFLP, hypertension, and proteinuria are not present. Risk factors may be identified for hepatitis, including drug exposure or known hepatitis exposure. Finally, hepatitis does not have a predilection for the third trimester.

Both hemolytic uremic syndrome (HUS) and thrombotic thrombocytopenic purpura (TTP) share some features with AFLP, including thrombocytopenia, renal insufficiency, microangiopathic anemia, and alterations in mental status. However, the coagulopathy, which is a hallmark of AFLP, is not found in TTP or HUS cases, in which the prothrombin time and fibrinogen levels are normal. In addition, antithrombin III activity is normal in TTP and HUS.

Management

The most critical component of caring for a woman with AFLP is the delivery of her fetus. There is no clear benefit to immediate cesarean delivery versus induction of labor and vaginal delivery with meticulous supportive care. In fact, in one report of 28 patients with AFLP, almost all of the maternal hemorrhagic complications occurred in association with surgical trauma. However, factors such as known fetal growth restriction and uteroplacental insufficiency, nonreassuring fetal status by fetal heart rate monitoring, and early gestational age with a markedly unfavorable cervix may appropriately influence a decision to choose cesarean section over vaginal delivery. Coagulation parameters should be corrected prior to surgical delivery, and consideration given to a vertical midline incision, avoiding the dissection associated with a Pfannenstiel incision. The use of an intraperitoneal, closed suction drain, as well as a similar subcutaneous drain (or delayed secondary closure) should also be considered. If vaginal delivery can be accomplished, avoidance of episiotomy in the presence of a coagulopathy is suggested. Anesthesia should be carefully planned, and regional anesthesia considered if coagulation abnormalities can be corrected. If not, and general anesthesia is chosen, inhalation agents with the potential for hepatotoxicity (such as halothane) should be avoided. The use of isoflurane has been described. In addition, the dose of narcotics, which are metabolized by the liver, should be adjusted.

Additional supportive care for AFLP includes monitoring for hypoglycemia, treatment of coagulopathy with transfusion when clinically indicated, optimizing nutrition, and surveillance for infection. Although transfusion with antithrombin III has been suggested in the light of its severe depression in patients with AFLP, this approach is not known yet to be of clinical benefit. Although there are several reported cases of liver transplantation for patients with ongoing liver failure in the immediate postpartum period, it has been argued that with ongoing supportive care, all patients with AFLP will ultimately experience complete resolution of the liver failure. Importantly, AFLP has been recognized to recur in subsequent pregnancy, in a small number of cases. At least one such case was associated with LCHAD heterozygosity in the patient. Table 15-7 presents the cornerstones of supportive care for patients with AFLP.

TABLE 15-7 Management Cornerstones for Acute Fatty Liver of Pregnancy by Affected System

General

Admit to ICU

Consulation as needed with gastroenterology/hepatology, critical care specialist, nephrology

Respiratory

Secure airway if comatose and ventilate, supplemental oxygen otherwise as needed. Evaluate for pulmonary edema

Central nervous system

Minimize encephalopathy

  Decrease endogenous ammonia

    Protein restrict diet, gradually add back as improved clinically

Neomycin orally 6–12 g/day to decrease ammonia producing intestinal bacteria

    Lactulose orally 30–45 mL q 6–8 h to evacuate colon

  Avoid hepatic metabolized medication (certain inhalation anesthetics, narcotics)

Bleeding/coagulopathy

Transfuse

  FFP, cryoprecipitate, packed red cells, platelets

GI protection

  H2 blockers (ranitidine 50 mg IV q 8 h, famotidine 20 mg IV q 12 h)

  Or sucralfate (1 gm po q 6 h or one hour before meals when eating)

Renal/electrolytes

Avoid hypovolemia

Correct electrolyte abnormalities

Surveillance for hypoglycemia

  Maintain glucose >60 mg%

  Dextrose 20% solution, at 125 cc/h provides about 2000 calories/day

Synthetic dDAVP if diabetes insipidus

Infection surveillance

Culture/treat if evidence of pneumonia (ventilator/aspiration), urosepsis (bladder catheter), bacteremia (IV lines), wound (if post operative)

SUGGESTED READING

Bacq Y, Riely CA: Acute fatty liver of pregnancy: the hepatologist's view. *The Gastroenterologist* 1993;1:257–264.

Castro MA, Fassett MJ, Reynolds TB, et al.: Reversible peripartum liver failure: a new perspective on the diagnosis, treatment, and cause of acute fatty liver of pregnancy, based on 28 consecutive cases. *Am J Obstet Gynecol* 1999;181:389–395.

Pereira SP, O'Donohue J, Wendon J, et al.: Maternal and perinatal outcome in severe pregnancy-related liver disease. *Hepatology* 1997;26:1258–1262.

Porter TF: Acute fatty liver of pregnancy. In: Clark SL, Cotton DD, Hankins GD, et al. (eds), *Critical Care Obstetrics, 3rd edn.* Boston: Blackwell Science, 1997.

Usta IM, Barton JR, Amon EA, et al.: Acute fatty liver of pregnancy: an experience in the diagnosis and management of fourteen cases. *Am J Obstet Gynecol* 1994;171:1342–1347.

Yang Z, Yamada J, Zhao Y, et al.: Prospective screening for pediatric mitochondrial trifunctional protein defects in pregnancies complicated by liver disease. *JAMA* 2002;288:2163–2166.

16 Neurologic Emergencies During Pregnancy

William H. Clewell

INTRODUCTION

A patient with a neurological emergency does not present with a diagnosis but rather with one or several clinical manifestations. The nature of the presentation, sequence of events, and constellation of signs and symptoms suggests a differential diagnosis. Starting from the presentation, the physician must select diagnostic tests and procedures and then, once a diagnosis is made, initiate treatment. The differential diagnosis may be altered by pregnancy and diagnostic procedures employed may be different from those one would use for nonpregnant patients. We will consider the following presentations: headache, seizures, altered state of consciousness, and motor or sensory changes. This signs and symptoms approach was chosen because patients do not usually come to the physician with a diagnosis but with a change in their condition, appearance of symptoms and the need for care.

HEADACHE

Headache is a common complaint in pregnancy. Patients who report having had the same problem for some time prior to pregnancy do not usually have a neurological emergency. Chronic and recurrent headaches may be due to tension, migraine, sinusitis, pseudotumor cerebri or in many cases be unexplained. Migraine headaches are relatively common in reproductive age women and often become less frequent and severe in pregnancy. In a minority of migraine sufferers, however, they may present for the first time or become more severe in pregnancy. They must be distinguished from other more immediately dangerous conditions. Many patients who think they have migraines do not have the classical pattern of aura, headache, and nausea. Headaches which, aside from frequency, are similar to those the patient has experienced in the past can generally be considered to not represent a neurological emergency and can be managed symptomatically. Medications used for the treatment of migraine headache are listed in Table 16-1. If headaches become more frequent and severe or have accompanying neurologic manifestations, then they require further evaluation.

Onset of a new headache or the occurrence of a headache with a different location, quality, or accompanying neurologic symptoms demands further evaluation. Figure 16-1 and Table 16-2 outline an approach to the evaluation of headache in pregnancy. The sudden onset of headache requires immediate evaluation and perhaps admission to the hospital. Headache is a common feature of preeclampsia which must be considered in any patient in the second half of pregnancy. Since preeclampsia consists of a constellation of clinical and laboratory abnormalities, appropriate clinical and laboratory evaluation should be able to determine if it is a likely diagnosis in a specific patient (see Chap 5).

The differential diagnosis of sudden, severe headache in pregnancy is the same as that for the nonpregnant patient with the addition of preeclampsia.

TABLE 16-1 Medications for Migraine

Medication	Class	Dosage	Route of administration	Safety in pregnancy
Acetaminophen	Pain reliever	4 g/day max	PO or PR	Yes
Codeine	Narcotic	30–90 mg q 3–4 h	PO	Yes
Meperidine (Demerol)	Narcotic	25–100 mg q 3–6 h	PO, IM, or IV	Yes
Ibuprofen	Nonsteroidal	3200 mg/day (divided doses)	PO	Avoid in late pregnancy
Fioricet[a]	Sedative, pain reliever, vasoconstrictor	2 tabs q 4 h, 6 per day max	PO	Yes
Midrin[b]	Vasoconstrictor, sedative, pain reliever	2 caps, then 1 q h, no more than 5 in 12 h	PO	Yes
Caffeine	Vasoconstrictor	500 mg in 50 mL IV, may repeat	PO or IV	Yes
Imitrex[c]	Vasoconstrictor	PO 300 mg/day SC 6 mg (max, 12 mg/day)	PO, SC, nasal spray	Yes
Ergotamine and caffeine	Vasoconstrictor	2 mg + 200 mg, then 1 mg + 100 mg 2 caps 30 min	PO or PR	No
Nortriptyline	TCA (prophylaxis)	25–100 mg qhs	PO	Yes
Amitriptyline	TCA (prophylaxis)	50–100 mg qhs	PO	Yes
Sertraline	SSRI (prophylaxis)	50–100 mg qhs	PO	Probably yes
Fluoxetine	SSRI (prophylaxis)	20–40 mg qhs	PO	Probably yes
Propranolol	β-Blocker (prophylaxis)	80–120 mg qd	PO	Low risk of IUGR
Nadolol	β-Blocker (prophylaxis)	20–80 mg qd	PO	Risk of IUGR
Atenolol	β-Blocker (prophylaxis)	25–100 mg qd	PO	Risk of IUGR
Carbamazepine	Anticonvulsant (prophylaxis)	Up to 1200 mg/day	PO	Risk of malformations

TCA, Tricyclic antidepressant; SSRI, Selective serotonin reuptake inhibitor.
[a]Butalbital (50 mg), acetaminophen (325 mg), caffeine (40 mg).
[b]Isometheptene mucate (40 mg), dicloralphenazone (100 mg), acetaminophen (325 mg).
[c]Sumatriptan.

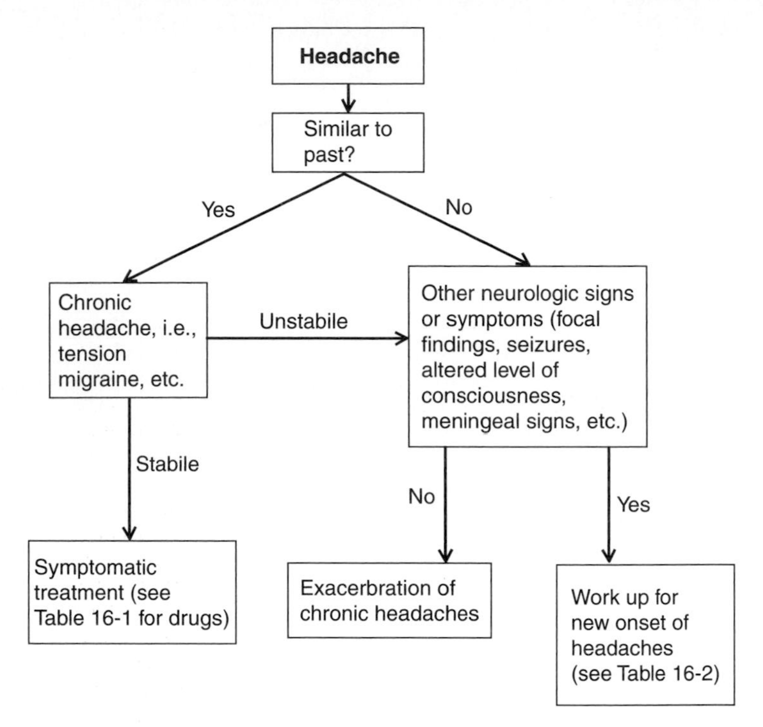

FIG. 16-1 Workup of headache.

It includes subarachnoid hemorrhage, intracerebral hemorrhage, cortical vein thrombosis, meningitis, and mass lesions (tumors or abscesses). Subarachnoid hemorrhage can be due to ruptured cerebral aneurysms, arteriovenous malformations (AVM) or, rarely, preeclampsia or eclampsia.

Cerebral aneurysms usually occur on the vessels of the circle of Willis or the proximal portions of the vessels arising from it. These saccular or berry aneurysms can be found in any patient but are more common in patients with Marfan's syndrome or familial polycystic kidneys. Bleeds from aneurysms are more common in older patients (generally over age 30) and tend to occur in late pregnancy. In contrast, hemorrhage from an AVM tends to occur in

TABLE 16-2 Workup for New Headaches

Rule out preeclampsia
Clinical evaluation (BP, edema, proteinuria)
Laboratory
Rule out mass lesions
MRI, CT, or MRA
Rule out infection
LP
Clinical evaluation
Rule out AVM or aneurysm
MRI, CT, or MRA

TABLE 16-3 CNS Hemorrhage Condition at Presentation (Hunt and Botterell Scale)

Grade	Hemorrhage condition
I	Alert, with/without nuchal rigidity
II	Drowsy/severe headache No CNS deficit except cranial nerves
III	Focal CNS deficits (mild hemiparesis)
IV	Stupor with severe CNS deficit
V	Moribund

younger patients (peak between 15 and 20 years) and is equally likely at all gestational ages. There is no way to clinically distinguish between bleeding from an AVM, a berry aneurysm, or preeclampsia. These patients all present with sudden onset of severe headache, nausea and vomiting, and meningeal signs. They may have focal neurological deficits, altered state of consciousness, seizures, and hypertension. The condition of the patient at presentation is the most important prognostic feature (see Table 16-3).

The diagnosis of possible subarachnoid hemorrhage in pregnancy starts with a high index of suspicion raised by the presentation. Clinical and laboratory evaluation for possible preeclampsia/eclampsia must be accomplished since it is the more common diagnosis and if confirmed requires specific therapy and possible delivery as the definitive treatment. If eclampsia is ruled out, the cornerstone of evaluation is CNS imaging with CT, MRI, or MRA. Imaging contrast dyes may be used in pregnancy to help determine the nature of the hemorrhage and its source. Cerebral angiography may also be used to pinpoint the site of bleeding. Spinal tap will serve to confirm the presence of subarachnoid blood and rule out meningitis as the cause of the headache. Simultaneously, with the initiation of the diagnostic workup, neurological and neurosurgical consultation should be obtained.

Surgical management of both AVM and berry aneurysms can be accomplished in pregnancy but if the patient is near term, consideration of delivery prior to or simultaneously with the surgical repair should be considered. Surgery under hypotensive anesthesia or hypothermia can be well tolerated by the fetus. Continuous fetal heart rate monitoring is needed during and after surgery. Anesthetic medications generally suppress fetal heart rate variability and can make monitor interpretations more difficult. If fetal bradycardia occurs, it is desirable to raise the maternal blood pressure to improve uteroplacental perfusion. Careful attention to maternal oxygenation will improve fetal condition. Almost all women known to have an AVM or berry aneurysm deliver by cesarean section. If the lesion has been surgically treated by excision in the case of AVM or clipping in the case of aneurysm, then vaginal delivery can be safely conducted.

SEIZURE

When a pregnant woman presents with a seizure, the first question to ask is whether she has a seizure disorder. The second question to ask oneself is whether this represents eclampsia (Fig. 16-2). Seizure disorders occur in approximately 0.5 percent of the population and are the most common neurologic complications of pregnancy. There appears to be an increase in

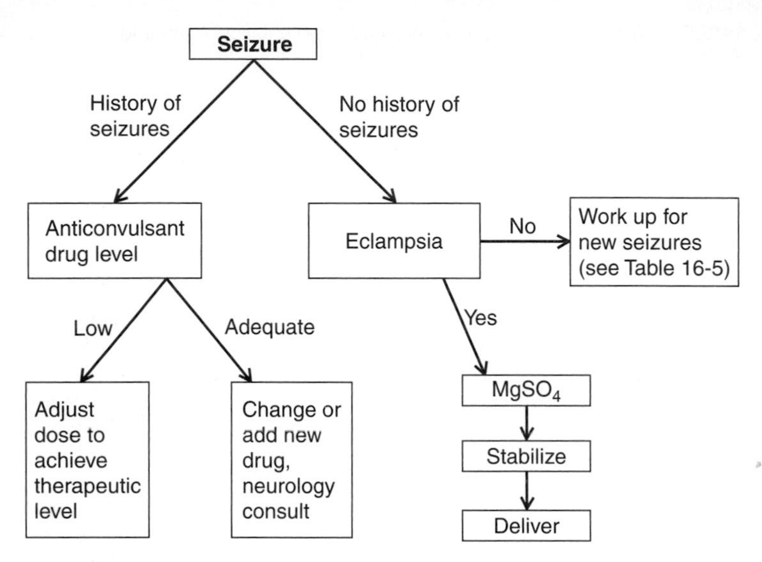

FIG. 16-2 Workup for seizures.

seizure frequency in pregnancy, but it is unclear how much of this increase is due to increased susceptibility to seizures and how much is due to declining blood drug levels. Both the volume of distribution and hepatic clearance of anticonvulsant drugs are increased in pregnancy. This can be especially dramatic in the case of phenytoin. The renal clearance of phenobarbital also increases in pregnancy. These physiologic changes result in falling anticonvulsant levels while the patient is maintained on a constant dose.

A woman who, when not pregnant, experienced at least one convulsion per month can expect an increase in seizure frequency during pregnancy. When a pregnant woman, whose seizures have been well controlled prior to conception, presents with a recurrence of seizures, one must confirm adequate blood levels of her anticonvulsant medication. Infants of epileptic women have a higher incidence of birth defects than the general population. This risk is present for women not on medication as well as those on anticonvulsants. The magnitude of the risk increases with the severity of the maternal condition and the number of drugs required to control the seizures. A variety of malformations have been associated with maternal anticonvulsant use. Dysmorphic facial features are seen with a variety of agents. Distal digital hypoplasia occurs in 15 to 30 percent of infants exposed to phenytoin and carbamazepine. Neural tube defects appear in 1 to 2 percent of infants exposed to valproic acid in the first trimester. It is unclear whether the anomalies seen with anticonvulsant therapy are due to the direct embryotoxic effect of drugs or relative folate deficiency or antagonism. Dietary supplementation with folic acid in doses of 0.5 to 1 mg per day, starting prior to conception, seems reasonable but direct proof of efficacy is lacking.

Use of anticonvulsants in the third trimester may contribute to bleeding problems in the fetus and newborn. While the mother's clotting system appears to be unaffected by anticonvulsants, about one-half of exposed newborns have a deficiency of vitamin K-dependent clotting factors. Maternal vitamin K supplementation of 20 mg per day, for two weeks prior to delivery, results in normal clotting parameters in the newborn. In case of preterm labor, a single 10 mg intramuscular dose to the mother should be adequate. Since most infants receive 1 mg of vitamin K intramuscularly at birth, clinical hemorrhagic disease of the newborn is quite rare even in patients on anticonvulsants.

The new onset of seizures, especially in the third trimester or postpartum, should be considered to be due to eclampsia until proven otherwise. The initial treatment should be magnesium sulfate as outlined in Chap 5. Earlier in pregnancy or with eclampsia ruled out, the initial therapy can be with phenytoin. If the patient is in status epilepticus, this can be accomplished with an intravenous loading dose of 18 to 20 mg/kg with a maximum rate of 50 mg/ min. Transient hypotension and heart block can occur with rapid intravenous infusion of phenytoin. The patient should be on a cardiac monitor during this therapy. For patients not in status epilepticus, oral treatment is appropriate and safer.

Status epilepticus is a life-threatening emergency and treatment must be initiated immediately to preserve both maternal and fetal well being. Prolonged seizure activity can lead to lactic acidosis, cardiovascular instability, and irreversible brain injury. Initial steps in therapy are to establish an airway and venous access. The Epilepsy Foundation of America has published a timetable for the treatment of status epilepticus (Table 16-4).

Once the acute seizure is controlled, the patient must be evaluated for etiology. Potential causes include trauma, infection, metabolic disorders, space-occupying lesions, central nervous system bleeding, and drug use. Neurological consultation should be obtained as soon as the work-up is started (see Fig. 16-2 and Table 16-5).

A pregnant woman with a seizure disorder may be on one or several of the commonly used anticonvulsants. While none have been shown to be completely safe for the fetus, uncontrolled seizures are unequivocally dangerous to both the mother and fetus. Table 16-6 lists the doses, therapeutic blood levels, and side effects of the commonly used drugs.

ALTERED STATE OF CONSCIOUSNESS AND FOCAL NEUROLOGIC SIGNS

When a patient presents with altered state of consciousness, it is often accompanied or preceded by seizure, headache, or focal neurologic signs. When it occurs without these other features, one must consider drug exposure or a catastrophic intracerebral event such as massive hemorrhage or stroke. In these latter conditions, the onset of the event may not have been witnessed and only the fully developed situation observed. The evaluation of patients with altered consciousness is similar to that for new onset of seizures. Often the patient has had a seizure which was not witnessed and she is found in the postictal state. Because of its serious consequences and relatively high prevalence, eclampsia must be considered in any patient with altered consciousness. Once eclampsia is eliminated and a thorough neurologic examination completed, the cornerstone of evaluation is brain imaging

Table 16-4 Suggested Timetable for the Treatment of Status Epilepticus

Time (Min)	Action
0–5	Diagnose status eplilepticus by observing continued seizure activity or one additional seizure. Give oxygen by nasal cannula or mask: position patient's head for optimal airway patency, consider intubation if respiratory assistance is needed. Obtain and record vital signs at onset and periodically thereafter; control any abnormalities as necessary; initiate EEG monitoring. Establish IV line; draw venous blood samples for glucose level, serum chemistries, hematologic studies, toxicology screens, and determination of antiepileptic drug levels.
6–9	If hypoglycemia is established or a blood glucose determination is not available, administer glucose. In adults, give 100 mg of thiamine followed by 50 mL of 50% glucose by direct push into the IV. In children, the dose of glucose is m mg/kg of 25% glucose.
10–20	Administer either 0.1 mg/kg of diazepam at 5 mg/min by IV. If diazepam is given, it can be repeated if seizures do not stop after 5 min. If diazepam is used to stop the status, phenytoin should be administered next to prevent recurrent status.
21–60	If status persists, administer 15–20 mg/kg of phenytoin no faster than 50 mg/min in adults and 1 mg/kg/min in children by IV; monitor ECG and blood pressure during infusion. Phenytoin is incompatible with glucose-containing solutions. The IV should be purged with normal saline before the phenytoin infusion.
>60	If status does not stop after 20 mg/kg of phenytoin, give additional doses of 5 mg/kg to a maximum dose of 30 mg/kg. If status persists, give 20 mg/kg of phenobarbital by IV at 100 mg/min. When phenobarbital is given after benzodazepine, the risk of apnea is great and assisted ventilation is usually required. If status persists, give anesthetic dose of drugs such as phenobarbital or pentobarbital; ventilatory assistance and vasopressors are virtually always necessary.

Source: From Epilepsy Foundation of America. Treatment of status epilepticus. *JAMA* 1993;270:854–859.

Table 16-5 Workup of New Onset Seizures

Rule out CNS bleeding
- MRI, CT, or MRA
- LP
- Neurologic and/or neurosurgical consultation

Rule out CNS infection
- LP

Rule out metabolic disorder
- Electrolytes
- BUN/creatinine
- Calcium
- Glucose

Rule out drug exposure
- Urine drug screen (cocaine, methamphetamine, etc.)

Neurologic examination for focal signs

EEG

TABLE 16-6 Anticonvulsants Commonly Used in Pregnancy

Drug	Maternal effects	Fetal effects	Usual dosage	Therapeutic levels (μg/mL)
Carbamazepine (Tegretol)	Drowsiness, leucopenia ataxia hepatotoxicity	Possible craniofacial and neural tube defects	400–1200 mg in divided doses	4–10
Ethosuximide (Zarontin)	Nausea, hepatotoxicity, leucopenia, thrombocytopenia	Possible teratogenesis	500 mg/day	40–100
Gabapentin (Neurontin)	Leukopenia, drowsiness, ataxia	Too little data to report	900–1800 mg/day in divided doses	Not followed
Phenobarbital	Drowsiness, ataxia	Possible teratogenesis, coagulopathy, neonatal depression, withdrawal	60–240 mg/day as single dose	10–35
Phenytoin (Dilantin)	Nystagmus, ataxia, gingival hyperplasia, megaloblastic anemia	Possible teratogenesis, coagulopathy, hypocalcemia	300–600 mg/day as single dose	10–20 (free phenytoin, 1–2)
Primidone (Mysoline)	Drowsiness, ataxia, nausea	Possible teratogenesis, coagulopathy, neonatal depression	750–2000 mg/day, divided	5–12
Valproic acid	Ataxia, drowsiness, alopecia, hepatotoxicity, thrombocytopenia	Neural tube defects, possible craniofacial and skeletal defects	12–15 mg/kg/day, divided doses	50–100

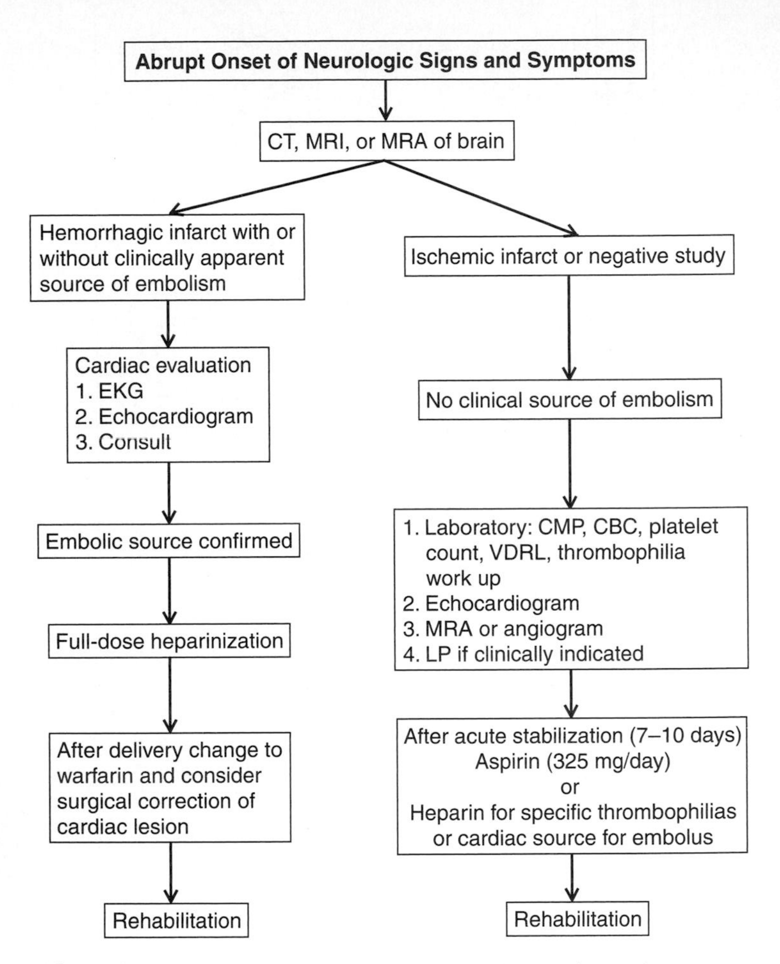

FIG. 16-3 Evaluation and management of altered state of consciousness.

by MRI or CT. Figure 16-3 outlines the initial steps in evaluation and management of this emergency.

Thrombotic Stroke

Thrombotic stroke is relatively rare in the reproductive age group. The overall incidence is one per 20,000 live births. About half of the pregnancy-associated events occur in the immediate postpartum period. The other half occurs predominantly in the late second and third trimesters. Certain conditions predispose to it including hypertension, diabetes, hyperlipidemias, smoking, collagen vascular disease, and some thrombophilias. During the first 24 hours, attention should be paid to maintaining normal blood sugar and adequate arterial pressure to assure cerebral perfusion. Bed rest assists in cerebral perfusion by avoiding orthostatic changes in blood pressure. Heparin appears to play a minor role in the acute phase but in certain circumstances it is useful in preventing recurrence. Intracranial hypertension may develop and must be controlled with dexamethasone and osmotic diuresis with mannitol. In the absence of vascular instability, maternal stroke poses little threat to the fetus. If associated with thrombophilia, this condition may pose an independent threat to fetal well being.

Embolic Stroke

Embolic stroke usually occurs in the settings of known valvular heart disease, cardiomyopathy, or arrhythmia. For these reasons, cardiac evaluation is essential to the evaluation of maternal stroke. Once the diagnosis of embolic stroke is confirmed, the management is similar to thrombotic stroke with the exception of anticoagulation. As with thrombosis, heparin does little to improve the acute condition but is useful to prevent recurrence. In many cases anticoagulation should be delayed for 7 to 10 days to avoid converting an infarct into a hemorrhagic infarct.

17 Cardiopulmonary Resuscitation of the Pregnant Patient

Thomas M. Bajo   Robert Raschke

INTRODUCTION

A number of textbook chapters and review articles discuss cardiopulmonary resuscitation (CPR) of pregnant patients. This chapter is similar to those, but emphasizes the resuscitation of the hospitalized gravid patient whose fetus is of sufficient gestational age to survive outside the mother. A simplified approach to ACLS is included.

Cardiopulmonary arrest is uncommon during pregnancy, reportedly occurring once in every 30,000 pregnancies. Events so uncommon have resulted in no published randomized controlled clinical trials of CPR during pregnancy. Hence, much of the information on the subject comes from animal model studies and from years of accumulated anecdotal human cases. Advanced cardiac life support (ACLS) guidelines have been developed principally for sudden death from ischemic heart disease, a relative rarity during pregnancy. Although underlying medical illness may increase the risk of sudden death, intrapartum death most often occurs in previously healthy women and is related to embolism, complications of anesthesia, or cerebrovascular accidents. The unpredictability and rarity of sudden death during pregnancy make preparation difficult. Thus, the single most important factor for improving the survival chances of mother and baby is an organized, time-conscious team approach.

CODE ARREST TEAM

Cardiopulmonary arrest in the labor and delivery area tends to be a chaotic event. It is imperative that there be an organized team approach with tasks performed in a time-conscious manner. The code team should have, at minimum, these members:

- Code team leader
- Airway person
- Chest compression person
- Vascular access person
- Drug preparation person
- Drug administration person
- Event recorder
- Physician to perform cesarean delivery
- Neonatologist/pediatrician

Each individual on the team must understand his or her particular assignment. The equipment needed is that which is necessary to sustain ACLS, to perform cesarean delivery, and to resuscitate the newborn infant. It is the responsibility of the code team leader to direct team members according to the situation and to be cognizant of time since the mother's death.

PATHOPHYSIOLOGY OF CARDIOPULMONARY ARREST IN PREGNANCY

Cardiopulmonary arrest results in maternal and fetal injury secondary to the precipitating illness and to the dramatic decrease in oxygen supply, the latter being associated with tissue injury. Cardiopulmonary adaptations to pregnancy allow a balanced delivery of oxygen (DO_2) to the mother's tissues and uterus. Likewise, fetal cardiovascular adaptations allow balanced delivery of oxygen (DO_2) to fetal tissues and delivery of blood to the umbilical and placental circulation. Adequate maternal and fetal tissue oxygen consumption (VO_2) to maintain tissue viability depends on maintenance of adequate gas exchange from mother to fetus and maintenance of adequate oxygen delivery (DO_2) to the tissues. Clinical experience and animal experimentation indicate that, during normal pregnancy, maternal systemic and uterine oxygen delivery exceed the minimal level necessary to sustain maternal and fetal life, thereby compensating for conditions that may decrease maternal tissue and uterine oxygen delivery.

During cardiopulmonary arrest, oxygen delivery to maternal tissue and the uterus is dramatically reduced or eliminated completely. There are few maternal or fetal adaptations to such severe reductions in oxygen delivery sufficient to sustain tissue viability. Tissue death begins in minutes.

GOALS OF CARDIOPULMONARY RESUSCITATION (CPR) DURING PREGNANCY

The principal goal of CPR is to restore spontaneous breathing and circulation quickly. This can be viewed as a two-step process, although the actual events often occur simultaneously. Once a stable rhythm is achieved, emphasis shifts to oxygen delivery (cardiac output × arterial oxygen content) so that both maternal and fetal oxygen consumption can be maintained (Table 17-1). Typically, the cause of cardiopulmonary arrest during pregnancy is difficult to determine initially. As stated previously, ACLS guidelines have been designed principally for resuscitation after sudden death caused by ischemic heart disease. By contrast, the arrested gravida is best viewed as having a severe form of shock, often with moderate or severe hypoxemic lung disease. Using the broad categories of shock (cardiogenic, hypovolemic, obstructive, or distributive) provides a quick method for determining the genesis of arrest. It also provides an opportunity to modify the ACLS guidelines based on the perceived precipitating event.

TABLE 17-1 Goals of CPR-ACLS[a]

Establish stable rhythm	
Drugs	
Cardioversion	
Electrical pacing	
Maintain oxygen delivery (cardiac output × CaO_2)	
Think	Treatment
Cardiogenic	Fluids
Hypovolemic	Drugs
Obstructive	Chest compression
Distributive	Airway/oxygen
	Other

[a]CPR: cardiopulmonary resuscitation; ACLS: advanced cardiac life support.

TABLE 17-2 Pregnancy CPR (Ideal)

1. ACLS maneuvers should benefit mother and baby.
2. Fetal monitoring should be available.
3. Continue ACLS and deliver baby to improve maternal and fetal survival based on responses to airway, breathing and circulation (ABC's)

CPR, cardiopulmonary resuscitation; ACLS, advanced cardiac life support.

The success rate of CPR during pregnancy is not known. In nonpregnant patients, chest compression is estimated to produce cardiac output approximately 30 percent of normal. In late pregnancy, the supine position results in decreased maternal stroke index. This is probably secondary to inferior vena cava compression by the gravid uterus. Therefore, chest compression in the supine pregnant patient can result in dramatic decreases in oxygen delivery to maternal tissues. Additionally, aortic compression by the uterus results in decreased uteroplacental oxygen delivery. Thus, manual displacement of the uterus to the left, or placing the patient in a 15 to 30 degree left lateral tilt position, is advised. The latter movement makes chest compression more difficult and probably less effective; however, ideal CPR of the pregnant patient is tempered by the reality of the situation (Tables 17-2 and 17-3).

PERIMORTEM CESAREAN SECTION

The interval over which CPR can be continued without severe injury to the mother and fetus is not known. If spontaneous circulation with adequate arterial oxygenation is not achieved within minutes of cardiopulmonary arrest, consideration needs to be given to perimortem cesarean delivery (Fig. 17-1), which is performed to save the life of both mother and child. Review of the published literature (Table 17-4) shows that the fetus has the greatest chance of being delivered intact if it is born within 5 minutes of the mother's cardiopulmonary arrest. Additionally, both animal experimental and human clinical experience have shown that a mother's cardiovascular function can improve dramatically after emergency delivery. Currently, the recommendation is to complete delivery of the baby by emergency cesarean no more than 5 minutes after spontaneous circulation ceases.

MEMORY AID: THE FOUR-FIVE RULE

Begin the perimortem cesarean 4 minutes after the mother's cardiac arrest to have the baby delivered no later than 5 minutes after cessation of spontaneous circulation.

TABLE 17-3 Pregnancy CPR (Reality)

- Cardiac arrest is a rare event.
- The precipitating event is often difficult to identify.
- It is difficult to predict mother's response to ACLS. No systematic studies of CPR/ACLS on pregnant animals or humans.
- Fetal monitoring is difficult.
- There is a need for *time-dependent decisions* to optimize chances of fetal-maternal viability.

CPR, cardiopulmonary resuscitation; ACLS, advanced cardiac life support.

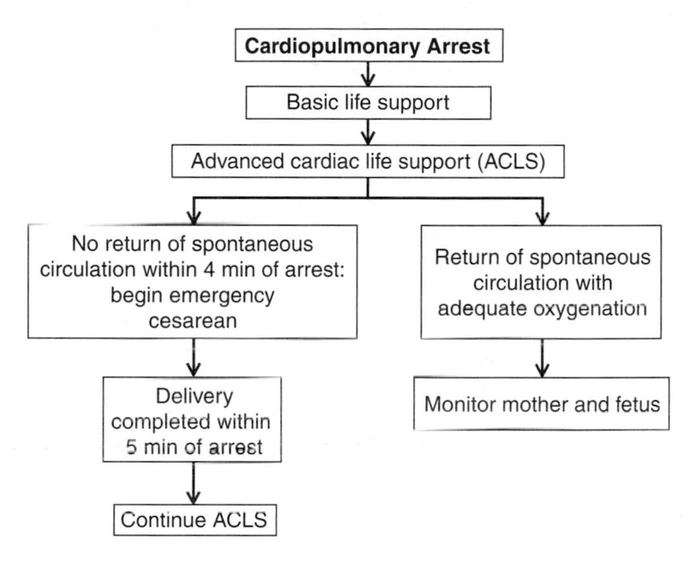

FIG. 17-1 Management of a pregnant woman in cardiopulmonary arrest.

Algorithm for Management of a Pregnant Woman in Cardiopulmonary Arrest (the Patient is Pulseless and not Breathing)

Note: This algorithm takes a somewhat different cognitive approach than those presented in the ACLS 2000 guidelines. The content is consistent, but simplified for the sake of practicality. The reader should refer to the ACLS 2000 guidelines for full details (see Appendices A to D).

1. *Note time of arrest* and mentally plan to initiate emergent cesarean within 4 minutes, if pulse not established.
2. *Instruct airway team to proceed with intubation*
3. *Assess CPR.* Ensure manual displacement of uterus to the left
4. *Establish central venous access* (large bore catheters such as a 9 French introducer preferred)

TABLE 17-4 Interval from Death of Mother until Perimortem Cesarean Delivery of Surviving Infants: 1900 to 1985

Interval (min)	Patients (no.)	Percent
0–5	42 normal infants	70
6–10	7 normal infants	13
	1 mild neurologic sequela	
11–15	6 normal infants	12
	1 severe neurologic sequela	1.7
16–20	1 severe neurologic sequela	
21+	2 severe neurologic sequelae	
	1 normal infant	3.3

Source: Adapted from Katz VL, Dotters DJ, Droegemueller W: Perimortem cesarean delivery. *Obstet Gynecol 1986*;68(4):571.

TABLE 17-5 If Pulselessness is Caused by a Fast Heart Rhythm, Proceed Stepwise Until Successful

Supraventricular tachycardia or atrial fibrillation
- DC shock at 100 J
- DC shock at 200 J
- DC shock at 300 J
- DC shock at 360 J

Ventricular fibrillation or pulseless ventricular tachycardia
- DC shock at 200 J (150 J biphasic)
- DC shock at 300 J (150 J biphasic)
- DC shock at 360 J (150 J biphasic)
  - Administer vasopressin, 40 units IV & shock at 360 J
  - Administer amiodarone, 300 mg IV & shock at 360 J

Note: See Appendices for greater detail.

5. *Assess team resources.* Are team members present to perform cesarean delivery and to resuscitate baby, if necessary?
6. Assess the rhythm
   - *Is pulselessness caused by a fast heart rhythm?* If a fast rhythm is causing pulselessness—typically ventricular fibrillation or ventricular or supraventricular tachycardias with rates of 180 or greater—shock the patient (Table 17-5).
   - *Is the heart rhythm too slow?* If the heart rate is slow, atropine, 1 mg IV (may repeat to cumulative maximum of 3 mg), or transcutaneous pacing may be tried.

     Typically, a slow heart rate will not cause pulselessness, unless the patient is asystolic. Slow rhythms are often associated with diseases in the differential of fulminant shock/pulseless electrical activity (Table 17-6).
   - *Is the QRS complex wide?* Consider the possibility of hypermagnesemia or hyperkalemia. Give CaCl, 5 meq IV and repeat, if warranted.

     A wide complex QRS may be seen with tachycardic or bradycardic rhythms, and is associated with poor prognosis if there is no response to CaCl.
7. Support the circulation
   - Epinephrine, 1 mg IV, Q5 min
   - Aggressive fluid resuscitation
   - Vasopressor/inotropic drugs

     Consider the full differential diagnosis of fulminant shock/pulseless electrical activity listed in Table 17-6. Only tension pneumothorax and tamponade require specific therapy not listed in the algorithm above.
8. *If no pulse is established by 4 minutes, proceed to emergent cesarean.* This approach applies to the most common causes of arrest in pregnant patients, including: catastrophic hemorrhage, primary respiratory arrest with secondary cardiovascular collapse, amniotic fluid embolism, massive pulmonary embolism, and adverse effects of anesthetic agents or intravenous magnesium infusions. In the case of suspected pulmonary embolism, anticoagulant agents appropriate for use in nonpregnant patients will generally be contraindicated by the proximity of probable birth.

TABLE 17-6 Differential of Cardiac Arrest in Pregnant Patients

Extreme rhythm disturbances
Ventricular fibrillation
Ventricular tachycardia
Very fast supraventricular tachycardias
Severe brady arrhythmias/asystole
Arrhythmias associated with hyperkalemia or hypermagnesemia
Hypovolemia
Abruptio placentae
Bleeding associated with placenta previa/acreta/increta/coagulopathy
Subcapsular hepatic hematoma
Cardiogenic shock
Hypoxemia from primary respiratory failure vascular collapse is secondary
Obstructive shock
Pulmonary embolism
Abdominal compartment syndrome
Tension pneumothorax
Tamponade
Venous gas embolism
Distributive/vasogenic shock
Amniotic fluid embolism
Overdose of spinal anesthetic agents

9. *The hour after the code.* Considerations for the patient who regains a pulse, but remains unstable
   - Resuscitated patients often have suffered massive hemorrhage associated with consumptive and dilutional coagulopathy: consider nonclosure of the abdominal incision if cesarean was necessary. This will facilitate direct access to maternal vessels and allow for cross clamping of the aorta, in extreme cases.
   - Massive transfusions, first with O negative blood, then with cross-matched blood are most rapidly administered with a rapid transfuser through a large bore catheter. Aggressive transfusion of fresh frozen plasma, platelets, or cryoprecipitate is often necessary to repair coagulopathy (see Chap. 2). This magnitude of transfusion therapy may be associated with complications such as hydrostatic pulmonary edema, transfusion-related lung injury, and hypocalcemia from citrate toxicity.
   - Rewarming of the hypothermic patient may improve hemostasis.
   - Embolization of uterine or hepatic arteries is sometimes helpful in patients with hemorrhage from either of these sources. Intraabdominal hemorrhage can lead to abdominal-compartment syndrome, whereby high intraabdominal pressure leads to shock. This syndrome may be treated by laparotomy.
   - In cases of massive pulmonary embolism, surgical thrombectomy can be life-saving.

Remarkable neurologic recovery has been observed in pregnant patients who have survived prolonged cardiopulmonary arrest. Thus, we advocate an appropriately aggressive approach in the hours and days after a cardiac arrest.

APPENDIX A: VENTRICULAR FIBRILLATION (VF)/PULSELESS VENTRICULAR TACHYCARDIA (VT) ALGORITHM

Primary ABCD Survey

Focus: basic CPR and defibrillation

- Check responsiveness
- Activate emergency response system
- Call for defibrillator

A. **Airway:** open the airway
B. **Breathing:** provide positive-pressure ventilations
C. **Circulation:** give chest compressions
D. **Defibrillation:** assess for and shock VF/pulseless VT, up to three times (200 J, 200–300 J, 360 J, or equivalent biphasic energy) if necessary

↓

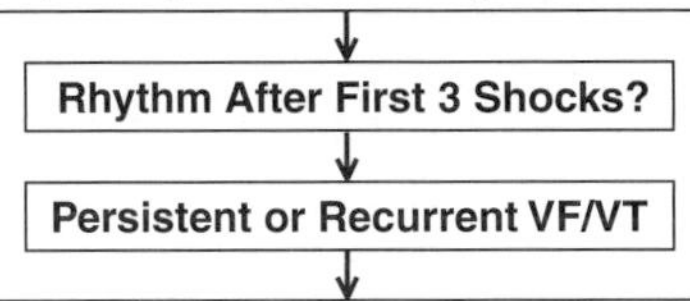

↓

Secondary ABCD Survey

Focus: more advanced assessments and treatments

A. **Airway:** place airway device as soon as possible
B. **Breathing:** confirm airway device placement by exam plus confirmation device
B. **Breathing:** secure airway device; purpose-made tube holders preferred
B. **Breathing:** confirm effective oxygenation and ventilation
C. **Circulation:** establish IV access
C. **Circulation:** identify rhythm → monitor
C. **Circulation:** administer drugs appropriate for rhythm and condition
D. **Differential Diagnosis:** search for and treat identified reversible causes

↓

Epinephrine 1 mg IV push, repeat every 3 to 5 min
or
Vasopressin 40 U IV, single dose, 1 time only

↓

Resume attempts to defibrillate
1 × 360 J (or equivalent *biphasic*) within 30 to 60 s

↓

Consider antiarrhythmics:

- Amiodarone, lidocaine,
- Magnesium if hypomagnesemic state,
- Procainamide for intermittent/recurrent VF/VT,

Consider buffers

↓

Resume attempts to defibrillate

Adapted from *Circulation* 2000;102(Suppl I):I-136–I-165. Please refer to this article for situation-specific details. Reprinted with permission of the American Heart Association, Inc.

APPENDIX B: PULSELESS ELECTRICAL ACTIVITY ALGORITHM

Pulseless Electrical Activity
(PEA = Rhythm on monitor, without detectable pulse)

↓

Primary ABCD Survey
Focus: basic CPR and defibrillation

- Check responsiveness
- Activate emergency response system
- Call for defibrillator

A. **Airway:** open the airway
B. **Breathing:** provide positive-pressure ventilations
C. **Circulation:** give chest compressions
D. **Defibrillation:** assess for and shock VF/pulseless VT

↓

Secondary ABCD Survey
Focus: more advanced assessments and treatments

A. **Airway:** place airway device as soon as possible
B. **Breathing:** confirm airway device placement by exam plus confirmation device
B. **Breathing:** secure airway device; purpose-made tube holders preferred
B. **Breathing:** confirm effective oxygenation and ventilation
C. **Circulation:** establish IV access
C. **Circulation:** identify rhythm → monitor
C. **Circulation:** administer drugs appropriate for rhythm and condition
C. **Circulation:** assess for occult blood flow (pseudo-EMT)
D. **Differential Diagnosis:** search for and treat identified reversible causes

↓

Review for most frequent causes

- Hypovolemia
- Hypoxia
- Hydrogen ion – acidosis
- Hyper-/hypokalemia
- Hypothermia
- Tablets (drug OD, accidents)
- Tamponade, cardiac
- Tension pneumothorax
- Thrombosis, coronary (ACS)
- Thrombosis, pulmonary (embolism)

↓

Epinephrine 1 mg IV push,
repeat every 3 to 5 min

↓

Atropine 1 mg IV (if PEA rate is slow),
Repeat every 3 to 5 min as needed, to a total
Dose of 0.04 mg/kg

Adapted from *Circulation* 2000;102(Suppl I):I-136–I-165. Please refer to this article for situation-specific details. Reprinted with permission of the American Heart Association, Inc.

APPENDIX C: ASYSTOLE ALGORITHM

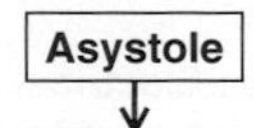

Primary ABCD Survey

Focus: basic CPR and defibrillation

- Check responsiveness
- Activate emergency response system
- Call for defibrillator

A. **Airway:** open the airway
B. **Breathing:** provide positive-pressure ventilations
C. **Circulation:** give chest compressions
C. **Confirm:** true asystole
D. **Defibrillation:** assess for VF/pulseless VT; shock if indicated

Rapid scene survey: any evidence personnel should not attempt resuscitation?

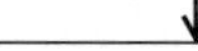

Secondary ABCD Survey

Focus: more advanced assessments and treatments

A. **Airway:** place airway device as soon as possible
B. **Breathing:** confirm airway device placement by exam plus confirmation device
B. **Breathing:** secure airway device; purpose-made tube holders preferred
B. **Breathing:** confirm effective oxygenation and ventilation
C. **Circulation:** confirm true systole
C. **Circulation:** establish IV access
C. **Circulation:** identify rhythm → monitor
C. **Circulation:** give medications appropriate for rhythm and condition
D. **Differential Diagnosis:** search for and treat identified reversible causes

Transcutaneous pacing
If considered, perform immediately

Epinephrine 1 mg IV push
repeat every 3 to 5 min

Atropine 1 mg IV,
repeat every 3 to 5 min,
up to a total of 0.04 mg/kg

Asystole persists

Withhold or cease resuscitation efforts?

- Consider quality of resuscitation?
- Atypical clinical features present?
- Support for cease-efforts protocols in place?

Adapted from *Circulation* 2000;102(Suppl I):I-136–I-165. Please refer to this article for situation-specific details. Reprinted with permission of the American Heart Association, Inc.

APPENDIX D: BRADYCARDIA ALGORITHM

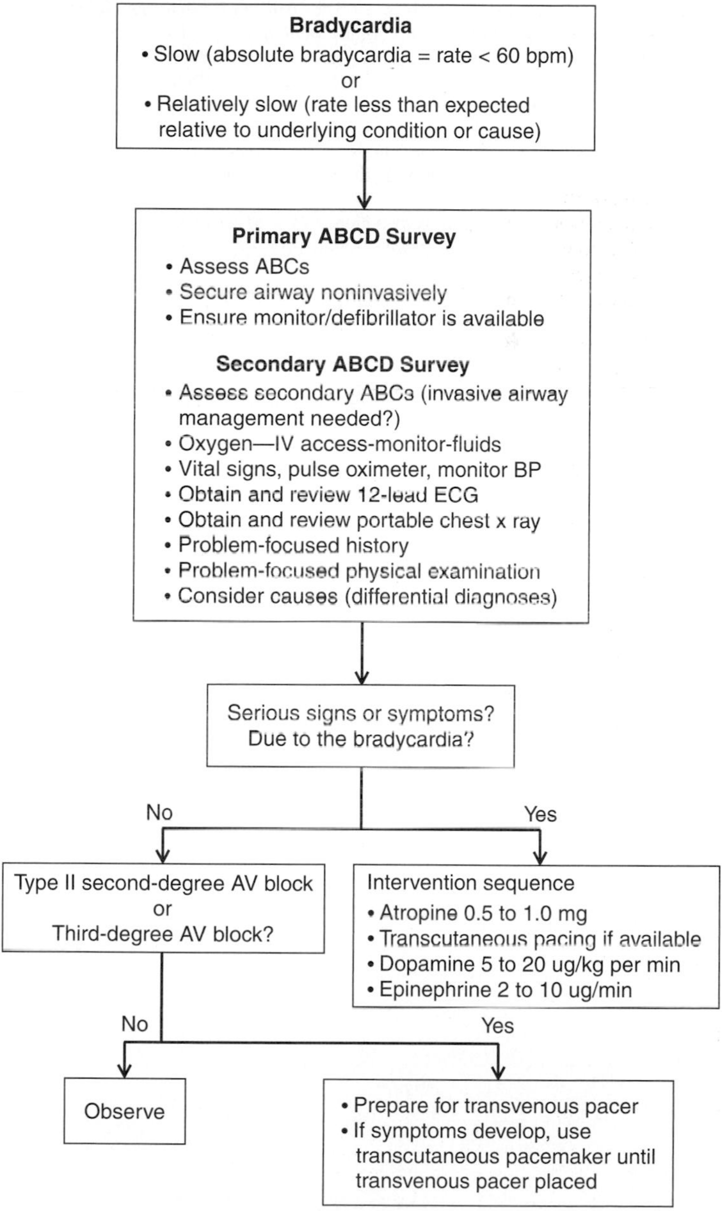

Bradycardia

- Slow (absolute bradycardia = rate < 60 bpm)

or

- Relatively slow (rate less than expected relative to underlying condition or cause)

↓

Primary ABCD Survey

- Assess ABCs
- Secure airway noninvasively
- Ensure monitor/defibrillator is available

Secondary ABCD Survey

- Assess secondary ABCs (invasive airway management needed?)
- Oxygen—IV access-monitor-fluids
- Vital signs, pulse oximeter, monitor BP
- Obtain and review 12-lead ECG
- Obtain and review portable chest x ray
- Problem-focused history
- Problem-focused physical examination
- Consider causes (differential diagnoses)

↓

Serious signs or symptoms?
Due to the bradycardia?

No →

Type II second-degree AV block
or
Third-degree AV block?

- No → Observe
- Yes →
  - Prepare for transvenous pacer
  - If symptoms develop, use transcutaneous pacemaker until transvenous pacer placed

Yes →

Intervention sequence

- Atropine 0.5 to 1.0 mg
- Transcutaneous pacing if available
- Dopamine 5 to 20 ug/kg per min
- Epinephrine 2 to 10 ug/min

Adapted from *Circulation* 2000;102(Suppl I):I-136–I-165. Please refer to this article for situation-specific details. Reprinted with permission of the American Heart Association, Inc.

SUGGESTED READING

American Heart Association: Guidelines 2000 for cardiopulmonary resuscitation and emergency cardiovascular care. ACLS 2000. *Circulation* 2000;102(Suppl 1):I1–I384.

Creasy RK, Resnick R: Placental respiratory gas exchange and fetal oxygenation. In: Creasy RK, Resnick R (eds), *Maternal-Fetal Medicine: Principles and Practice.* Philadelphia: W.B. Saunders, 1994.

Elkayam U, Gleicher N: *Cardiac Problems in Pregnancy: Diagnosis and Management of Maternal and Fetal Disease,* 2nd edn. New York: Alan R. Liss, 1990; p. 809.

Katz VL, Dotter DJ, Droegemueller W: Perimortem cesearan delivery. *Obstet Gynecol* 1986;68(4):571.

Meschia G: Safety margin of fetal oxygenation. *J Reprod Med* 985;30(4):308.

Strong TH, Lowe RA: Perimortem cesarean section. *Am J Emerg Med* 1989;7:489–494.

18 Trauma and Pregnancy

Cathleen M. Harris

TRAUMA AND PREGNANCY

Epidemiology

Trauma complicates one in 12, or about 8 percent, of pregnancies. Two-thirds of all trauma cases among pregnant women are due to motor vehicle crashes, with other common causes including falls, burns, penetrating wounds, and bites. One to twenty percent of gravidas experience domestic abuse, and up to 60 percent of victims report two or more assaults during pregnancy. Physical violence during the 12 months before delivery is common, and is associated with an increased likelihood of admission for pregnancy complications such as kidney infections, premature labor, and trauma due to falls or blunt abdominal trauma.

Admission to the ICU, for severe trauma, occurs in about 3 in 1000 pregnancies, and the maternal death rate due to trauma is estimated to be 1.9 per 100,000 live births. Indeed, trauma is the leading cause of nonobstetric maternal death. With regard to pregnancy outcomes, it is estimated that 1300 to 3900 pregnancies are lost due to maternal trauma annually. Mild maternal injuries carry a 1 to 5 percent pregnancy loss rate, while life-threatening trauma is associated with fetal losses of 40 to 50 percent. Because most women experience mild trauma during pregnancy, a majority of fetal losses actually take place after only minor maternal injury.

A recent review of fetal death certificate data from 16 states indicated that vehicle crashes are the leading cause of fetal deaths due to maternal trauma, accounting for 82 percent of cases. Other important causes included firearm injuries and falls. In that study, the overall rate of fetal deaths was 3.7 per 100,000 live births. Placental injury occurred in 42 percent of fetal deaths, and maternal death was noted in 11 percent of cases. A peak rate of 9.3 fetal deaths per 100,000 live births was seen in women aged 15 to 19 years old.

Physiological Changes of Pregnancy

It is important to understand the normal physiological adaptations to pregnancy, since they have a direct bearing on how pregnant women respond to trauma, and how providers should interpret examination findings and laboratory values. Table 18-1 provides a summary of pertinent changes.

Type of injury and pregnancy risk are influenced greatly by the trimester of gestation during which injury takes place. For example, in the first trimester, the risk of direct trauma to the uterus and its contents is very low, since the uterus is protected within the bones of the pelvis. After mid-pregnancy (20 weeks), abdominal organs are displaced by the growing uterus, and uteroplacental circulation can be compromised in the supine position due to aortocaval compression. In late pregnancy, the risk of direct injury to the uterus, fetus, and placenta is at its greatest. After approximately 23 to 24 weeks, the OB provider needs to consider fetal viability when making decisions regarding pregnancy evaluation and treatment plans.

TABLE 18-1 Trauma-related Maternal Adaptations to Pregnancy

Category	Adaptation	Clinical consequences
Cardiovascular system	Cardiac output increases 30–50% Pulse increases (105 bpm normal) Blood pressure declines	Adaption to tolerate blood loss
Hematological system	Plasma volume increases 40–50% RBC mass increases 30%	Dilutional anemia Circulating blood volume 6 L
Pulmonary system	Minute ventilation increases 30–40% FRC[a] decreases 20%	Respiratory alkalosis is normal Decreased pCO_2 Rapid hypoxemia when supine or apneic At risk for aspiration
Uterus and Placenta	20–30% shunt Marked increase in uterine size Placental flow high flow and low resistance circuit	Potential rapid blood loss Abdominal organs displaced Supine hypotension
Gastrointestinal system	Slowed stomach emptying Organ displacement	Increased risk of aspiration Location of injury influences organ damage

[a]FRC, Functional residual capacity.

Types of Trauma

Blunt abdominal trauma represents the most common mechanism of injury during pregnancy, accounting for two-thirds of cases. Up to 25 percent of all trauma patients with severe blunt trauma experience significant injuries to the liver or spleen. Upper abdominal pain, referred shoulder pain, and elevated liver function tests are suggestive of injuries to these organs. Focused assessment using sonography for trauma (FAST US), CT scan, or diagnostic peritoneal lavage (DPL) may aid in the diagnosis. FAST US is the method of choice for pregnant women, and will be discussed below. If DPL is necessary, an open technique is suggested for pregnant women.

Penetrating trauma during pregnancy typically involves gunshot wounds or stabbings. There is a very high rate of fetal loss due to direct injury to the fetus, cord, or placenta in late pregnancy. Paradoxically, the patient's outcome is more favorable than for pregnant versus nonpregnant patients, since vital maternal organs are protected by the uterus and its contents, which absorb energy from projectiles. The severity and type of injury depends on the size and velocity of the projectile, the anatomic region penetrated, the angle of entry and distance from which a projectile originates, and the size and position of the uterus in the abdomen.

Pelvic fractures represent serious injuries, since hypovolemic shock occurs frequently due to retroperitoneal or intraabdominal hemorrhage. Injuries to the bladder and urethra are common, and examining for hematuria is important. Pelvic fractures themselves are not a definite contraindication to vaginal delivery, but severely disclocated or unstable fractures may be a reason to consider cesarean as the route of delivery.

Maternal and Fetal Outcomes after Trauma

Abruptio placentae is one of the most common and feared complications of blunt abdominal trauma. The risk of abruption is between 1 and 5 percent after minor trauma, but approaches 50 percent or more after severe injury. Risk markers for abruption after motor vehicle crashes include low education level, nonwhite race, lack of seatbelt use, and high-speed collision. Other risk markers for abruption include maternal tachycardia, abdominal pain, vaginal bleeding, premature rupture of membranes (PROM), uterine contractions, and abnormal fetal heart rate.

Fetomaternal hemorrhage (FMH) describes the phenomenon of fetal bleeding into the maternal bloodstream. FMH is found in up to 30 percent of severe trauma cases. The clinical consequences can be severe, such as fetal death due to acute hemorrhage, fetal anemia leading to hydrops, and maternal sensitization to RhD or other minor antigens. Fortunately, the mean fetal blood loss is typically low, with 98 percent of cases less than 30 mL. For Rh negative women, administering 300 μg of RhIG after trauma will protect against nearly all cases of Rh sensitization, since it is adequate to cover 30 mL of bleeding. Additional Rhogam can be given to women with more than 30 mL of fetal bleeding. This calculation can be determined based on the KB screen.

(no. of fetal cells/no. of adult cells) × maternal RBC volume (~75 cc/kg)
= fetal cells in maternal circulation

Preterm birth after trauma could take place for a variety of reasons, including refractory preterm labor, abruption, or intervention for nonreassuring fetal status. Rarely, will delivery occur due to injury to the uterus or fetus or in response to deterioration in maternal condition. Preterm contractions are common after trauma in the third trimester. In 90 percent of cases, contractions cease spontaneously. If tocolytic therapy is considered after trauma, it should be approached with caution, as the safety and efficacy of this intervention has not been evaluated.

Direct fetal trauma complicates less than 1 percent of all pregnancies following trauma. Most cases result from serious maternal injury or from penetrating trauma. Uterine rupture is estimated to occur in 0.6 percent of all maternal traumas. Usually, uterine rupture is the result of direct abdominal impact with high force. The extent of injury and clinical presentation are highly variable. Seventy-five percent of cases involve the fundal region of the uterus, and fetal death is common. Among cases of uterine rupture after trauma, maternal death was seen in 10 percent—much higher than for cases of uterine rupture due to other causes. Clinical features include uterine pain or tenderness, nonreassuring fetal monitoring, abdominal distension, peritoneal signs, and minimal vital sign changes to hypovolemic shock.

Uncommon types of maternal injuries reported in published literature include rupture of the thoracic aorta, and liver rupture. Unusual fetal consequences of trauma have been reported to include limb-body wall complex after trauma in early pregnancy, fetal subdural hemorrhage, and fetal CNS damage, such as hydrocephalus or cerebral palsy. Cases of uterine rupture with fetal death and fetal spinal fracture have been reported, even with seat belt use (Table 18-2).

Evaluation and Treatment

The ideal setting for the evaluation and treatment of pregnant trauma victims is the level I trauma unit. The trauma team is composed of ER and trauma physicians and nurses as well as anesthesia personnel. An obstetrician and

TABLE 18-2 Risk Markers for Adverse OB Outcomes

Demographic characteristics
Young maternal age 15–19 years
Nonwhite gravidas
Low education level
Incident characteristics
Vehicle speed
Lack of safety restraints
Ejection from vehicle
Motorcycle or pedestrian
Penetrating wound to abdomen
Domestic abuse
Repeated trauma episodes
Trauma to breasts and abdomen common
Severe maternal trauma
Hemodynamically unstable
Maternal tachycardia
Multiple injuries
OB symptoms
Over 4–6 contractions in first 4 h
ROM or vaginal bleeding
Decreased fetal movement
Abnormal FHR tracing
Fetal tachycardia or bradycardia
Late decelerations
Decreased variability
Abnormal laboratory data
Elevated WBC
Decreased fibrinogen
Positive Kleihauer-Betke test

OB nurse should both be present if possible, and persons able to perform neonatal resuscitation, as well as delivery and neonatal equipment should be immediately available.

The initial assessment of pregnant trauma patients is no different from any other patient. It is important to stabilize the mother first, then turn attention to the pregnancy and fetus. The primary evaluation follows the ABCDEF format as described below

A—Airway	Consider placing laryngeal mask airway (LMA) or endotracheal tube (ETT) if necessary
B—Breathing	Supplemental oxygen in most cases
C—Circulation	Assess hemodynamic stability. Establish 2 large bore IV lines and replete blood loss with isotonic crystalloid solution in a 3:1 ratio.
D—Disability	Assign an injury severity score (ISS), Glasgow coma scale (GCS) score, or assess the patient in terms of alertness (alert, responds to voice, responds to pain, unresponsive). ISS scores have a similar predictive value for pregnant women as compared to nonpregnant individuals.

E—Expose the patient	Remove all clothing and inspect the entire body
F—Fetal basic assessment	Measure fundal height, fetal heart monitoring, gestational age determination

Secondary Assessment of Maternal Status

After primary assessment and initial stabilization, a secondary assessment for specific injuries and pregnancy status can begin. Secondary assessment for the mother may include Emergency Department or inpatient hospital observation, laboratory studies, and radiological evaluation. Routine laboratory studies include complete blood count, comprehensive metabolic panel, urinalysis, urine drug screen, and serum ethanol level. Additional tests that should be considered for pregnant women include blood type and Rh, Kleihauer-Betke, clotting panel, and a confirmatory pregnancy test (Table 18-3).

For the adult patient, CT-scan, DPL, and ultrasound are used regularly in the evaluation of blunt abdominal trauma. CT-scan is the primary method of assessment for patients with stable abdominal injury at many institutions. However, focused assessment using sonography for trauma patients (FAST US) is an alternative approach that has recently gained popularity. FAST US involves performing a bedside ultrasound examination for signs of intraperitoneal hemorrhage. FAST US is a technique that is ideal for the pregnant trauma victim. Its advantages are that it is portable, rapid, noninvasive, and can be performed equally well by ER or trauma physicians. FAST US is especially well suited for the gravid patient, since reducing ionizing radiation exposure is desirable.

However, FAST US is less sensitive than CT or DPL, as occasional false negatives occur when initial evaluation shows no free fluid. A repeat examination in 30 minutes may decrease false negative results. The sensitivity (about 80 percent) and specificity (98 percent) of FAST US are similar in pregnant versus nonpregnant patients. In reproductive aged women, small amounts of free fluid in the cul-de-sac are normal, but patients with fluid elsewhere are likely to have injury (PPV 61 percent and NPV 99 percent).

At one Level I trauma unit, 2.9 percent of all female trauma patients aged 15 to 40 years were pregnant, and 11 percent of pregnancies were incidentally found on ultrasound. The total radiation exposure to the conceptus among women with incidental pregnancy was more than 5 rad in 85 percent of cases. Using FAST US to identify pregnancies, providers were able to decrease the amount of radiation exposure to fetuses compared to patients diagnosed only by serum HCG.

TABLE 18-3 Suggested Laboratory Studies for Pregnant Trauma Patients

- Complete blood count
- Comprehensive metabolic panel
- Urinalysis
- Urine drug screen
- Type and screen
- Kleihauer-Betke
- Fibrinogen/disseminated intravascular coagulopathy panel
- Basic obstetric ultrasound for: number of fetuses, fetal heart tones, position, amniotic fluid volume, placental location and appearance, gestational age assignment, basic anatomy, and radiological studies as clinically indicated

Radiation Exposure

Fetuses exposed to x rays in the uterus have varying levels of risk. An "all or none" effect occurs if the pregnancy is less than four weeks menstrual age, while embryo/fetuses at 4 to 16 menstrual weeks have a small increased risk for malformations or mutagenesis at 2 to 3 percent above background rates when exposed to high levels. There is a slight increased risk for development of childhood cancers for infants exposed in utero. Providers should be able to discuss the risks of medical radiation with pregnant trauma victims. Consideration should be given to formal radiation exposure assessment when provisional estimates are greater than 10 mGy. This can be done by the hospital's radiation safety officer.

Radiation Risk Categories

Low risk	<10 mGy
Intermediate risk	10–250 mGy
High	>250 mGy

Secondary OB Assessment

The purpose of the secondary OB assessment is to look for clinical signs of abruption, preterm labor, fetomaternal hemorrhage, uterine rupture, and direct uterine or fetal injury. Also, gaining additional information about the pregnancy will aid in making decisions about the management of maternal injuries as well as determining if delivery is warranted.

The diagnosis of abruption is a clinical one, based on the triad of vaginal bleeding, abdominal pain and uterine contractions, and nonreassuring fetal heart rate patterns. Cardiotocography (CTG) is the most sensitive clinical tool for diagnosing abruption. Among women with contractions at more than every 10 minutes, the risk of abruption is about 20 percent. The most sensitive laboratory indicator of abruptio placentae is a decreased fibrinogen content. The sensitivity of ultrasound for diagnosing abruption has been disappointing. Obstetric ultrasound is best used to identify the presence of a live fetus, gestational age, the general appearance of the placenta and the amniotic fluid volume, and to do a basic anatomy survey and assess for any direct injury to the pregnancy. This information will help guide management decisions for the pregnancy overall. Additional pregnancy-related evaluation could include Kleihauer-Betke testing for fetal-maternal hemorrhage, but this is not readily available at all hospitals. Flow cytometry and fluorescence microscopy represent alternative laboratory methods to diagnose fetomaternal hemorrhage.

Otherwise, observation for signs of preterm labor and fetal well being involves serial vital sign measurements, serial examination, and continuous fetal monitoring for a period of at least 4 to 6 hours. Numerous studies have evaluated the optimal observation period for pregnant women after trauma. For most women who experience minor trauma, 4 to 6 hours is sufficient, but several factors may prompt a more prolonged observation period. Four to six hour observation (including serial vital signs, examination, and continuous fetal monitoring) is recommended if

- Maternal trauma is minor
- Hemodynamically stable mother
- Primary evaluation is negative

- FAST US is negative
- Patient is asymptomatic regarding obstetric complaints
- Less than six contractions per hour during the first 4 to 6 hours
- Normal FHR pattern on CTG
- Normal examination and laboratory data

Must do a 24 to 48 hour OB evaluation if

- Multiple or severe maternal injuries
- Mother hemodynamically unstable
- Obstetric symptoms are present (bleeding, ROM)
- Contractions more than 6 per hour during first 4 to 6 hours
- Abnormal FHR pattern on CTG
- Abnormal examination (e.g., fundal tenderness)
- Abnormal lab data (e.g., +KB, abnormal fibrinogen)

Suggested management algorithms for pregnant women experiencing blunt abdominal trauma are depicted in Figs. 18-1 and 18-2. These algorithms incorporate primary and secondary evaluation strategies for mother and fetus.

Cardiopulmonary Resuscitation (CPR) and Perimortem Cesarean Delivery

CPR During Pregnancy (see Chap. 17)

Rarely, a pregnant woman is sufficiently unstable to require CPR and advanced cardiac life support (ACLS) procedures. In order to use CPR effectively, for women in late pregnancy, it is important to recall that aortocaval compression by the gravid uterus decreases cardiac output by 25 percent, and that supine hypotension is common. Indeed, a study of CPR in animal models with partial cava ligation showed that successful resuscitation took 10 times longer with more medication needed.

Left lateral displacement of the uterine fundus (15 to 30 degree left lateral tilt or placing a wedge under the right hip) will improve maternal hemodynamics. The force of chest compressions is somewhat decreased using this method, but overall CPR efficiency may be maximized. Case reports of women, with an improvement in cardiopulmonary function after emergent cesarean during CPR, support the notion that correcting the effects of aortocaval compression may have a beneficial effect on resuscitation efforts in some cases. In rare cases, open cardiac massage has been employed to improve the cardiac index, but there is little data to support its use.

Cesarean Delivery after Trauma

There is a clear role for cesarean delivery in the case of the perimortem gravida or nonreassuring fetal testing in fetuses above the age of viability. With regard to perimortem cesarean Katz and coworkers reported on infant survival rates after maternal death and performance of perimortem cesarean. In their review of cases from 1900 to 1985, 70 percent of infants delivered within 5 minutes of maternal death survived, and all were normal, whereas survival and normal development decreased as the interval from maternal death to delivery increased. Current recommendations are, that if a pregnant woman with a live fetus at or above viability does not respond to CPR efforts within 4 minutes, cesarean delivery is indicated in order to achieve optimal maternal and fetal outcomes. This is contingent on adequate

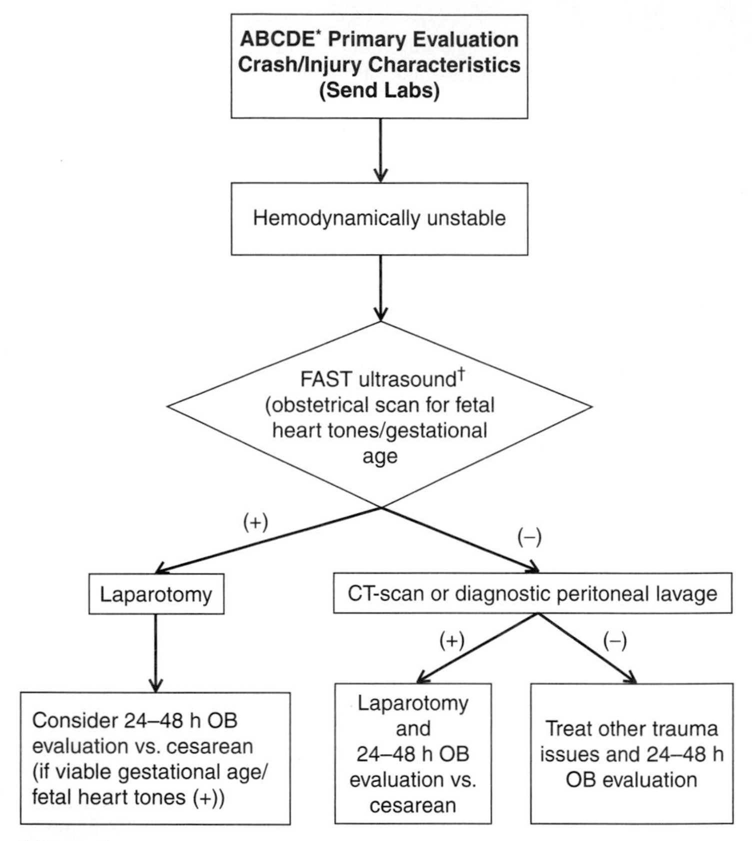

*See text.
†Focused assessment using sonography for trauma patients.

FIG. 18-1 OB trauma (unstable).

OB/Pediatric/ ER/Trauma infrastructure to perform a cesarean delivery in the Emergency Department and provide neonatal resuscitation (Table 18-4).

Cesarean delivery also may have a place in the management of selected cases of maternal trauma. Morris and others reported on the use of cesarean delivery in 9 Level I trauma centers from 1986 to 1994. Thirty-two of 441 pregnant women delivered by cesarean section, due to fetal or maternal distress. Salvageable fetuses included those at 26 weeks or greater, with fetal heart tones present. Overall, the fetal survival rate was 45 percent, while the maternal survival was 72 percent. Of interest, 13 women had a cesarean section when fetal heart tones were absent, and none of these infants survived. However, among the 20 fetuses with fetal heart tones and gestational age over 26 weeks the survival rate was 75 percent. Five infant deaths were thought to be due to delayed recognition of fetal distress, and 60 percent were in mothers with mild to moderate injuries. Of interest, fetal survival

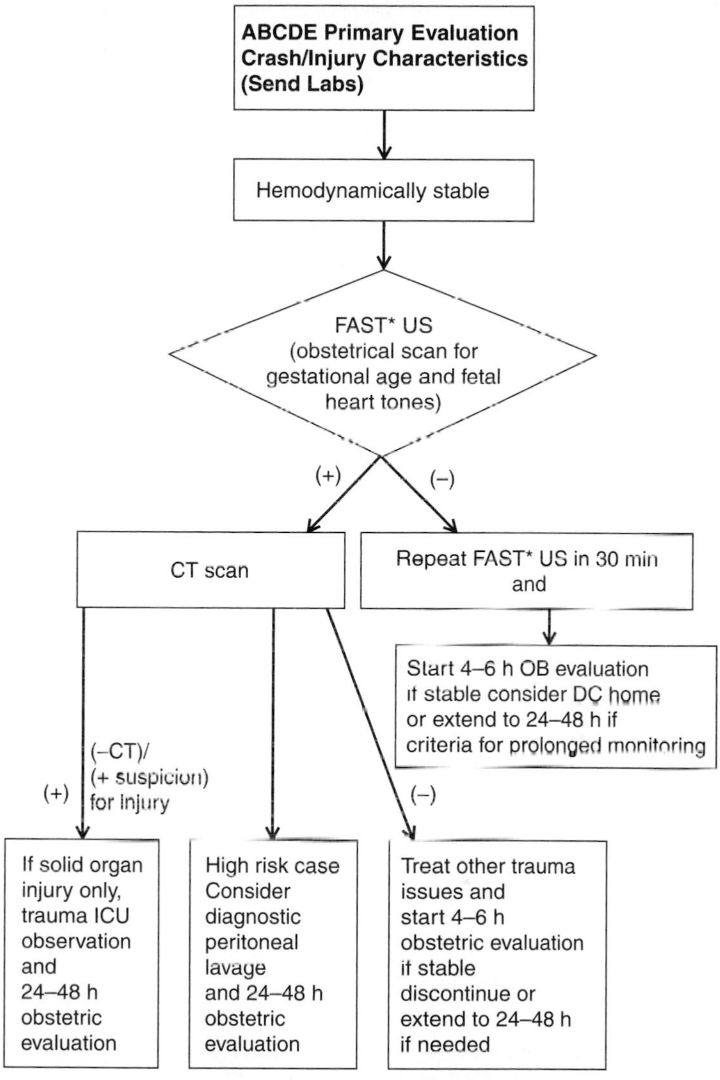

FIG. 18-2 OB trauma (stable).

rate was 78 percent among fetuses born to mothers with an injury severity score of greater than 25, while maternal survival was only 44 percent. By contrast, among women with an injury severity score under 16, maternal survival was 100 percent, but fetal survival was only 73 percent, giving support to the concept that even minor maternal injury places fetuses at risk.

TABLE 18-4 Interval from Death of Mother Until Perimortem Cesarean Delivery of Surviving Infants: 1990 to 1985

Interval	Patients	Percent
0–5 min	42 normal infants	70
6–10 min	7 normal infants 1 mild neuro sequela	13
11–15 min	6 normal infants 1 severe neuro sequela	12
16–20 min	1 severe neuro sequela	1.7
≥21 min	2 severe neuro sequela 1 normal infant	3.3

Source: Katz VL et al.: *Obstet Gynecol* 1986;68(4):511–518.

In summary, routine cesarean delivery after maternal trauma is not necessarily beneficial, but cesarean delivery may be clearly indicated when certain situations occur:

1. Fetal heart tones are present, and the fetus is at a viable gestational age (23 to 24 weeks or greater)
2. Adequate facilities and personnel are immediately available to perform fetal assessment, cesarean delivery, and neonatal resuscitation
3. Maternal CPR is given with no response within 4 minutes
4. Abnormal FHR patterns—fetal bradycardia, prolonged decelerations, or repetitive late decelerations
5. Severe maternal illness—profound hypotension or cardiovascular instability
6. Direct uterine or fetal injury

Discharge from Hospital after Trauma—Special Considerations

- Consider follow-up with obstetrical provider within 48 to 72 hours
- Consider fetal kick counts twice a day or follow-up nonstress test
- Counsel patients about signs and symptoms of preterm labor and abruption
- Rhogam 300 μg IM within 72 hours for any Rh negative woman who is unsensitized
  (Larger dose of RhIG if KB positive—calculate dose based on percentage)
- Tetanus prophylaxis is similar to that for nonpregnant patients
- Reinforce recommendations about proper use of safety restraints

Use of Restraints and Airbags

The American College of Obstetricians and Gynecologists recommends that every pregnant woman use safety restraints. The proper positioning is to wear the lap belt low across the hips, below the belly, and to wear the shoulder harness across the center of the chest, between the breasts. The lap belt should never be used across the fundus and the shoulder belt should never be placed under the arm. Based on current data, although limited, airbag deployment is not associated with adverse OB outcomes.

Research supports the idea that using seatbelts saves fetuses as well as mothers. In one case-control study, lack of proper restraints and high estimated speed (>30 mph) were associated with abruption after motor vehicle crashes. Unfortunately, as many as one third of pregnant women do not use safety restraints during pregnancy. When surveyed, reasons women gave for not using seat belts included discomfort or inconvenience, a habit of never using, and fear of hurting the baby. Programs to educate pregnant women about proper seat belt use have been shown to improve maternal use of restraints. Among women who used restraints properly, 73 percent experienced an acceptable fetal outcome after trauma, in contrast to 38 percent of improperly restrained women.

Key Concepts

Trauma is common—1 in 12 pregnancies
Motor vehicle accidents are the leading cause, accounting for two-thirds of cases
Always consider domestic violence—present in 1 to 20 percent of gravidas
Blunt abdominal trauma is most common mechanism—two-thirds of cases
Pregnancy loss in 1 to 5 percent of minor trauma, and 40 to 50 percent of major trauma
Primary assessment ABCDEF, then secondary OB assessment when stable
FAST US is an excellent modality for maternal and fetal assessment after blunt abdominal trauma
Obstetrical management depends on establishing fetal viability
Fetal evaluation consists of examination, CTG for either 4 to 6 or 24 to 48 hours (for pregnancies >20 weeks), and laboratory data
CTG is most sensitive indicator of abruption
KB is most sensitive test of fetomaternal hemorrhage
All pregnant women should use seat belts and airbags
All pregnant women who are Rh negative and not sensitized should receive rhogam after blunt abdominal trauma or significant vaginal bleeding
Tetanus prophylaxis is safe
Maternal resuscitation is best done in left lateral tilt in the third trimester
Perimortem cesarean should be instituted if no response to CPR after 4 minutes

SUGGESTED READING

Baerga-Verela Y, Zietlow SP, Bannon MP, et al.: Trauma in pregnancy. *Mayo Clin Proc* 2000;75:1243–1248.

Bochicchio GB, Haan J, Scalea TM: Surgeon-performed focused assessment with sonography for trauma as an early screening tool for pregnancy after trauma. *J Trauma* 2002;52(6):1125–1128.

Cokkinides VE, Coker AL, Sanderson M, et al.: Physical violence during pregnancy: maternal complications and birth outcomes. *Obstet Gynecol* 1999;93(5):661–666.

Corsi PR, Rasslan S, Becheeli de Oliveira L, et al.: Trauma in pregnant women: analysis of maternal and fetal mortality. *Injury* 1999;30(4):239–243.

Curet MJ, Schermer CR, Demarest GB, et al.: Predictors of outcome in trauma during pregnancy: identification of patients who can be monitored for less than 6 hours. *J Trauma* 2000;49(1):18–25.

Dahmus MA, Sibai BM: Blunt abdominal trauma: are there any predictive factors for abruptio placentae or maternal-fetal distress? *Am J Obstet Gynecol* 1993;169:1054–1059.

Gochicchio Gb, Napolitano LM, Haan J, et al.: Incidental pregnancy in trauma patients. *J Am Coll Surg* 2001;192:566–569.

Goodwin H, Holmes JF, Wisner DH: Abdominal ultrasound examination in pregnant blunt trauma patients. *J Trauma* 2001;50(4):689–694.

Goodwin TM, Breen MT: Pregnancy outcome and fetomaternal hemorrhage after non-catastrophic trauma. *Am J Obstet Gynecol* 1990;162(3):665–671.

Horon IL, Cheng D: Enhanced surveillance for pregnancy-associated mortality—Maryland, 1993–1998. *JAMA* 2001;285(11):1455–1459.

Johnson HC, Pring DW: Car seatbelts in pregnancy: the practice and knowledge of pregnant women remain causes for concern. *Obstet Gynecol Surv* 2000;55(11):675–677.

Lanoix R, Akkapeddi V, Goldfeder B: Perimortem cesarean section: case reports and recommendations. *Acad Emerg Med* 1995;2:1063–1067.

Leggon RE, Wood GC, Indeck MC: Pelvic fractures in pregnancy: factors influencing maternal and fetal outcomes. *J Trauma* 2002;53:796–804.

Nagy KK, Roberts RR, Joseph KT, Smith RF, et al.: Experience with over 2500 diagnostic peritoneal lavage. *Injury* 2000;31:479–482.

Pape HC, Pohlemann T. Gansslen A. et al.: Pelvic fractures in pregnant multiple trauma patients. *J Orthop Trauma* 2000;14(4):238–244.

Pearlman MD, DeSantis Klinich K, Schneider LW, et al.: A comprehensive program to improve safety for pregnant women and fetuses in motor vehicle crashes: a preliminary report. *Am J Obstet Gynecol* 2000;182:1554–1564.

Pearlman MD, Tintinalli JE, Lorenz RP: A prospective controlled study of outcome after trauma during pregnancy. *Am J Obstet Gynecol* 1990;162(6):1502–1510.

Reis PM, Sander CM, Pearlman MD: Abruptio placentae after auto accidents. A case-control study. *J Reprod Med* 2000;45(1):6–10.

Rogers FB, Rozycki GS, Osler TM, et al.: A multi-institutional study of factors associated with fetal death in injured pregnant patients. *Arch Surg* 1999;134:1274–1277.

Schultze PM, Stamm CA, Roger J: Placental abruption and fetal death with airbag deployment in a motor vehicle accident. *J. Obstet Gynecol* 1998;92(4 Pt 2):719.

Segui-Gomez M: Driver air bag effectivess by severity of the crash. *Am J Public Health* 2000;90(10):1575–1581.

Sirlin CB, Casola G, Brown MA, Patel N, et al.: Use of blunt abdominal trauma: importance of free pelvic fluid in women of reproductive age. *Radiology* 2001;219:229–235.

Van Hook JW: Trauma in pregnancy. *Clin Obstet Gynecol* 2002;45(2):414–424.

Weiss HB, Songer TJ, Fabio A: Fetal deaths related to maternal injury. *JAMA* 2001;286(15):1863–1868.

19 Transport of the Critically Ill Obstetric Patient

John P. Elliott

INTRODUCTION

The broad framework of regionalization is based on the notion that sophisticated perinatal care should be available to every patient within a designated region, even if it is not specifically available at each hospital within the region. The level of care provided within individual hospitals is determined by the availability of technology, skilled nursing and medical personnel, and other related support services. Thus, when transport becomes necessary, it is to match a patient to the level of technology and support she and her baby need.

Indication for Maternal Transport

Maternal transport to a tertiary facility should be considered when the facility at which a patient is located does not have the capacity to manage actual or anticipated complications of either mother or child. For example, Low analyzed 463 maternal transports in the United States over a 6-month period, noting prematurity as the primary reason for transport in 330 (71 percent) cases, hemorrhage in 79 (17 percent), pregnancy induced hypertension in 41 (9 percent), and eclampsia in 8 (2 percent). In a study done by the author, acute maternal medical complications were the indication for transport in 360 of 1541 (23.4 percent) maternal patients transported in Arizona over an 18-month period. Fifty-two percent had hypertensive crises, 36 percent had hemorrhage, 6 percent were trauma victims, and 3 percent had respiratory compromise.

Obstetric Intensive Care During Transport

In general, critical care obstetric patients should be stabilized at the referring hospital prior to transport. Hypertensive emergencies such as severe preeclampsia should be treated with magnesium sulphate to stabilize the neuromuscular irritability that can lead to eclamptic seizures. In addition, diastolic hypertension should be lowered to 100 to 105 mmHg by cautious administration of intravenous hydralazine or labetalol. Third trimester bleeding due to placenta previa or abruptio placentae can cause hypovolemic shock and disseminated intravascular coagulopathy (DIC). Thus, the estimated blood loss should be replaced with a crystalloid solution such as normal saline or lactated Ringer's solution in a 3:1 ratio (3 mL of crystalloid for each milliliter of blood loss). Because maternal intravascular volume increases by about 50 percent during pregnancy, signs and symptoms of shock may not be apparent until blood loss approaches 2000 to 2500 mL. Magnesium sulfate may also be used as a tocolytic. DIC is treated with blood component therapy (see Chap. 2). During transport, left-side recumbent positioning should be utilized to optimize uteroplacental function as described below. Table 19-1 illustrates an example of typical maternal transport standing orders.

TABLE 19-1 Maternal Transport Standing Orders

Premature labor and/or rupture of membranes (PROM), multiple pregnancy, abnormal presentations

Prior to transport

1. Assess blood pressure (BP), temperature, pulse, respiratory rate and fetal heart tones
2. Assess contractions (frequency, duration, quality), status of membranes; time of PROM (if applicable), color and if PROM was confirmed by nitrazine or ferning. If membranes intact, may perform vaginal exam as indicated by the patient's labor pattern/affect. If PROM, do not do digital exam. Sterile speculum exam only if in active labor and delivery is deemed imminent
3. Administer medications as ordered by medical director
4. Start IV (if absent) with 18 or 16 g catheter; 1000 mL LR at 50–150 mL/h. Fluid restrict, when necessary, for tocolytic drugs
5. Left/right lateral uterine displacement
6. Record above data, obtain consent for transport and obtain copies of the patient's chart
7. Assess maternal/fetal condition and call perinatologist, if necessary, for consultation and further orders
8. Help facility prepare for birth, if imminent, and notify dispatch if neonatal transport team is needed

During transport

1. Vital signs with fetal heart tones q15 min
2. Administer tocolytics and other meds p.r.n.
3. Record above information
4. Explain procedures to patient and family; reassure patient

Emergency medications

- Terbutaline: 0.25 mg SQ when contraction frequency is more than q10 min, providing there are no contraindications such as maternal heart disease, maternal diabetes mellitus, shortness of breath, tachycardia or heavy maternal bleeding. May repeat every 1/2 to 1 h if pulse <120
- Meperidine: 25–50 mg IVP for labor pain. May repeat every hour. Observe BP closely. For other causes of pain, speak with medical director before administering
- Magnesium sulfate: IVPB 40 g/1000 mL LR or 20 g/500 mL LR. Bolus 6 g over 10 to 15 min. Follow with 3 g per hour via infusion pump to suppress contractions—adjust as needed. Note: 6 g bolus diluted to not greater than 10% solution. May use 100 mL bag of LR or NS for $MgSO_4$ bolus
- Antidote for magnesium toxicity: Calcium gluconate lg IV push, slowly over 3 min. Observe BP closely
- Continually assess for adequate urine output, deep tendon reflexes, and respiratory rate/effort

Preeclampsia/eclampsia

Prior to transport

1. Assess vital signs, fetal heart tones and deep tendon reflexes
2. Assess contractions (frequency, duration, quality), status of membranes (see PROM/premature labor orders)
3. Right/left lateral uterine displacement
4. Start IV. Mainline 1000 mL LR, infuse at 0–100 mL/h as indicated by hydration, cardiopulmonary status, etc. (hold total fluids at 75 mL/h, if possible)

(continued)

TABLE 19-1 (*continued*) Maternal Transport Standing Orders

Preeclampsia/eclampsia (*continued*)

5. Mix $MgSO_4$ 40 g/1000 mL LR (6 g bolus diluted to not greater than 10% IV solution). May use 100 mL bag of NS or LR for $MgSO_4$ bolus
6. Administer meds as indicated by condition:
   $MgSO_4$ 4–6 g IV bolus over 10–15 min, considering patient's weight, urine output and deep tendon reflexes. $MgSO_4$—continuous infusion of 2–3 g/h via infusion pump
7. Foley catheter if patient cannot void
8. Record above information, obtain copy of chart, obtain consent to transport
9. Assess maternal/fetal condition for transport and call perinatologist for consultation or further orders

During transport
1. Take vital signs with fetal heart tones q15 min
2. Administer medicines p.r.n.
3. Explain procedures to patient and family
4. Foley catheter p.r.n.

Emergency medications
- Hydralazine: First choice for hypertension. May require hydration before medicating. Give when diastolic ≥110 mmHg. Give 2–10 mg IV push every 15–20 min until BP begins to decrease. Stop when diastolic blood pressure is 100–105 mm Hg or a total of 30 mg given. Consult medical director
- Labetalol: Give when diastolic ≥110 mmHg. 10 mg (4 mL) over 2 min IV push. If desired effect not reached after 10 min, give 20 mg (8 mL) IV push. Call medical director
- Oxygen: 12 L by nonrebreathing mask p.r.n.
- Morphine: 2–5 mg slow IV push for acute pulmonary edema
- Furosemide: 20–40 mg slow IV push over 2–3 min for acute pulmonary edema

Eclampsia

- Establish airway: Provide supplemental oxygen. Assist with bag/mask or endotracheal intubation for hypoventilation
- If seizure persists: Rebolus with two additional grams $MgSO_4$ (total bolus should not exceed 8 g)
- If seizure persists after second $MgSO_4$ bolus: Sodium amobarbital IV push 250 mg over 3–5 min (discuss with medical director)

Hemorrhage (General)

Prior to transport
1. Assess vital signs and fetal heart tones
2. Assess contractions, status of membranes, extent of bleeding, number of bleeding episodes, and amount of blood loss (weigh pads, when possible)
3. O_2 12 L/non-rebreathing mask
4. Start IV with 16 g needle. Infuse 1000 mL LR using blood transfusion tubing at 125 mL/h or as necessary to maintain adequate blood pressure and urine output greater than 30 mL/h
5. With active bleeding or suspected abruption, place a second IV line. Use 16 g catheter
6. Check hemoglobin/hematocrit, type and cross (or screen)
7. May travel with blood infusing. Use NS to clear tubing
8. Administer medications as ordered (IV ritodrine and terbutaline are contraindicated). See Premature Labor, PROM Section for tocolytics

(*continued*)

TABLE 19-1 (*continued*) Maternal Transport Standing Orders

Hemorrhage (General) (*continued*)
9. Foley catheter p.r.n.
10. Assess maternal-fetal condition for transport and call perinatologist p.r.n.
11. Record above information, obtain copy of chart and permit for transport
12. No vaginal exam unless placenta previa has been ruled out; then, if necessary, perform gentle vaginal exam or sterile speculum exam to document cervical status prior to departure
During transport
1. Check vital signs and fetal heart tones q15 min or more often, as deemed necessary
2. Check blood loss, keep pad count
3. Record above information
4. Reassess the patient and call perinatologist for consultation or further orders
Acute hemorrhage with hypoperfusion
1. O_2 12 L/nonrebreathing mask
2. Start additional IV lines and increase IV fluids, as needed
3. Military antishock trousers (MAST) application as indicated (see Chap. 18)
4. Left/right lateral uterine displacement
5. Elevate feet
6. If hypotensive, consider ephedrine 5–25 mg slow IV. Observe BP closely. Call medical director
Acute postpartum hemorrhage
1. Oxytocin 20–30 u/L NS, 125–150 mL/h
2. Methylergonovine 0.2 mg IM. Contraindicated in the presence of maternal hypertension or sepsis
3. 15-Methyl $F_{2\alpha}$ 0.25 mg IM. Contraindicated in the presence of maternal asthma or pulmonary hypertension. Call medical director
Excessive nausea and vomiting
• Promethazine 25 mg IV
Emergency delivery
1. Perform emergency delivery whenever imminent during transport
2. May perform small midline episiotomy, as necessary, to prevent laceration
3. Cut and clamp the umbilical cord 1/2 in from stump
4. Administer oxytocin 10–20 units IM or added to full IV bag after placenta is delivered
5. Obtain cord blood when time permits
6. Resuscitate newborn (see Chap. 26) provide warmth, O_2 by bag and mask, with intubation p.r.n. If estimated time of arrival is greater than 20 min and situation permits, obtain chem strip for glucose
7. For neonatal glucose less than 40 mg/dL give dextrose 10% IV or gavage, if necessary. Give 2–4 mL/kg over 3–5 min

Maternal Trauma

Transport of the pregnant trauma victim requires special knowledge and skills by the transport team. The uterus may be injured without signs of direct physical trauma. Abrupt deceleration with resulting contra-coup forces can be harmful to both the fetus and the placenta. In most cases of maternal trauma, every effort should be made to stabilize serious maternal injuries prior to transport. All pregnant patients beyond 20 weeks gestation

TABLE 19-2 Maternal Flight Nurse Skills and Qualifications

Skills

1. Vaginal speculum exam; digital cervical exam
2. Vaginal delivery
3. Advanced cardiac life support—certified
4. Intubation—maternal and/or neonatal

Qualifications/requirements

1. Basic and advanced cardiac life support capable
2. Neonatal resuscitation capable
3. National certification in obstetrics
4. Three years of tertiary obstetric experience
5. Successful completion of maternal flight nurse course/exam

should be transported in left lateral tilt position to prevent hypotension from aorto-caval compression. Supine hypotension may significantly compromise the maternal cardiac output and placental perfusion. Should the patient require a backboard for neck or back stabilization, the entire backboard can be tilted to the left by placing rolled sheets or towels under the right side of the board. The fetal heart rate should be auscultated in all maternal traumatic injuries. The absence of fetal heart tones may be associated with placental abruption and/or fetal death. The uterus should also be examined carefully for evidence of tenderness or rigidity. Vaginal bleeding should be ruled out in all gravid trauma patients.

The Emergency Medical System (EMS) in the United States is efficient at triaging trauma victims to designated trauma centers. However, when considering transport of a pregnant woman from an accident scene, the EMS system often fails to recognize that the fetus/neonate also needs to be treated at an appropriate level facility. Level I trauma patients in the second or third trimester of pregnancy ideally should be transported to a hospital that combines Level I trauma capabilities with Level III obstetric and neonatal facilities.

The Obstetrical Transport Crew

Transport of the critically ill obstetric patient often requires personnel with skills beyond that of the typical advanced life support/emergency medical ambulance crew. These care providers may be cross-trained adult trauma nurses or dedicated obstetrical nurses. They must have an excellent working knowledge of maternal physiology and the process of labor. Experience with obstetric drugs and fetal monitoring is also essential. The ability to perform advanced cardiac life support, to interpret electrocardiograms and to perform successful endotracheal intubation, if necessary, are important skills for a perinatal flight nurse to possess (Table 19-2). Table 19-3 lists the recommended equipment for perinatal transport along with a detailed plan for equipment organization/flight-kit planning.

The comprehensive care of the critically ill obstetric patient during transport requires care providers that have a detailed knowledge of maternal physiologic adaptations and a comprehensive understanding of the disease processes unique to obstetrics. The combination of perinatal regionalization and a skilled perinatal transport service may simultaneously improve survival and reduce morbidity for both mother and baby.

TABLE 19-3 Equipment for Maternal Transport

Contents of maternal flight nurse delivery bag[a]	
Ob delivery kit	
• Bulb syringe	• 1 chux
• Suction trap	• Sterile gloves (latex and nonlatex)
• Self-inflating resuscitation bag	• Cord clamp (2)
• Infant and newborn mask	• Scissors (curved/straight) (2)
• Infant hat	• Curved Kelly clamp
• Pediatric stethoscope	• Short ring forceps
• Infant blanket pack	• Plastic placenta bag
• Portawarm mattress	• 2 cloth towels
• Sterile gloves (latex and nonlatex)	• Sterile 4 × 4 in gauze (2)
	• Bulb syringe

Contents of maternal flight nurse pharmacy bag[a]		
$MgSO_4$ 10 g (2) Furosemide 20 mg (2) Oxytocin 10 U (3) $MgSO_4$ 10 g (3) Normal saline 10 mL (3)	Ephedrine 50 mg (3) Dextrose 50% 50 mL Hydralazine 20 mg (2) $D_{10}W$ vial 5 mL (2) Hep-lock	Methylergonovine 0.2 mg (2) Labetalol 100 mg (2) Terbutaline 1 mg (3) Ammonium salts (2) Promethazine HCl 25 mg (2) Albuterol, unit dose 2.5 mg (2)
Thermometer TB syringe (2) 3 mL syringe (2)	Band-aids Needles 19 g (3) 22 g (3) Filter (3)	Alcohol swabs Labels Hep-lock cap
Dimenhydrinate (2) Narcotic sheets	Cord clamp (2) Aspirin (2) Tylenol (2)	Drug labels (4) Inventory
Bretylium 500 mg (2) Verapamil 5 mg (3)	Epinephrine 1:1000 (3)	Atropine 1 mg (2) Lidocaine 1 g/50 cc (1) Sodium amobarbital 250 mg (1)
Epinephrine 1:10,000 (2) Calcium gluconate 10% (1) Diphenhydramine (2)	Sodium bicarb 50 cc jet (1) 2% lidocaine 100 mg jet (2) Procainamide 1 g (1)	
		Meperidine 100 mg (1) Diazepam 10 mg (4) Morphine 10 mg (1) Naloxone 0.4 mg (2)

(continued)

TABLE 19-3 (*continued*) Equipment for Maternal Transport

Contents of top portion maternal flight nurse medical bag[a]		
3-mL syringe (2)		Alcohol wipes
Tuberculin syringe (2)		Virowipes
Insulin syringe (1)		
Stopcock		
19-gauge needles		
Syringes	100 mL normal saline (2)	
10 mL		
20 mL		
30 mL		
60 mL		
	Bite stick	
	Drug bag	
Contents of base portion maternal flight nurse medical bag[a]		
250 mL D_5W	1000 mL LR	Sterile speculum
500 mL NS	500 mL LR	
Cardiac electrodes		
Orange	**Green**	**Yellow**
Laryngoscope handle and bulb	In self-seal bags	IV start kit
Blades	Chemstrips	Nonsterile gloves (latex and nonlatex)
McIntosh (3, 4)	Alcohol wipes	Mainline tubing
Miller (0, 1, 3)	Lancets	IV Catheters
Spare "C" batteries (2)	Cotton balls	16 gauge (3)
Xylocaine gel	KY jelly	18 gauge (3)
Benzoin (2)	Betadine jelly	24 gauge (2)
1-in adhesive tape	Nitrazine paper	23-gauge butterfly
10-mL syringe	Tape-measure	T connector
	Blood tubes	Tourniquet
	Purple (2)	
	Red (2)	
	Vacutainer	
	Alcohol	
	Band-Aids	
	Tourniquet	
	Needles	
	Small self-seal bag (2)	
	Urine dipstick	
	Plastic bags (2)	
	Flashlight	
	Peri pads (2)	
Sterile gloves (latex and nonlatex)		

(continued)

TABLE 19-3 (*continued*) Equipment for Maternal Transport

Contents of outside pockets maternal flight nurse medical bag[a]		
Left side	**Top handle pocket**	**Right side**
Micro drip extension set	Micro drip extension set	Stylette
Blood tubing with pump	Stopcock	Adult
Salem pump	60-mL syringe	Pediatric
	needles	End-tidal CO_2 detector
	Top center	**Zipper bag**
	Stethoscope	PEEP valve
	Doppler and gel	Magill forceps
	BP cuff (regular and oversized)	Oral airways
		Medium adult
	Bottom center	Small adult
	Emesis bag	Infant
	Adult BVM oxygen bag	ET tubes
	Leg BP cuff	2.0
	Charts (3)	2.5
	Self-inflating Ambu-bag	3.0
	Red isolation bag (1)	3.5
		7.0
		7.5
		8.0
		7.0 Endotrol
		Beck Airways Airflow Monitor

[a]Description of some components of the maternal flight nurse bag by brand name does not necessarily infer endorsement of that brand

SUGGESTED READING

Baxt WG, Moody P.: The impact of a rotorcraft aeromedical emergency care service on trauma mortality. *JAMA* 1983;249:3047–3051.

Elliott JP, Foley MR, Young L, et al.: Transport of obstetrical critical care patients to tertiary centers. *J Reprod Med* 1996:41;171–175.

Elliott JP.: Magnesium sulfate as a tocolytic agent. *Am J Obstet Gynecol* 1983; 147:277–284.

Elliott JP, O'Keeffe DF, Freeman RK. Helicopter transportation of patients with obstetric emergencies in an urban area. *Am J Obstet Gynecol* 1982;143:157–162.

Elliott JP, Sipp TL, Balazs KT.: Maternal transport of patients with advanced cervical dilatation—to fly or not to fly? *Obstet Gynecol* 1992;79:380–382.

Elliott JP, Trujillo R.: Fetal monitoring during emergency obstetric transport. *Am J Obstet Gynecol* 1987;157:245–247.

Kanto WP, Bryant J, Thigpen J, et al.: Impact of a maternal transport program on a newborn service. *South Med J* 1983;76:834–837.

Katz VL, Hansen AR.: Complications in the emergency transport of pregnant women. *South Med J* 1990;83:7–10.

Knox GE, Schnitker KA. In-utero transport. *Clin Obstet Gynecol* 1984;27:11–16.

Low RB, Martin D, Brown C.: Emergency air transport of pregnant patients: the national experience. *J Emerg Med* 1988;6:41–48.

Tsokos N, Newnham JP, Langford SA.: Intravenous tocolytic therapy for long distance aeromedical transport of women in preterm labour in Western Australia. *Asia-Oceania J Obstet Gynaecol* 1988;14:21–25.

20 Anesthesia for the Complicated Obstetric Patient

Lisa A. Dado

INTRODUCTION

A thorough understanding of the nature of the parturient's pain is the first aspect in providing optimal obstetric anesthetic care. Once the biology and pathophysiology of this special acute pain is discussed, then the benefits of analgesia for this pain will appropriately follow. Pharmacology of local anesthetics and related drugs will be reviewed, with special emphasis on complications associated with their administration. A variety of techniques including epidural, subarachnoid and other regional techniques will be discussed with benefits and complications reviewed. General anesthesia for cesarean section delivery will be outlined. A variety of special consideration patients will be addressed including: (1) The preeclamptic patient, (2) preterm birth patient on tocolytics, (3) HIV positive mothers, (4) coagulopathies, (5) cardiac disease, and (6) pulmonary disease.

Nature of the Patient's Pain

The current concept of pain focuses on the peripheral nervous system relaying a stimulus to the central nervous system for interpretive evaluation—the somatosensory system (Fig. 20-1). The peripheral system consists of afferent neurons which are embedded in body tissues awaiting nociceptive (painful) stimuli. These afferent neurons are termed Ad (A-delta) and C-fibers. These fibers transverse into the spinal segments and synapse at the dorsal spinal ganglion. Here, substance-P is released causing the painful effect to be initiated. From each spinal segment stimulated, these messages ascend through one of two pathways to the thalamus for further modulation: the lateral spinothalamic tract or the medial lemniscus tract. Once at the thalamus, adjustment and regulation from inherent emotional and psychological factors occurs. The data supports the emphasis on the importance of perceptual factors that influence a patient's total pain experience (Table 20-1). The psychodynamics of prior experience, motivation, anxiety, anticipation of pain, attention, personality, and ethnic and cultural factors all influence the modulation of substance-P release, affecting the pain experience. From the thalamus, this information is synthesized in the sensory cortex for relay to the many effector sites which contribute to the pain response. Once pain has been perceived, there is an initiation of the pain response which has neuroendocrine, behavioral and psychological implications.

In humans, there is a 300 to 600 percent increase in epinephrine and 200 to 400 percent increase in norepinephrine levels produced during severe pain experienced in active labor. There is a 200 to 300 percent increase in cortisol levels, as well as, increases in corticosteroid and adreno-cortictropic hormone

Schematic of the somatosensory system.

1. A-delta (Ad) and C fibers in body tissues, afferent nociceptor fibers.
2. Spinal ganglion. Substance P is released at receptor. Its function is to cause a "pain" affect.
3. Medial lemniscus tract (anterior ascending tract).
4. Lateral spinothalamic tract (anterior ascending tract).
5. Thalamus, the relay center for incoming sensory input from Ad and C fibers and psychological and emotional factors.
6. Cerebral cortex integrating center from sensory input.

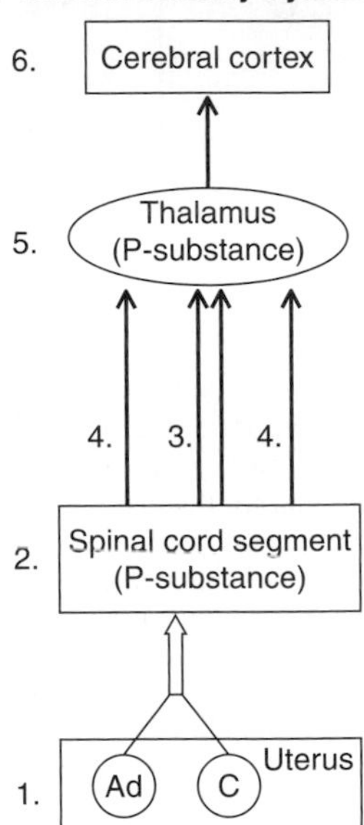

FIG. 20-1 Schematic of the somatosensory system. **1.** A-delta (Ad) and C fibers in body tissues, afferent nociceptor fibers. **2.** Spinal ganglion. Substance P is released at receptor. Its function is to cause a "pain" affect. **3.** Medial lemniscus tract (anterior ascending tract). **4.** Lateral spinothalamic tract (anterior ascending tract). **5.** Thalamus, the relay center for incoming sensory input from Ad and C fibers and psychological and emotional factors. **6.** Cerebral cortex integrating center from sensory input.

levels reaching their peaks at or after delivery. During labor the cardiac output increase is 40 to 50 percent with a further 20 to 30 percent increase during painful contractions. The systolic and diastolic blood pressures also increase by 20 to 30 mmHg. These increases in cardiac output (CO) and systolic blood pressure (SBP) lead to a significant increase in left ventricular stroke work that may be harmful to patients with preeclampsia, hypertension, cardiac valvular disease, pulmonary hypertension, or severe anemia.

With the sympathetic-induced lipolytic metabolism, increases in free fatty acids and lactate produce relative maternal acidosis. Increased sympathetic activity increases metabolism and oxygen consumption, and decreases gastrointestinal and urinary bladder motility. Respiratory rate is increased with resultant respiratory alkalosis. The kidney compensates by excreting HCO_3^-. Diminished $PaCO_2$ levels below 25 to 27 mmHg may result in increased uteroplacental resistance and reduced oxygen delivery to the fetus.

During peak contractions, there is a reduction of intervillous blood flow leading to a significant decrease in placental gas exchange. This exaggerates the already dramatic reduction in uterine blood flow, secondary to the increases in norepinephrine and cortisol.

TABLE 20-1 Pain Perception

Psychological	Anxiety, fear, emotional arousal
Behavioral	Verbalization, motor activity
Neuro-endocrine	Hyperventilation—maternal respiratory
	Endocrine (stress) response
	↑ adrenocorticotropic hormone (ACTH), ↑ cortisol
	↑ epinephrine, norepinephrine
	↑ lipolytic metabolism—metabolic acidosis
	Cardiovascular Response
	↑ systemic vascular resistance
	↑ cardiac output
	↑ blood pressure
	↑ oxygen consumption
	↑ left ventricular stroke work
	Gastrointestinal function
	↓ gastric motility
	↑ risk for gastroesophageal reflux/aspiration
	↑ nausea and vomiting
	Urinary function
	↓ emptying—urinary retention
	oliguria
Fetal effects	↓ uterine blood flow
	↑ fetal heart rate alterations

Effects of Analgesia

By blocking nociceptive input, there is a reduction in the release of cathecholamines, adrenal corticotropic hormone and cortisol in the parturient (Table 20-2). Effective analgesia significantly reduces pain related hemodynamic changes. Maternal cardiac output fluctuations are modulated and oxygen consumption is reduced. Gastric and bladder motility is not adversely affected by neuroblockade. Cautious epidural analgesia has been reported to provide a vasomotor blocking effect which increases intervillous blood flow and oxygen delivery to the fetus.

The first stage of labor refers to the beginning of cervical dilation and effacement until its completion. The second stage of labor extends from complete cervical dilation until delivery of the infant. The third stage is the delivery of the placenta.

TABLE 20-2 Analgesic Effects

Psychological	↓ Anxiety, ↓ fear, ↑ emotional stability
Behavioral	↓ Motor activity
Neuroendocrine	↓ Respiratory alkalosis (maternal)
	↓ Catechol release
	↓ Cortisol
	↓ Adrenocorticotropic hormone (ACTH)
	↓ Metabolic acidosis (maternal)
	↓ Cardiac output
	↓ Oxygen consumption
	↓ Left ventricular stroke work
	Normal gastrointestinal function
	Normal urinary function
Fetal effects	↑ Uterine blood flow
	More stability in fetal heart rate tracing

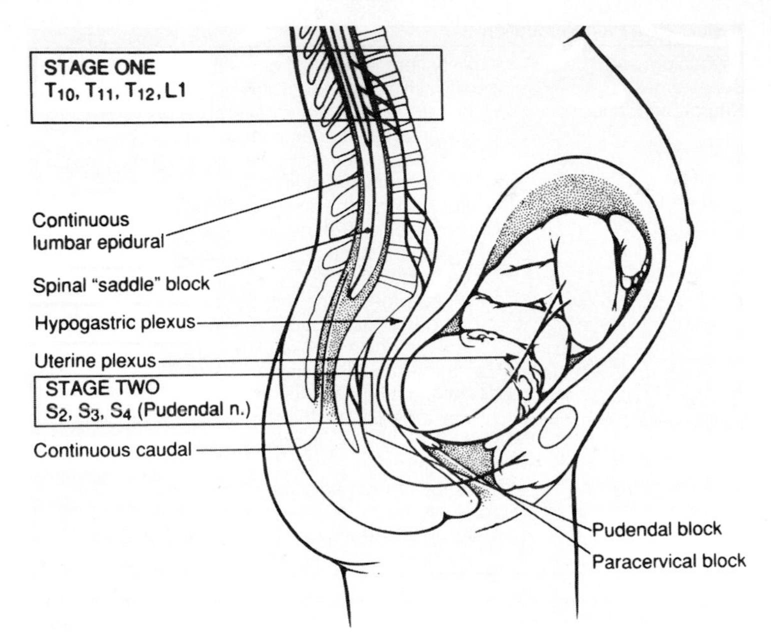

FIG. 20-2 Note the completely separate pain fibers responsible for pain in the first and second stages of labor: T_{10}-L_1 versus S_2-S_4 (*Reproduced with permission from Principles and Practice of Obstetric Analgesia and Anesthesia, John J. Bonica, 2nd edn. Baltimore, MD: Williams & Wilkins.*)

Transmission of pain during the first stage of labor is from spinal segments (pain fibers) T_{10}, T_{11}, T_{12}, and L_1 and the second and third stage of labor is from S_2, S_3 and S_4 (Fig. 20-2). It is important for the care provider to understand the differences between the pain conduction (spinal levels) during the first stage of labor, as compared with the second and third stage, in order to provide appropriately directed analgesia. It is also important to consider that pain may also be due to the pathology of the gestation, such as abruptio placenta, infection, adnexal torsion, or appendicitis, and these may be *masked* if total neuroblockade is achieved from T_4-S_5 at the onset of labor. Only segments necessary for the specific pain of labor should be blocked (Table 20-3). Relatively decreased fetal perfusion has been reported to occur both in the presence and absence of overt maternal hypotension secondary to a sympathectomy mediated reduction in uterine blood flow.

Pharmacology of Local Anesthetics and Related Drugs

The desired action of all local anesthetics is the reversible blockade of nerve conduction and, therefore, the cascade of events producing perception of pain. These drugs prevent the development of an action potential in a nerve by blocking sodium channels responsible for propagating a response in the nerve fiber (Fig. 20-3). Local anesthetics exist in both charged and uncharged form. The uncharged state of the drug crosses the lipid nerve membrane and enters the cell. Once in the cell, it reequilibrates into the charged form that is

TABLE 20-3 Innervation of Pelvic Viscera

Uterus	Motor fibers from parasympathetic pelvic nerves from S_2, S_3, S_4, and sympathetic sensory
Tubes/ovaries	Motor fibers from parasympathetic pelvic nerves from S_2, S_3, S_4, and sympathetic sensory fibers via the ovarian plexus from T_{12}, L_1
Broad ligament	Motor fibers from parasympathetic pelvic nerves from S_2, S_3, S_4, and sympathetic sensory fibers via the hypogastric plexus from T_{12}, L_1
Cervix	Motor fibers from parasympathetic pelvic nerves from S_2, S_3, S_4, and sympathetic sensory fibers via the hypogastric plexus from T_{12}, L_1
Vagina	Motor fibers from parasympathetic pelvic nerves from S_2, S_3, S_4, and sympathetic sensory fibers via the hypogastric plexus from T_{12}, L_1
Vestibule/hymen	Erectile vasodilator fibers from parasympathetic pelvic nerves from S_2, S_3, S_4
Labia	Posterior labial nerve S_2, S_3, and perineal branch of the posterior femoral cutaneous nerve S_1, S_2, S_3
Clitoris	Erectile vasodilator fibers from parasympathetic pelvic nerves from S_2, S_3, S_4
Perineum	Motor and sensory innervation from the pudendal nerve arising from S_2, S_3, S_4
Bladder	Sympathetic fibers from T_{11}, T_{12}, L_1, L_2 via the superior/inferior hypogastric plexuses control the sphincter and parasympathetic fibers from S_2, S_3, S_4 control filling/emptying of the bladder
Anus	Motor and sensory innervation from the pudendal nerve arising from S_2, S_3, S_4

Note: Reproduced with permission from *Principles and Practice of Obstetric Analgesia and Anesthesia*, John J. Bonica, 2nd edn. Malvern, Pennsylvania: Williams & Wilkins.

readily dissolved in water. This charged form now reaches the sodium channels and blocks them from the inside.

Ionization

The capacity for an uncharged species to assume a charged form, is the essential property of all local anesthetics. They are a combination of a weak base and a strong acid.

$$B + H^+ \neq BH^+$$

As a general principle, lowering the pH will increase the ionized percentage of the drug, and raising the pH will increase the uncharged form of the drug. Since the local anesthetics are usually supplied in an acidic medium, the addition of $NaHCO_3$ will increase the relative uncharged portion allowing the drug to cross the nerve membrane more readily resulting in a quicker onset of block.

Usual doses

0.1 cc $NaHCO_3$/10 cc bupivicaine
1.0 cc $NaHCO_3$/10 cc lidocaine

Precipitation of the local anesthetic will occur if too much $NaHCO_3$ is added. Comparative properties of lidocaine and bupivacaine are outlined in Table 20-4.

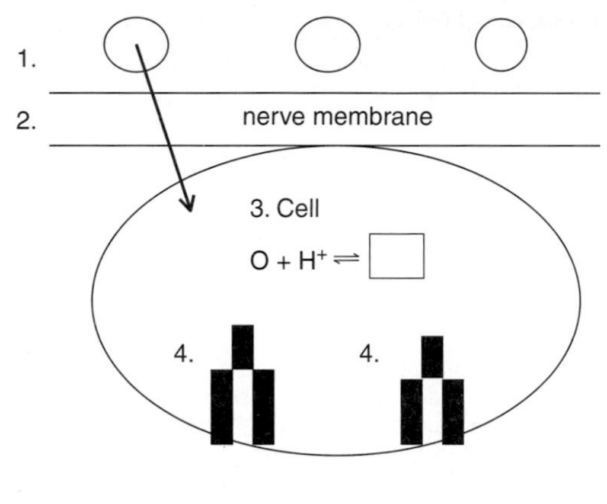

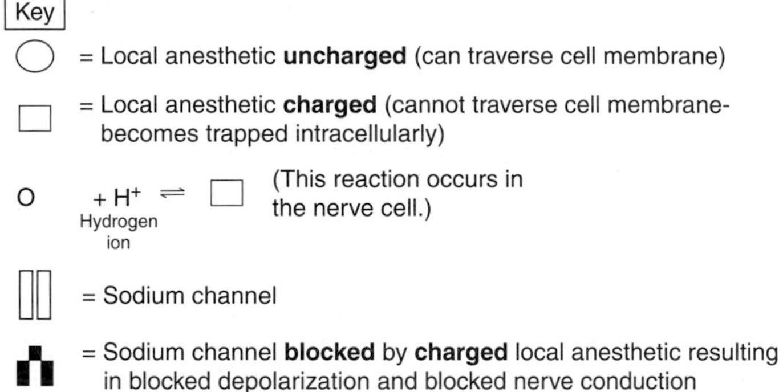

FIG. 20-3 *Uncharged* **(1)** local anesthetic passes through the *nerve membrane* **(2)** into the *cell* **(3)** where the local anesthetic gains a H^+ (hydrogen ion) to become charged *blocked Na^+-channel* **(4)** in the nerve cell by the *charged* local anesthetic does not allow the nerve to propagate a nerve impulse.

Protein Binding

Protein binding is another property important to understand. All local anesthetics bind to albumin and μ-1-acid glycoprotein (AAG). It is the free—portion of the drug that is responsible for toxicity. In pregnancy, albumin levels are depressed, so AAG binding becomes most important. AAG is released in response to surgery, trauma, infection, and inflammation. Once AAG sites are saturated with local anesthetics, the free drug levels progressively increase. Protein binding also decreases with decreasing pH. Therefore, in an acidotic environment a high proportion of free drug with the potential for cardiac or neurotoxicity should be anticipated.

Absorption

Absorption of local anesthetics refers to the movement of the drug from the site of injection to the bloodstream. Therefore, the more vascular the area and the larger the total dose of anesthetic used, the higher the resulting serum level of the drug. The addition of a vasoconstrictor (epinephrine) to

TABLE 20-4 Properties of Lidocaine, Bupivacaine and Ropivacaine

Property	Lidocaine	Bupivacaine	Ropivacaine
Molecular weight	234	288	274
pK_a	7.7 (at pH 7.4, more drug in basic form)	8.1	8.0
Lipid solubility (directly related to speed of onset)	↑↑↑↑↑	↑↑	↑↑↑
Protein binding	64%	95%	94%
Elimination $T_{1/2}$ (h)	1.6	2.8	1.9
Maximum dose[a]	5 mg/kg (350 mg in a 70 kg patient) (7 mg/kg with epinephrine)	2–3 mg/kg (175 mg in a 70 kg patient)	>2 mg/kg
Toxicity	Seizures	Cardiac arrest	Seizures with much larger doses

a1% = 10 mg/cc; 0.25% bupivacaine = 2.5 mg/cc; 0.2% ropivacaine = 2.0 mg/cc.

the local anesthetic can decrease the absorption and therefore, *toxicity* of the drug used.

Toxicity

Local anesthetic toxicity may manifest with central nervous system or cardiac effects. As the doses increase, disinhibition and CNS excitation occurs producing seizures. Local anesthetic bind and inhibit cardiac Na^+, Ca^{2+} and K^+ channels as concentrations increase causing cardiac arrest. Treatment of adverse reactions depends on the severity of their effects from spontaneous recovery, to supportive care with oxygen and maintaining the airway, to ACLS.

New Medication

Ropivacaine

Ropivacaine is a relatively new local anesthetic with similar characteristics to bupivicaine. This is produced solely as the S-enantiomer, whereas bupivicaine is a mixture of the S and R forms. This S-form has less ability to bind Na–channels in the myocardial conduction system. Therefore, there is less risk of cardio toxicity with ropivacaine. As seen in Table 20-4. Ropivacaine and bupivicaine have very similar physical properties except for the margin of safety, in ropivacaine, which produces less toxic side effects. There also appears to be *less of a motor block* compared to bupivicaine improving patient satisfaction during the laboring process.

Epidural Analgesia/Anesthesia

Lumbar epidural block is the most common form of analgesia used to provide relief from the nociceptive pathways during the stages of labor. The epidural space is the interval superiorly bounded by the foramen magnum, inferiorly by the lower end of the dural sac, anteriorly by the posterior longitudinal ligament and posteriorly by the ligamentum flavum. The approach to the

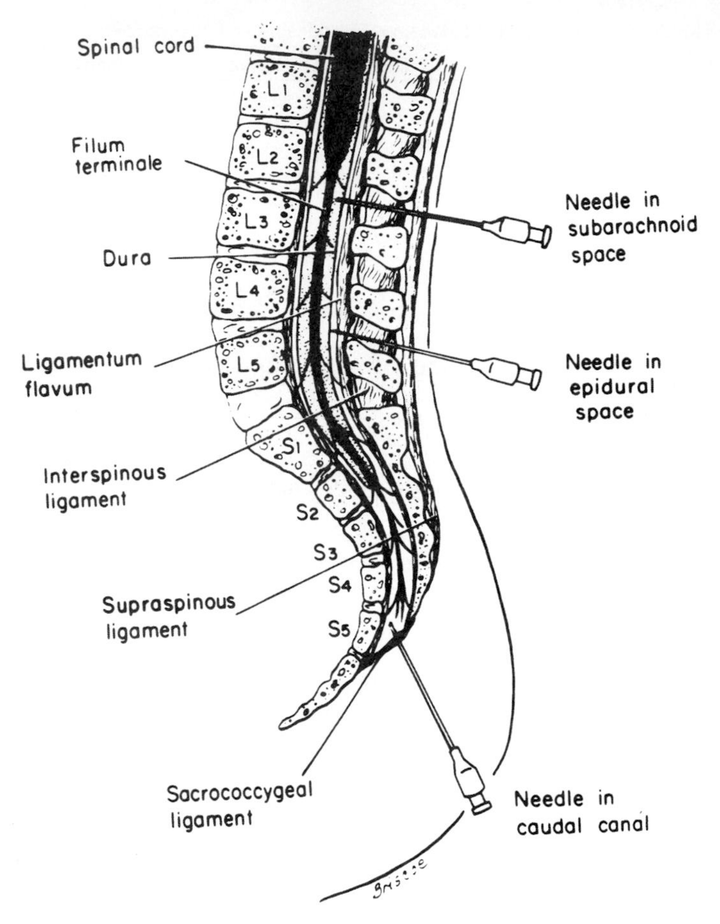

FIG. 20-4 Lumbosacral anatomy showing needle depth for epidural and subarachnoid injections. (*Reproduced with permission from Anesthesia for Obstetrics, Sol M. Shnider, 3rd edn. Baltimore, MD: Williams & Wilkins.*)

epidural space is posteriorly through the skin, subcutaneous fat, supraspinous ligament, interspinous ligament, ligamentum flavum and into the epidural space (Fig. 20-4).

The size of the epidural space varies along its course with the largest diameter existing at the L_2 interspace with a range of 4 to 9 mm. A simple maneuver which helps to open up the bony entrance to the epidural space is flexion of the lumbar spine (Fig. 20-5).

The contents of the epidural space include fat, vertebral venous plexus, lymphatics, arteries, and dural spinal nerve projections. In pregnancy, with the increase in intraabdominal pressure, the venous plexus becomes distended. This phenomenon, and the accompaning increase in epidural fat that

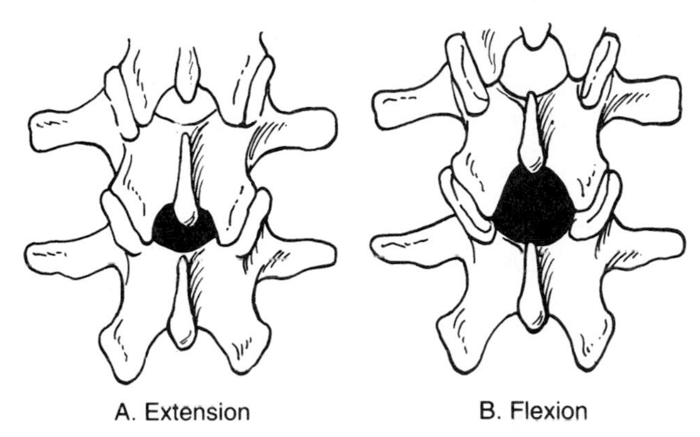

FIG. 20-5 Lumbar vertebrae. When patient is fixed, the interlaminar space enlarges, increasing the ability to enter the epidural/subarachnoid space. (*Reproduced with permission from Principles and Practice of Obstetric Analgesia and Anesthesia, John J. Bonica, 2nd edn. Pennsylvania: Williams & Wilkins, Malvern.*)

occurs during pregnancy, functions to substantially reduce epidural volume. Therefore, pregnant patients usually require less volume of local anesthetic, as compared to nonpregnant controls, to produce a similar level of blockade.

Once the epidural catheter is in place, local anesthetic is administered according to the appropriate pain pathway and corresponding stage of labor. In the first stage of labor, T_{10} block is sufficient. In the late first stage and second stage of labor the nerves to be blocked include the sacral area so the parturient should be dosed in the semi-Fowler's position to allow downward spread of the local anesthetic. Finally, for predelivery and the third stage of labor, the parturient may be seated upright (with a vena cava tilt) to secure sacral root spread of the drug (Fig. 20-6). This blockade may be achieved by intermittent bolus injections or by continuous infusion of the drug with changes in patient positioning altering the level of blockade.

With the uppermost level of analgesia at T_{10}, the five lowermost vasomotor segments supplying the pelvis, lower trunk and limbs are interrupted causing a decrease in total peripheral resistance, venous return and cardiac output. In normal parturients, this insult induces a reflex cardiovascular response directed towards maintaining systemic blood pressure. Preload of an adequate intravenous crystalloid infusion, keeping the parturient on her side, and minimizing the dose of the local anesthetic all minimize the adverse decrease in blood flow to the pelvis and its structures.

High epidural anesthesia that extends to T_4-S_5 is associated with a significant interruption of vasomotor segments resulting in significant hypotension. Again, fluid preload and lateral tilt of the parturient can augment the reflex corrective responses of the cardiovascular system in this situation. Extending the epidural blockade above spinal level T_{10} is unnecessary and counterproductive for the normal laboring patient. If epidural analgesia needs to be changed to anesthesia for a cesarian section, then these risks are necessary and measures to prevent them should be instituted. In addition, ephedrine, in most

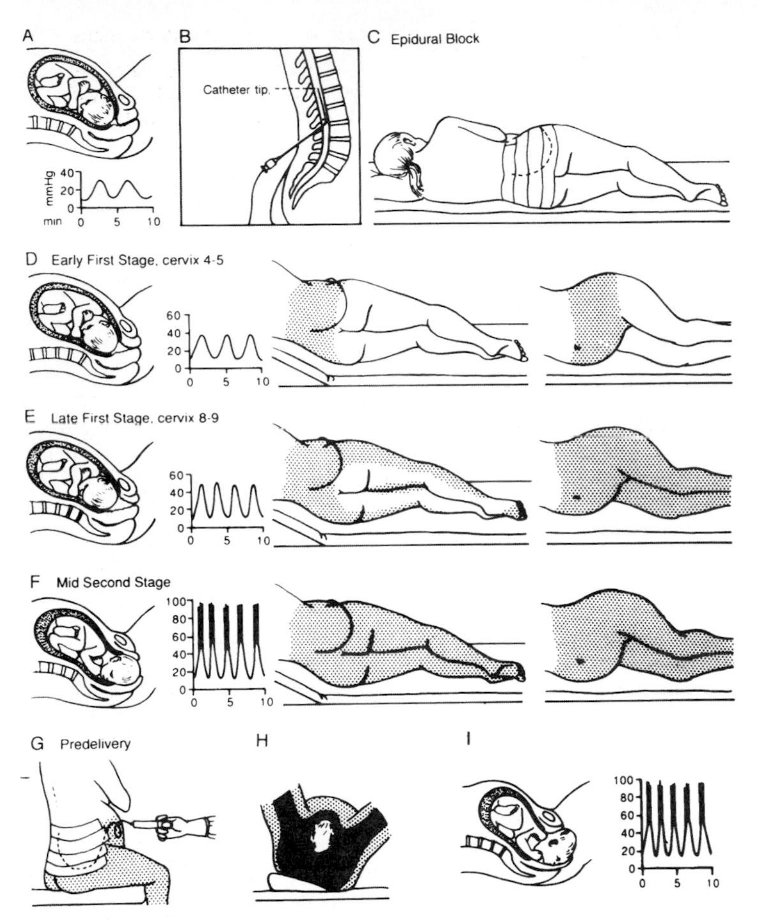

FIG. 20-6 Lumbar epidural analgesia. **A-C.** Epidural catheter may be placed early in the first stage of labor **D.** When the patient experiences labor pain, local anesthetic may be injected to achieve a T_{10}-L_1 neuroblockade. **E-F.** In late first stage and mid-second stage of labor—the patient should be elevated 15–20° to allow caudad spread of local anesthetic to achieve a T_{10}-S_5 block. **G-I.** To ensure sacral root dispersion of local anesthetic, once flexion and internal rotation of baby's head occurs, more local anesthetic can be injected with the patient in the seated upright position with a left tilt to the pelvis. (*Reproduced with permission from Principles and Practice of Obstetric Analgesia and Anesthesia, John J. Bonica, 2nd edn. Malvern, Pennsylvania: Williams & Wilkins.*)

circumstances, is the best vasopressor to augment blood pressure without reducing blood supply to the uterus.

Contraindications to lumbar epidural analgesia/anesthesia are reviewed in Table 20-5. The advantages and disadvantages of regional analgesia/anesthesia are outlined in Table 20-6.

TABLE 20-5 Contraindications to Lumbar Epidural Analgesia/Anesthesia

- Parturients who refuse the block or have great fear of puncture of the spine. In our experience, many patients who are concerned initially about epidural block will consent to be managed with this technique provided they are properly informed. However, if they still refuse, it is an absolute contraindication to the technique.
- Lack of skill by the administrator, not only in carrying out the procedure, but in the management of the parturient and in the prompt treatment of complications.
- Infection at the puncture site or in the epidural space.
- Severe hypovolemia from hemorrhage, dehydration, or malnutrition.
- Coagulopathies.
- Lack of resuscitation equipment in the immediate area ready for *prompt* use.
- In addition to the above, absolute contraindication to continuous caudal epidural anesthesia are infection or cyst in the area of the sacrococcygeal region and having the presenting part close to the perineum.

Relative Contraindications Include

- Lack of appreciation by the obstetrician as to how the procedure influences the management of labor.
- A very rapid or precipitate labor, or in any case which requires immediate anesthesia. On the other hand for the anesthesiologist who is very skilled and has had extensive experience, extension of the epidural block in patients who have had the catheter in place during labor can be done as rapidly as getting things ready for anesthesia.
- Cephalopelvic disproportion unless the block is used for a trial of labor prior to cesarean section.

Source: Reproduced with permission from *Principles and Practice of Obstetric Analgesia and Anesthesia*, John J. Bonica, 2nd edn, Malvern, Pennsylvania: Williams & Wilkins.

A combined spinal/epidural analgesia technique provides rapid onset of spinal opioid analgesia, plus the flexibility of the epidural blockade. Sufen tanil 10 μg or Fentanyl 25 μg injected spinally when the epidural catheter is inserted, can reliably give several hours of analgesia to patients in the early first stage of labor (<5 cm dilation). The continuous infusion of a weak local anesthetic (0.125 percent/0.0625 percent bupivicaine or 0.2 percent/0.1 percent ropivacaine) with a low dose narcotic (Sufentanil 1 to 2 μg/cc or Fentanyl 5 to 10 μg/cc) can provide good perineal analgesia for later stages of labor. If needed, higher concentrations of bupivacaine or lidocaine can be bolused for more complete nerve blockade. Less motor blockade, less hypotension, less local anesthetic administered with inherent toxicity risk, and faster onset of analgesia are all benefits of this combined technique.

The side effects of intrathecal opioids and corresponding treatment are listed in Table 20-7.

Other Regional Analgesic/Anesthetic Techniques

There are two important techniques to discuss that may be used by the obstetric care provider to provide analgesia when obstetrical anesthesia coverage is unavailable. Although these techniques are relatively easy to execute, a thorough knowledge of the anatomy, physiology, and effects of local anesthetics on mother and fetus is paramount.

TABLE 20-6 Advantages and Disadvantages of Regional Analgesia/Anesthesia

Advantages
• In contrast to opoids, regional analgesia produces complete relief from pain in most parturients.
• The hazards of pulmonary aspiration of gastric contents that is inherent in general anesthesia is diminished and can be even eliminated.
• *Provided it is properly administered* and no complications occur, regional analgesia/anesthesia causes no serious maternal or neonatal complications.
• Administered at the proper time, it does not impede the progress of labor at the first stage.
• Continuous techniques can be extended for delivery and may even be modified for cesarean section if this becomes necessary.
• Regional analgesia permits the mother to remain awake during labor and delivery so that she can experience the pleasure of actively participating in the birth of her child.
• Regional anesthesia for cesarean section also permits the mother to be awake and immediately develop bonding with the newborn.
• Provided the mother is doing well, the anesthesiologist can leave her and resuscitate the newborn if this is necessary.
Disadvantages
• Regional techniques require greater skill to administer than do administration of systemic drugs or inhalation agents.
• Technical failures occur even in experienced hands.
• Certain techniques produce side effects (e.g., maternal hypotension) that if not promptly and properly treated can progress to complications in the mother and fetus.
• Techniques that produce perineal muscle paralysis interfere with the mechanism of internal rotation and increase the incidence of posterior positions and thus require instrumental deliveries.
• These procedures can only be carried out in the hospital.

Source: Reproduced with permission from *Principles and Practice of Obstetric Analgesia and Anesthesia*, John J. Bonica, 2nd edn. Malvern, Pennsylvania: Williams & Wilkins.

TABLE 20-7 Intrathecal Opioids Side Effects and Recommended Treatment

Side effect	Treatment
Itching	Benadryl, 25 mg IV
	Propofol, 10 mg IV
	Naloxone, 40 μg IV
Nausea and vomiting	Reglan, 10 mg IV
	Propofol, 10 mg IV
	Naloxone, 40 μg IV
	Zofran, 4 mg IV
Hypotension	IV fluids
	Ephedrine
Urinary retention	Catheterization
	Naloxone, 400 μg IV

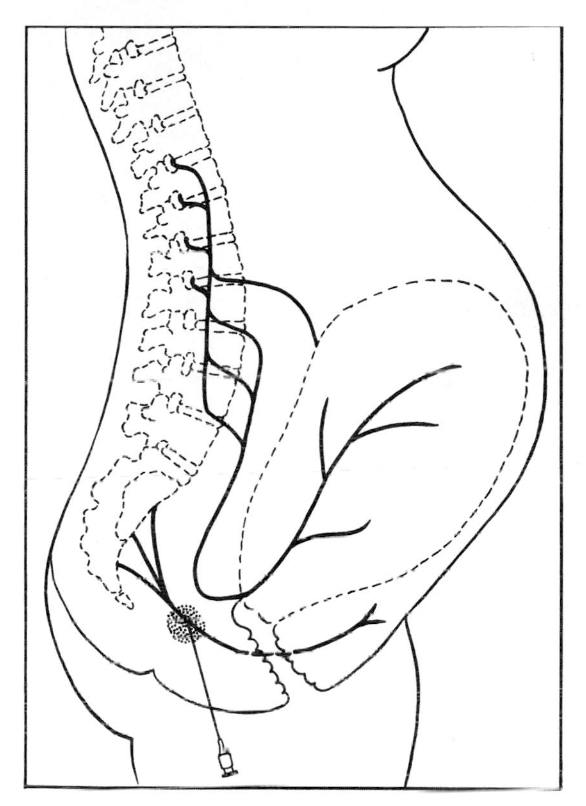

FIG. 20-7 Demonstration of the pudendal nerve block involving only S_{3-5} for the pain associated with the second stage of labor. (*Reproduced with permission from Principles and Practice of Obstetric Analgesia and Anesthesia, John J. Bonica, 2nd edn. Malvern, Pennsylvania: Williams & Wilkins.*)

Bilateral Pudendal Nerve Block

This block is an effective blockade for the second and third stages of labor, blocking the sacral nerves S_3-S_4-S_5 (Fig. 20-7). The transvaginal approach points the needle behind the sacrospinous ligament aiming toward the ischial spine. Up to 5 mg/kg of lidocaine (1 percent solution with or without 1:200,000 epinephrine) total dose, provides relief of perineal pain within 3 to 5 minutes (Figs. 20-8 and 20-9).

Bilateral Paracervical Block

Paracervical block interrupts uterine nociceptive pain pathways T_{10}-L_1, effecting complete relief from pain of the first stage of labor (Fig. 20-10). This does not, however, relieve any perineal pain of the second and third stages of labor. Using up to 5 mg/kg of lidocaine in a 1 percent solution total dose, will give good pain relief for approximately two hours. Associated transient fetal

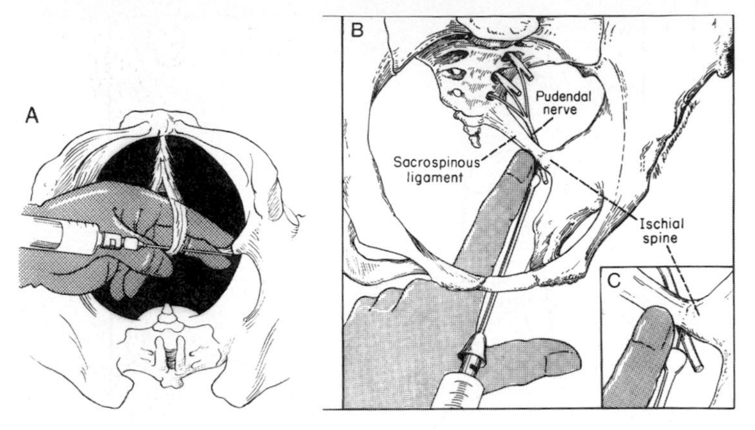

FIG. 20-8 The transvaginal approach to pudendal neuroblockade. **A-C.** This technique is performed bilaterally. The needle passes behind the sacrospinous ligament and posterior to the ischial spine. Aspiration, prior to injection of the local anesthetic drug, is prudent to avoid inadvertent intravascular administration. (*Reproduced with permission from Principles and Practice of Obstetric Analgesia and Anesthesia, John J. Bonica, 2nd edn. Malvern, Pennsylvania: Williams & Wilkins.*)

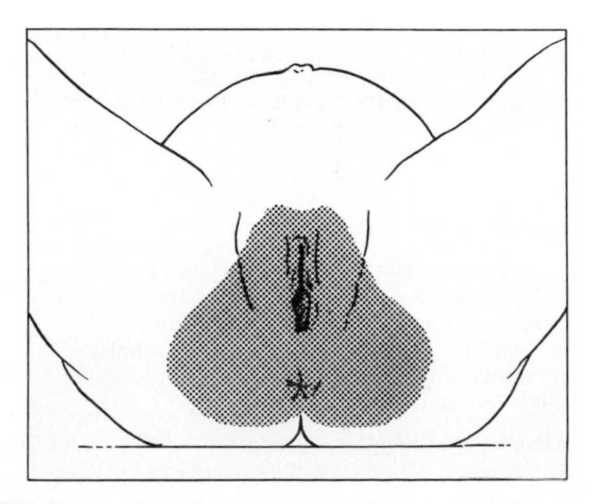

FIG. 20-9 Stippled area illustrates the extent of analgesia/anesthesia provided by pudendal neuroblockade—sufficient for the second stage of labor pain. (*Reproduced with permission from Principles and Practice of Obstetric Analgesia and Anesthesia, John J. Bonica, 2nd edn. Malvern, Pennsylvania: Williams & Wilkins.*)

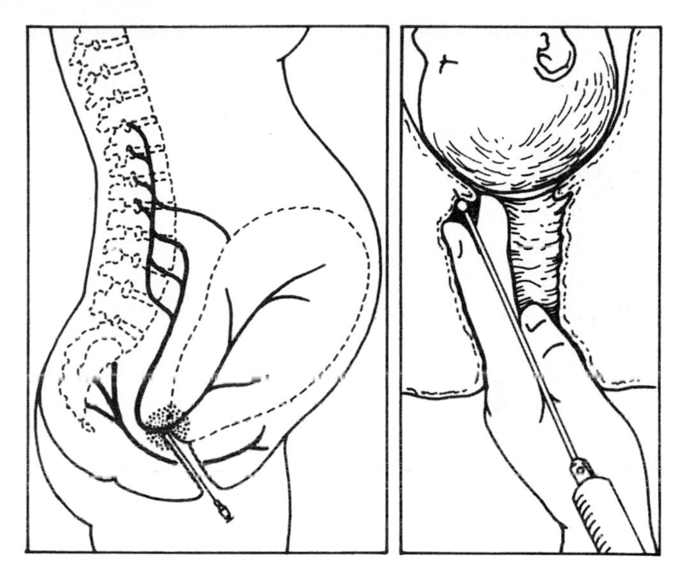

FIG. 20-10 A technique for bilateral paracervical block. Neuroblockade involving T_{10}-L_1 when accomplished is adequate for the pain associated with the first stage of labor. Injections are made into the bilateral fornices of the vagina. Note the proximity of the presenting part, as well as, the deeper pelvic plexus with uterine arteries and ureters. (*Reproduced with permission from Principles and Practice of Obstetric Analgesia and Anesthesia, John J. Bonica, 2nd edn. Malvern, Pennsylvania: Williams & Wilkins.*)

bradycardia has been reported with the use of paracervical blockade and therefore should be used with caution. Local anesthetics with epinephrine should not be used since the fetal head is so close to the injection site and the proximate location of the uterine artery and venous plexus that it may increase the risk of epinephrine uptake by mother and/or fetus.

Anesthesia for Cesarean Sections

Spinal Anesthesia

The advantages of spinal anesthesia responsible for its current popularity include, relative simplicity, rapidity, certainty, duration, low failure rate and minimal side effects. It also offers the lowest drug exposure since local anesthetic is being exposed directly to nerve fibers with minimal systemic uptake of the drug.

The primary disadvantages of spinal anesthesia are the effects of high $T_{2\text{-}4}$ blockade with maternal hypotension and postural puncture headaches (Table 20-8). The risk of the high spinal includes sympathectomy with resultant unopposed parasympathetic stimulation. This leads to hypotension, increased gastric motility, increased nausea/vomiting, and instability of uterine perfusion. In parturients with severe asthma or reactive airway disease, this may precipitate bronchospasm. Also, the high motor blockade may inhibit motor fibers of the respiratory muscles impairing normal ventilation.

TABLE 20-8 The Primary Disadvantages of the Use of Spinal Anesthesia and the Contraindications

Primary disadvantages
Frequency of hypotension
Postdural puncture headaches
Contraindications
Infection at the site of puncture
Disease of the central nervous system
Severe hypovolemia due to hemorrhage, dehydration or malnutrition
Feto-pelvic disproportion unless the block is used for a trial of labor prior to cesarean section
Parturient refusal or fear of the procedure, or emotional unsuitability for regional anesthesia
Severe hypotension or hypertension
Lack of skilled physicians
Lack of resuscitation equipment in the immediate area

Source: Reproduced with permission from *Principles and Practice of Obstetric Analgesia and Anesthesia*, John J. Bonica, 2nd edn. Malvern, Pennsylvania: Williams & Wilkins.

The postdural puncture headache risks are directly related to the size and type of needle used. With the 24/26 G Sprotte (blunted) needles now in use, the risk is <1 percent in this age group of patients. An important factor in the dispersion of the local anesthetic is the position of the patient. As shown in Fig. 20-11, the lowest point of the spine is T_5. Care therefore should be directed towards raising the patient's head in an effort to reduce the inadvertent cephalad spread of the drug. Complications of subarachnoid block include

- *Physiological:* hypotension, bradycardia or possible cardiac arrest
- *Nonphysiological:* respiratory arrest and toxicity reactions
- *Neurological:* paraplegia, arachnoiditis, or postdural puncture headache

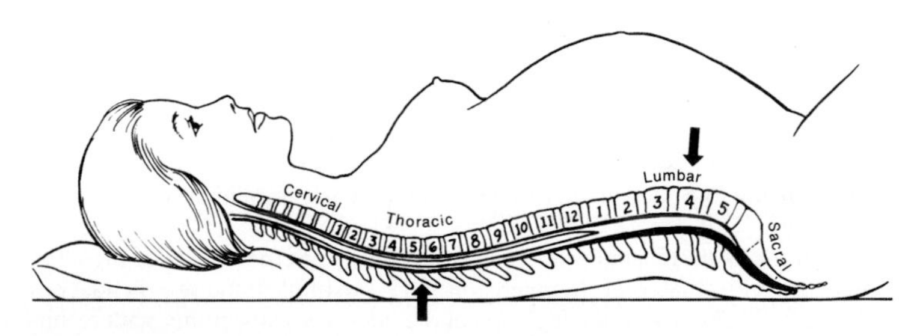

FIG. 20-11 The natural curves of the female spine in the supine position. Gravity tends to ascend the level of anesthetic spread to T_3-T_5, therefore, an early head-up tilt would assure a lower level of blockade. (*Reproduced with permission from Principles and Practice of Obstetric Analgesia and Anesthesia, John J. Bonica, 2nd edn. Malvern, Pennsylvania: Williams & Wilkins.*)

General Anesthesia for Cesarean Section

General anesthesia is reserved for life-threatening situations including severe fetal distress, cord prolapse, shoulder dystocia, intrauterine exploration for retained placenta or a twin, and replacement of an inverted uterus. In obstetrical anesthesia, the anesthesiologist is responsible for two lives: the mother and the baby.

Preanesthetic preparation includes a history and physical examination with emphasis on cardiac and pulmonary disease, evaluation of the airway, height/weight comparison, allergies, current medications, intravenous access and blood product availability. Every pregnant woman beyond the first trimester is considered to have a full stomach and is at risk for aspiration of gastric contents. This demands prophylaxis with a nonparticulate antacid, an H_2-blocker, and metochlorpropamide (Reglan). The most common cause of maternal death related to general anesthesia is aspiration pneumonia secondary to inability to secure the airway with an endotracheal tube.

Induction of Anesthesia

The patient should be placed on the operating table with a leftward pelvic tilt to prevent aorto-caval compression with monitors applied. She should receive a 500 cc to 1000 cc lactated Ringer's bolus while preoxygenation is performed. Cricoid pressure should be applied as the Sellick maneuver is achieved, to prevent regurgitation of stomach contents into the lung. The obstetrician who is prepared and ready to make an incision with one hand, may place the other hand on the patient's epigastric area. Intravenous induction with thiopental (3 to 5 mg/kg), propofol (1 to 2 mg/kg), ketamine (1 mg/kg), or Etomidate (0.2 to 0.3 mg/kg) may be used. Succinylcholine 1 mg/kg IV is given to achieve muscle relaxation to facilitate endotracheal intubation. Once the endotracheal tube is placed, the first breath given by the anesthesiologist should *not* be felt by the obstetrician's hand over the stomach. If a belch of air is perceived, the ETT may not, in fact, be in the trachea. This team approach assures maximal security of a protected, intubated airway, prior to surgical incision. Maintenance of a balanced general anesthesia with both inhalational agents and intravenous muscle relaxants is performed until delivery of the baby. At this time, narcotics may be given to reduce the concentration of inhalational drugs needed.

The patient should be completely awake and in control of her airway protective reflexes before extubation occurs. It is important to understand that the risk of aspiration at the end of surgery (extubation) is just as great as at the start (intubation).

Figure 20-12 is a guide to failed intubation events with/without a known difficult airway, with/without the ability to ventilate, and with/without fetal distress.

Special Considerations

Preeclampsia

Preeclampsia is a multisystem disease. Although its hallmarks are hypertension and proteinuria, patients may develop renal failure, thrombocytopenia, hemolysis, liver dysfunction and CNS involvement. For labor, epidural or epidural/spinal with narcotic/local anesthetic combinations are optimal to reduce the added stress related to pain. For cesarean section delivery, controversy

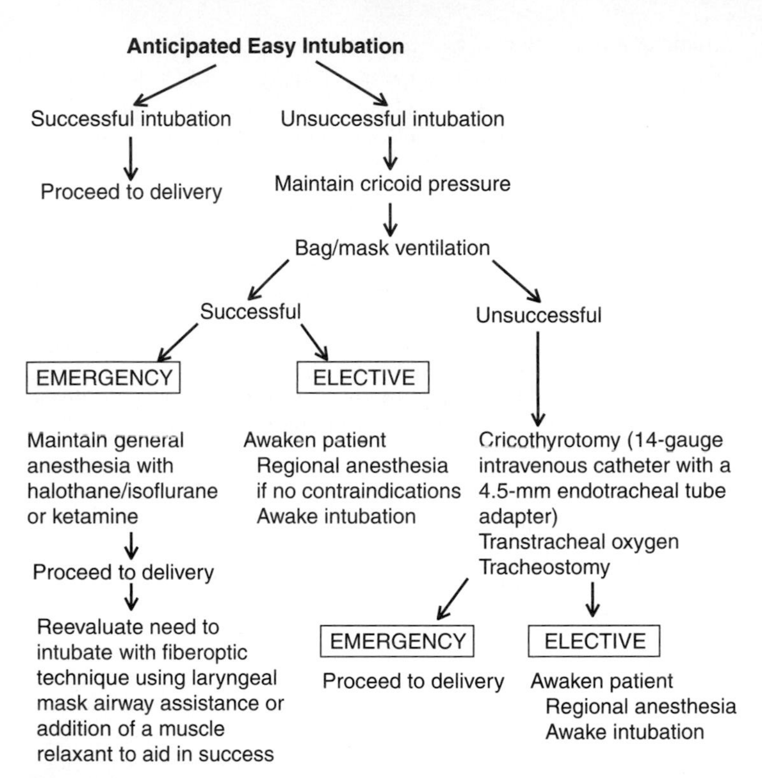

FIG. 20-12 Guide for failed intubation.

remains whether epidural or general anesthesia is best. Epidural anesthesia for cesarean section requires a high block-T_4 with the associated risk of maternal hypotension. General anesthesia requires intubation, which with tracheal stimulation may result in dangerous hemodynamic aberrations including hypertension, increased mean pulmonary artery pressure, and increased pulmonary capillary wedge pressure. With adequate invasive monitors such as an arterial line with or without a pulmonary artery catheter, careful hydration, use of Ephedrine and slow onset of the block, epidural blockade can be safely conducted. Also, the use of B-blocker agents (preinduction) or lidocaine to blunt the tracheal stimulation of intubation, can also be safe. Magnesium sulfate interacts with both depolarizing and nondepolarizing neuromuscular blocking drugs, so dosages must be altered accordingly. Close monitoring of the patient and open discussion of the patient's preoperative status with the obstetrician is helpful in determining the optimum anesthetic plan for mother and baby (see Chap. 5).

Preterm Birth

Patients with preterm labor, for whatever reason, will most likely have been on tocolytic drugs. If B-adrenergic drugs were used to secure uterine relaxation, care must be taken to observe for tachycardia, hypertension, chest pain, myocardial ischemia, arrhythmias, pulmonary edema, anxiety, nausea/vomiting, hyperglycemia, or hypokalemia that may be exaggerated by general anesthetics. In parturients on intravenous magnesium sulfate as a tocolytic agent, potentiation of muscle relaxant drug activity should be anticipated. Since preterm fetuses are often low birthweight, with diminished compensatory reserve, special attention should be directed at maintaining uteroplacental perfusion (see Chap. 22).

HIV-infected Parturients

Concern has been voiced in published literature that HIV positive parturients may not be candidates for regional anesthesia. The fear of spreading the infection to the central nervous system, adverse neurological sequelae, or attenuation of the immunological status of the patient has been questioned. To date, the available data support the use of epidural anesthesia in these patients with no substantiated evidence that these concerns are valid (see Chap. 26).

Coagulopathies

The preoperative laboratory tests recommended in a parturient with a suspected coagulopathy include: hemoglobin, hematocrit, platelet count, prothrombin time (PT), partial thromboplastin time (PTT), fibrinogen, and fibrin degradation products. There is no one source (authority) which specifies the best test or laboratory value in determining risk for epidural hematoma. The following are examples when epidural anesthesia is not recommended

- parturient on heparin therapy with elevated PTT or heparin level >0.24/mL
- parturient with known factor deficiency, for example. Von Willebrand's with low Factor 8 levels,
- parturient with severe HELLP syndrome
- parturient with disseminated intravascular coagulopathy
- parturient actively bleeding and hemodynamically unstable

Many examples of stable, but abnormal laboratory values may be amenable to an epidural technique. However, discussion with the obstetrician as to whether active bleeding is occurring and an overall risks versus benefits discussion of general anesthesia as compared to conduction anesthesia, in a given high risk circumstance, may help to determine the parturient's best overall anesthetic management.

Cardiac Disease—Congenital Heart Disease

The degree of shunting of blood in women with intracardiac defects is primarily determined by the balance of resistances in the systemic (systemic vascular resistance) and pulmonary vascular beds (pulmonary vascular resistance). During pregnancy, these resistances decline proportionally during the various stages of pregnancy. With atrial septal defect (ASD), ventricular septal defect (VSD), or patent ductus arteriosus (PDA) with a left to right shunt, these parturients usually tolerate pregnancy, anesthesia, and delivery well. Reminders are to be aware of arrhythmias, systemic embolism, right ventricular hypertrophy and failure, and pulmonary hypertension. These concerns are especially problematic in the postpartum period when placental shunting is gone (increased blood volume) resulting in an increased preload that places a strain on the shunt balance. Parturients with right to left shunts

TABLE 20-9 Causes of Pulmonary Edema

Cardiac (high pressures)	
Cardiac dysfunction	Decreased left ventricular contractility, mitral stenoses,
	Mitral regurgitation, intravascular volume overload, dysrhythmias
Pulmonary venous dysfunction	Venous occlusive disease, neurogenic pulmonary Vasoconstriction
Pulmonary embolization	Amniotic fluid, thrombus, fat, air
Airway obstruction	Edema, asthma, foreign body
Preeclampsia	Pulmonary hypertension
Miscellaneous	Pneumothorax, tumor, one lung anesthesia (down lung syndrome)
Noncardiogenic (permeability)	
Adult respiratory distress syndrome	
Aspiration syndromes	
Pulmonary embolization	
Abruptio placentae	
Dead fetus syndrome	
Sepsis	

Source: Reproduced with permission from *Principles and Practice of Obstetric Analgesia and Anesthesia*, John J. Bonica, 2nd edn. Baltimore, MD: Williams & Wilkins.

such as uncorrected Tetralogy of Fallot or Eisenmenger's syndrome, can be exacerbated by hypoxemia, hypercarbia and decrease in systemic vascular resistance.

In right or left ventricular outflow obstruction such as valvular stenosis or coarctation of the aorta, volume depletion, or decrease in systemic vascular resistance can significantly exacerbate symptoms. With careful monitoring and attention to the specifics of the cardiac lesion and resultant cardiopulmonary pathophysiology, anesthesia and analgesia can be safely conducted in the high risk parturient (see Chap. 8).

Pulmonary Disease—Pulmonary Edema

Pulmonary edema, when it occurs during pregnancy invariably has a predisposing etiology (Table 20-9). Basic management of this condition includes establishing the cause and reversing the effects of hypoxemia. The use of hemodynamic monitoring in the form of a pulmonary artery catheter and arterial line can be extremely useful in elucidating the etiology and most appropriate treatment for pulmonary edema (see Chap. 12).

Anesthetic management for delivery of the baby, in most circumstances, may be in the form of a conduction anesthetic. However, the parturient with severe respiratory failure may require general anesthesia with endotracheal intubation to obtain stability.

CONCLUSION

In conclusion, once an understanding of the nature of the parturient's pain is recognized, with techniques available to the anesthesiologist and obstetrician, an optimal care plan can be attained, even for high-risk parturients.

SUGGESTED READINGS

Avroy A. Fanacoff: *Neonatal-Perinatal Medicine: Diseases of the Fetus and Infant*, 5th edn. St. Louis, Missouri: Mosby, 1992.

Birnbach D. Ostheimer's *Manual of Obstetric Anesthesia*, 3rd edn. New York, New York: Churchill Livingstone, 2000.

Collis RE: Randomized comparison of combined spinal—epidural and standard epidural analgesia in labour. *Lancet* 1995;345(8962):1413–1416.

Dalton ME, Gross I: *Seminars in Perinatology*, April 2002, Vol. 26, No. 2. West Philadelphia, Pennsylvania: W.B. Saunders.

Donald Wallace, M.D: Randomized comparison of general and regional anesthesia for cesarean delivery in pregnancies complicated by severe preeclampsia. *Obstetrics & Gynecology* 1995;86(2):193–199.

Guyton and Hall: *Textbook of Medical Physiology*, 9th edn. West Philadelphia, Pennsylvania: W.B. Saunders, 1996.

Hughes S. Parturients infected with human immunodeficiency virus and regional anesthesia. *Anesthesiology* 1995;82(1):32–37.

IARS 2002 Review Course Lectures. Birnbaum, p. 12, Butterworth, pp. 22, 38, 54.

John J. Bonica: *Principles and Practice of Obstetric Analgesia and Anesthesia*, 2nd edn. Baltimore, Maryland: Williams & Wilkins, 1995.

Mark C. Norris, M.D: *International Anesthesiology Clinics*, Hagerstown, Maryland: Lippincott Williams & Wilkins, 1994;32(2):69–81.

Seminars in Perinatology, New Techniques & Drugs for Epidural Labor Analgesia, Philadelphia, Pennsylvania: W.B. Saunders, April 2002, p. 100, Table I.

Sol M. Shnider. *Anesthesia for Obstetrics*, 3rd edn. Baltimore, Maryland: Williams & Wilkins, 1993.

21 Special Considerations for the Patient with Multiple Gestations

John P. Elliott

INTRODUCTION

Human reproduction is most efficient when there is only one fetus in the uterus. Multiple gestations (Table 21-1) increase reproductive wastage and the incidence of complications for both mother and fetuses. They are complex pregnancies which need special consideration.

IMPORTANT PHYSIOLOGIC ADAPTATIONS WITH A MULTIPLE GESTATION

- In singletons, the cardiac output increases 30 to 50 percent over the non-gravid state; for twins the increase is 70 percent.
- Systemic vascular resistance falls incrementally more in multiple gestation as compared to singleton pregnancy.
- Renal plasma flow in pregnancy is 35 to 40 percent above non-pregnant levels and is probably further increased in multiple gestation.
- Hemodilution is more pronounced in multiple pregnancy than in singleton gestation.

THE IMPORTANCE OF PLACENTATION

Multiple gestation can result from the splitting of one zygote into two or more embryos, from multiple ovulations with fertilization of more than one egg, or a combination of the two processes. It is important to establish zygosity in a multiple gestation because it will affect pregnancy risk and management. Real-time ultrasonography is invaluable to classify placentation. Separate placentas or different sex fetuses will identify dichorionic/diamniotic gestation. When the placentas are fused, a thin, wispy membrane indicates monochorionic placentation, while a thicker, more echodense membrane would indicate dichorionic placentae. Placental tissue extending between the amnions (twin peak sign) would also indicate two chorions. Monochorionic placentation is associated with a higher rate of fetal loss and places that pregnancy at risk for twin-twin transfusion syndrome.

Two-thirds of twins are diamniotic/dichorionic, one-third are diamniotic/monochorionic, and 1 percent are monoamniotic/monochorionic. Monochorionic placentas are much less common among the high-order multiples, although the use of blastocyst transfer at about five days of life has increased the frequency.

COMPLICATIONS OF MULTIPLE GESTATIONS

Table 21-2 summarizes the rates of the most common complications in multiple pregnancy. With each additional fetus, complications tend to increase considerably.

TABLE 21-1 Incidence of Multifetal Gestations

	Spontaneous	Clomiphene (%)	Menotropins (%)	GIFT (%)[a]
Twins	1.2/100	8	18	22
Monozygotic	40/10,000			
Dizygotic	80/10,000			
Triplets	1/6889	0.5	3	4
Quadruplets	1/575,000	0.3	1.2	1.2
≥ Quintuplets	$1/47 \times 10^6$	0.13	—	—

[a]GIFT, gamete intrafallopian transfer.

CRITICAL CARE ENVIRONMENT FOR MULTIPLE GESTATIONS

Prematurity is the single most common complication of multiple gestation. Twins deliver at a mean gestational age of 36½ weeks, triplets at 33 weeks, quadruplets at 29½ weeks, and quintuplets at 27 to 28 weeks. Preterm labor occurs in over 40 percent of patients with twins and in 80 percent of triplets and quadruplets. Preterm labor in multiple gestation is a more formidable event than in a singleton pregnancy. The obstetrician must be prepared to use multiple tocolytic drugs, often at maximum doses, for three to four days before arresting the process. Magnesium sulfate is our tocolytic drug of choice. It is administered intravenously as a bolus (over 20 minutes) of 6 g, followed by a maintenance infusion of 3 to 5 g/h. Due to an increased creatinine clearance, higher infusion rates are often necessary to achieve therapeutic maternal serum levels of magnesium (6.5 to 8.0 mg/dL). It may be necessary to add terbutaline and/or indomethacin in selected cases. Should premature labor occur, corticosteroids are often administered to the mother to enhance the neonatal pulmonary function. However, they may also initiate labor when administered in triplet and quadruplet pregnancies.

Pregnancy-induced hypertension (PIH) is more frequent in multiple gestations; the consequences can engender critical care situations. PIH in multiple gestation tends to initiate earlier and to become more severe because the effort to prolong pregnancy in the name of fetal maturity allows the disease to worsen.

The physiology of multiple gestation, the complications it induces (abruptio placentae, diabetes, PIH, anemia), and the therapeutic interventions employed (tocolysis, corticosteroids) place these pregnancies at high risk for

TABLE 21-2 Pregnancy Complications of Multifetal Gestations

	Singleton (%)	Twin (%)	Triplet (%)	Quadruplet (%)[a]
Small for gestational age	4.6	17.4	30	10
Antepartum hemorrhage	2.0	2.8	6.7	10
Pregnancy induced hypertension	8.2	23	28	75
Anemia	3.5	2.5	19	40
Preterm labor	8.4	42.7	84	80
Fetal death >20 weeks	0.98	3.7	6.7	0

[a]Data from Phoenix Perinatal Associates, Phoenix, Arizona.

potentially disastrous complications. Hemorrhage can occur postdelivery from uterine atony due to the overly distended uterus.

Triplet and quadruplet pregnancies are at increased risk for pulmonary edema. In our (early) series of quadruplets, for example, 3 out of 14 developed the problem. All three patients had the combination of PIH with anemia, low colloid oncotic pressure, and the use of tocolytic agents. Pulmonary edema in these patients should be treated as follows:

- Oxygen should be administered.
- The patient should be placed in an upright position.
- Diuretic therapy should be vigorous with 40 to 80 mg of intravenous furosemide.

Another complication of multiple gestation is twin-twin transfusion syndrome (TTTS). Virtually all monochorionic pregnancies have vascular communications between the placentas. Artery-artery or vein-vein anastomoses do not result in hemodynamic changes, since the pressure in each vascular pairing is roughly equal. However, arteriovenous anastomosis can potentially direct blood from one baby (donor) into the placenta and circulation of the other (recipient). If this anastomosis is not balanced by a shunt of similar magnitude in the opposite direction, the volume overload in the recipient leads to polyhydramnios. The donor twin becomes hypovolemic and consequently develops severe oligohydramnios. Severe TTTS, or stuck twin syndrome, is a critical situation for the fetuses rather than the mother. Untreated, this syndrome has nearly 100 percent mortality. When one twin dies, the survivor remains at extreme risk of death or compromise due to volume shift from the survivor to the pressure sink created by the dead fetus, which offers no resistance to the blood pumped by the survivor.

Serial amnioreduction is the most widely used therapy for severe TTTS, with reported fetal survival rates of 60 to 80 percent. Amnioreduction is performed as soon as the diagnosis of TTS is made. Under local anesthesia, an 18-gauge spinal needle is transabdomenally inserted into the polyhydramnic sac. Extension tubing is attached to the needle and a Simms adapter connects to wall suction tubing, which is attached to wall suction (alternatively, vacuum bottles can be used). Amniotic fluid is withdrawn at a rate of about 1 L per 20 minutes. As much fluid is removed as possible with each procedure, with the goal of reducing the amniotic fluid volume into the normal or low normal range. The procedure is repeated as soon as the deepest fluid pocket in the recipient twin's sac exceeds 8 cm. Antibiotics are not used routinely. Tocolytics may be necessary to control preterm labor.

An alternative therapeutic intervention consists of laser ablation of the arteriovenous anastomosis between the twins. Laser coagulation is associated with approximately 70 percent survival, and with serious morbidity in 4 to 6 percent of survivors. The laser procedure is performed in only a few centers in the United States. Patients with acute TTTS with contractions and cervical change are not candidates for laser surgery. Yet another intervention is amniotic septostomy, whereby the intervening membrane is intentionally perforated. Two studies reported a mean pregnancy prolongation of eight weeks in 12 patients, with an 83 percent survival rate.

Among survivors, there can be complications: In the donor, hypovolemia can lead to hypoxic injury of the brain or kidney, with resultant hypoxic-ischemic encephalopathy or renal infarcts; cardiomyopathy can occur in the recipient from prolonged hypervolemia.

SUGGESTED READING

Deleia JE, Kuhlmann RS, Lopez KP: Treating previable twin-twin transfusion syndrome with fetoscopic laser surgery: outcomes following the learning curve. *J Perinatol Med* 1999;27:61–67.

Elliott JP, Radin TG: Serum magnesium levels during magnesium sulfate tocolysis in high order multiple gestations. *J Reprod Med* 1995;40:450.

Elliott JP, Radin TG: The effect of corticosteroid administration on uterine activity and preterm labor in high order multiple gestations. *Obstet Gynecol* 1995;85:250.

Elliott JP: Twin-twin transfusion syndrome: Role of therapeutic amniocentesis. *Contemp Obstet Gynecol* 1992;37:30–47.

Elliott JP, Urig MA, Clewell WH: Aggressive therapeutic amniocentesis in the treatment of acute twin-twin transfusion syndrome. *Obstet Gynecol* 1991;77:537.

Finberg HJ, Clewell WH: Definitive prenatal diagnosis of monoamniotic twins: swallowed contrast agent detected in both twins on sonographically selected CT images. *J Ultrasound Med* 1991;10:513.

Hecher K, Kiehl W, Zikulnig L, et al.: Endoscopic laser coagulation of placental anastamosis in 200 pregnancies with severe mid-trimester twin-twin transfusion syndrome. *E J Obstet Gynecol Reprod Biol* 2000;92:135–139.

Johnson J, Rossi K, O'Shaughnessy RW: Amnioreduction versus septostomy in twin-twin transfusion syndrome. *Am J Obstet Gynecol* 2001;185:1044–1047.

Kovacs BW, Kirschbaum TH, Paul RH: Twin gestations. I. Antenatal care and complications. *Obstet Gynecol* 1989;74:313.

Mahony BS, Petty CN, Nyberg DA, et al.: The "stuck twin" phenomenon: Ultrasonographic findings, pregnancy outcome, and management with serial amniocenteses. *Am J Obstet Gynecol* 1990;163:1513–1522.

Mari G, Detti L, Oz U, et al.: Long-term outcome in twin-twin transfusion syndrome treated with serial aggressive amnioreduction. *Am J Obstet Gynecol* 2000;183:211–217.

Saade GR, Belfort MA, Berry DL, et al.: Amniotic septostomy for treatment of twin oligohydramnios polyhydramnios sequence. *Fetal Diag Therap* 1998;13:86–93.

Veille JC, Morton MJ, Burry KJ: Maternal cardiovascular adaptation to twin pregnancy. *Am J Obstet* 1985;153:261.

22 Fetal Considerations in the Critical Care Patient

Thomas J. Garite

INTRODUCTION

Virtually any pathologic process which affects the mother has the potential to affect the fetus. The impact on the fetus will depend on many variables, including the duration of the insult, its effect on fetal oxygenation, and the caregiver's ability to intervene based on gestational age and the hemodynamic/respiratory status of the mother. Critical in these situations is a basic understanding of fetal physiology as it relates to these functions.

FETAL PHYSIOLOGY

The fetal impact of most critical maternal diseases will depend on how well the mother is able to deliver oxygen to the fetus while simultaneously compensating for her own condition. Fetal oxygen delivery depends on placental blood flow, differences in maternal and fetal partial pressures, oxygen carrying capacity of the mother's blood, and the placental surface area. It is inversely proportional to the thickness of the placental diffusing membrane. In diseases that primarily affect the mother (save for those that may lead to abruptio placentae), placental function remains constant; thus, the variables are uterine blood flow and uterine vascular oxygen pressure and content.

The fetus lives at a much lower oxygen tension than its extra-uterine counterpart. Its ability to do so is based on a hemoglobin/oxygen dissociation curve that is shifted to the left of its mother's (Fig. 22-1), allowing a considerably higher fetal oxygen saturation at lower partial pressures of oxygen. This is essential in the human placenta, which has a parallel flow mechanism. In this concurrent flow model (Fig. 22-2), the maximum fetal pO_2 is slightly less than that of the mother's venous pO_2, thereby allowing oxygen to be continually passed from mother to fetus. In the healthy, normally perfused placenta, fetal venous blood (the oxygenated side of the fetal circuit) will have a maximum pO_2 of about 35 torr, given a maternal venous pO_2 of 35 to 40 torr. At this pO_2, the fetal blood will be about 70 percent saturated with oxygen. The fetus will maintain aerobic metabolism at saturations above 30 to 35 percent, corresponding to a pO_2 of 15 to 20 torr. Maternal anemia can significantly alter the level at which anaerobic metabolism and acidosis may occur since reduced levels of hemoglobin will reduce the absolute amount of oxygen the blood can carry at a given saturation and pO_2. Even in the absence of maternal hypoxemia, the fetus may become hypoxic at severely low maternal hemoglobin levels (Fig. 22-3). The exact level at which this occurs is not well known, but is probably variable.

In critical care situations, uterine blood flow will have the greatest influence upon fetal oxygenation, and is generally a function of maternal cardiac output. During the late second and early third trimester, maternal cardiac output normally peaks at about 6 L/min. Maternal blood volume is also increased. Approximately 750 mL/min of maternal cardiac output flows through the low resistance placental bed. Utero-placental perfusion is critical to the maintenance

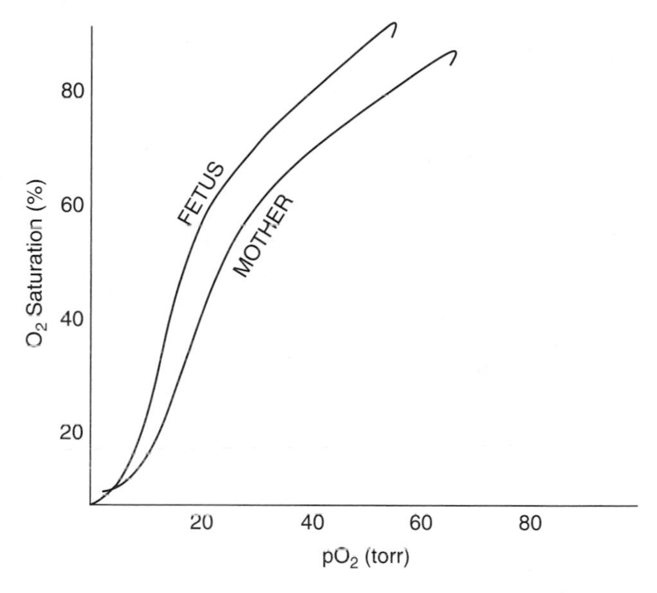

FIG. 22-1 The oxygen hemoglobin saturation curves for maternal and fetal blood (*Adapted from Hellegers AD, Schruefer JJ, Am J Obstet Gynecol,* 1961; 81:377).

of fetal oxygen levels; even minor alterations may result in fetal hypoxia. A variety of pathologic changes may occur in the critically ill mother that can result in decreased placental perfusion. For example, a large, occult blood loss (e.g., intraperitoneal hemorrhage) may not be as readily apparent in pregnancy due to the normal, pregnancy-induced increase in maternal blood volume and the ability of the mother to redistribute blood flow away from such nonessential organs as the uterus. As much as 2000 mL (30 percent) of maternal blood volume may be lost without significant changes in vital signs, as opposed to a margin of only 1000 mL (20 percent) in the nonpregnant state. The placental

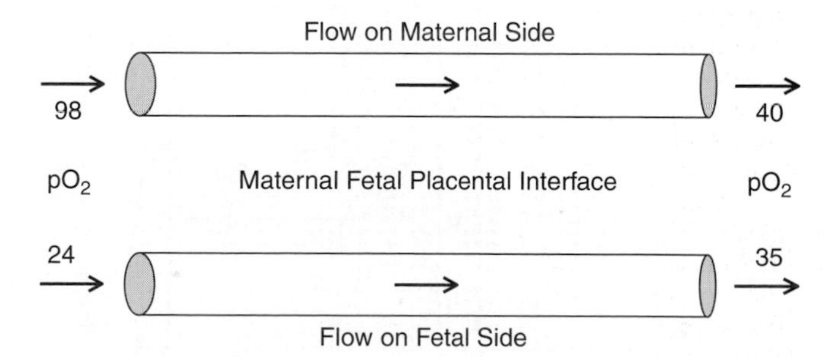

FIG. 22-2 Oxygenation based on concurrent model of maternal and fetal blood flow within the placenta, with actual values based on normals found at cordocentesis in the mid third trimester period (torr).

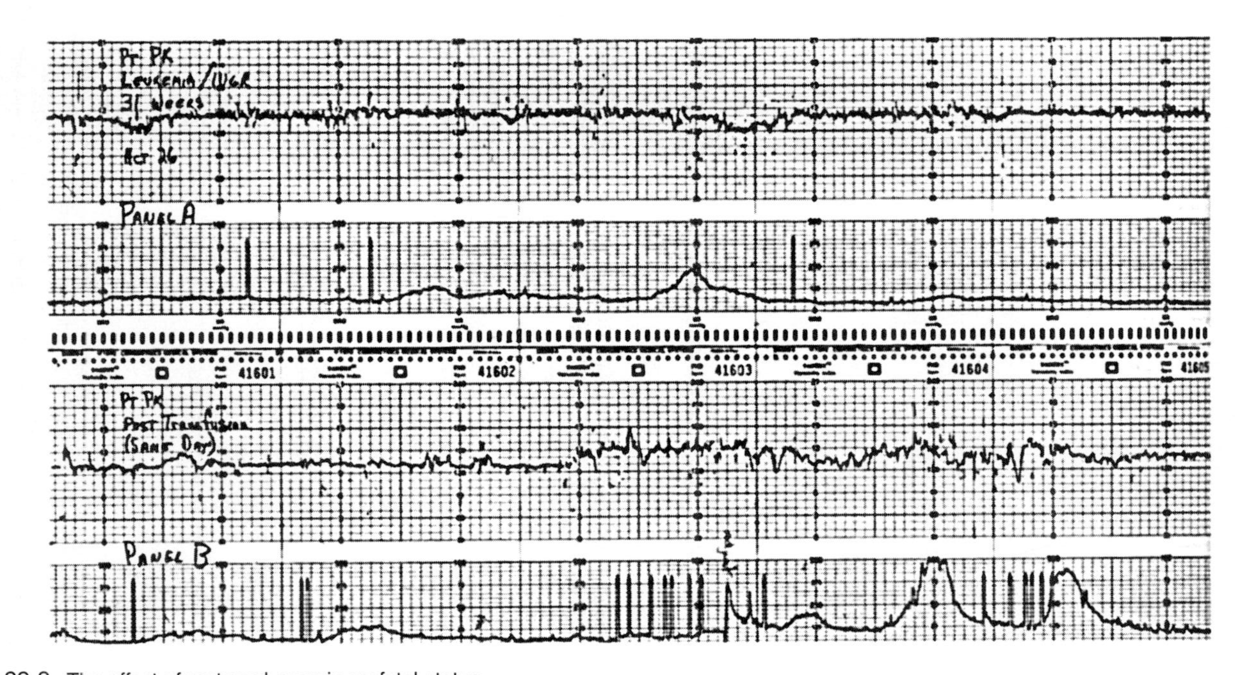

FIG. 22-3 The effect of maternal anemia on fetal status.

bed is neurologically linked to the maternal splanchnic bed; the physiologic response to decreased maternal blood volume is diversion of blood away from the placenta when higher priority maternal organs (e.g., brain, heart, adrenals) must be preserved. As a result, the fetus may become hypoxic in advance of maternal shock. Hypovolemia may result in decreased cardiac output, thereby further decreasing placental perfusion. Paradoxically, hypertension may also be associated with decreased placental perfusion. Indeed, the more severe the hypertension, the more likely one will encounter placental underperfusion and associated fetal hypoxia. Additionally, critical situations may be associated with premature onset of contractions, which further decrease uterine blood flow.

CRITICAL CARE PATIENTS WITH ACUTE INSULTS

While the fetus may demonstrate signs of hypoxia as a result of maternal illness, the temptation to proceed with delivery can sometimes result in destabilization of the mother, unnecessary intervention and the unnecessary delivery of an infant with the sequelae of prematurity. Usually, the better choice is to improve maternal condition so as to improve the fetal condition. One exception to this notion would be maternal cardio-pulmonary arrest, where delivery of the fetus may actually facilitate maternal resuscitation (see Chap. 17).

INITIAL EVALUATION AND CARE OF THE FETUS

There are some general considerations to be deliberated when evaluating and caring for the fetus of a critically ill mother. First, the gestational age and potential viability of the fetus should be determined, since all subsequent evaluation and management will depend on this issue. Second, to maximize fetal well being, ensure that there is some degree of left uterine displacement (usually best accomplished with a roll under the right maternal buttocks). Administer oxygen by face mask using a tight-fitting nonrebreathing mask, whenever possible. Determine the general condition of the mother, including her primary diagnosis and her vital signs as well as hemodynamic status and oxygen saturation via pulse oxymetry. Maternal evaluation also includes palpation of the uterus to determine its size, to ascertain fetal position and to detect tenderness or contractions. Maternal assessment may also include a perineal or pelvic examination to assess for bleeding, rupture of membranes, and cervical dilation. If the fetus is of a viable gestational age, cardiotachometry is the critical next step. This modality will help to determine fetal oxygen status and presence of uterine contractions. The ultrasound evaluation of the fetus should be reserved until fetal well being and uterine contraction status have been determined. Ultrasound will be important to rule out any obvious lethal anomaly (e.g., anencephaly) which would render further fetal evaluation moot. Ultrasound can also confirm gestational age so as to facilitate decisions regarding timing and route of delivery. Ultrasound may also be used as a tool to evaluate fetal condition if the fetal heart rate is not reassuring (i.e., biophysical profile, including amniotic fluid volume assessment). In some situations, more sophisticated fetal assessment such as Doppler flow studies may also be useful (Fig. 22-4).

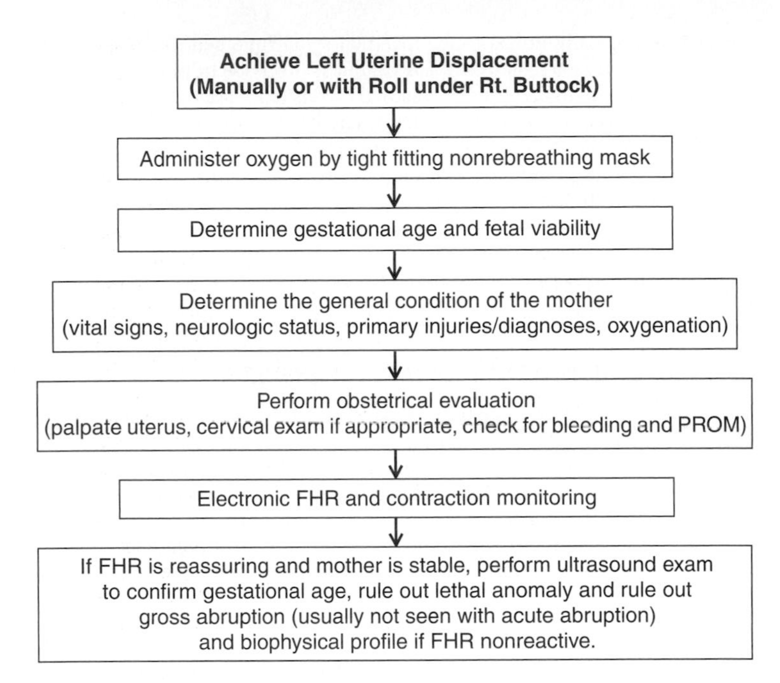

FIG. 22-4 Initial evaluation of the fetus in the critical care mother.

FETAL EVALUATION AND MANAGEMENT IN SPECIFIC CRITICAL SITUATIONS

Trauma

The initial evaluation and management is to ensure that the mother is appropriately assessed and stabilized. Major hemorrhage may lead to decreased placental perfusion and fetal hypoxia. As discussed earlier, occult intraabdominal hemorrhage may lead to diversion of blood away from the uterus. Late decelerations may be the earliest sign of this problem, even before significant changes in maternal vital signs become evident. Evaluation for intraabdominal hemorrhage is more difficult because the enlarged uterus causes tenting of the peritoneum; moreover, the anti-inflammatory effects of progesterone may dampen normal tenderness. Ultrasound can be useful in detecting intraperitoneal blood. Open peritoneal lavage has also been successfully used to make the diagnosis in pregnancy. In the patient who is tachycardic and hypotensive, aggressive fluid management is critical. In those patients where vasopressors are needed, one must consider their effects on the fetus. Low dose dopamine, for example, exerts its effect via increased cardiac output, but has been shown in animals to decrease uterine perfusion; thus, careful fetal monitoring is warranted if this drug is used. Norepinephrine and isoproterenol can have similar fetal effects. Ephedrine may be considered in that it is one agent that does not adversely affect uterine circulation.

The obstetric complications of major blunt trauma include abruptio placentae, fetal-maternal hemorrhage (with or without abruption), labor, and very rarely, uterine rupture and fetal trauma (see Chap. 18).

In patients without obvious clinical abruption (i.e., uterine contractions, pain, tenderness, and vaginal bleeding), the fetal heart rate (FHR) monitor may be the most sensitive tool to detect abruptio placentae. The characteristic findings with this modality include a tachysystolic contraction pattern and FHR decelerations (Fig. 22-5). Ultrasound will usually not reveal acute abruption, as the ultrasonic density of fresh blood is virtually identical to that of the placenta. Evaluation of the patient should also include laboratory assessment of hematocrit, fibrinogen, fibrin degradation products, and platelet count for retroplacental consumptive coagulopathy. Kleihauer-Bettke screening to rule out major fetal-maternal hemorrhage (and to determine whether and how much Rh negative immune globulin is needed) is also advised.

Delivery is generally the only option for patients with severe abruption. As a result, conflict can arise should the trauma team want to pursue additional diagnostic studies to rule out, for example, intracranial or other injuries. The obstetrician must become the advocate for the fetus. Open communication is essential. Tocolysis for premature labor associated with trauma-induced abruption should be approached with extreme caution. If considered at all, it should be limited to patients with very early gestational ages (i.e., <32 weeks) and who are hemodynamically stable with reassuring fetal status, no active bleeding and no coagulopathy. Corticosteroids for lung maturity should be used concurrently (Table 22-1).

Rarely, a patient will have a major fetal-maternal hemorrhage without significant clinical abruption. Fetal heart rate findings may include tachycardia, decreased variability, late decelerations, and/or sinusoidal patterns. A biophysical profile may reveal a depressed fetus. Kleihauer-Bettke screening can quantify the fetal hemorrhage. Whether middle cerebral artery Doppler studies will be diagnostic in this situation is presently unknown. In very early gestation, emergency intrauterine transfusion can be an alternative to delivery.

Following the initial evaluation, there should be a more prolonged interval of fetal heart rate and contraction monitoring (Fig. 22-6), the duration being dependent on the severity of injury, presence of contractions and/or vaginal bleeding, and other clinical findings. Following any significant abdominal trauma, the fetus should be observed on the FHR monitor for a minimum of 4 hours; if any signs of abruption exist, monitoring should be extended to at least 24 hours (Fig. 22-7).

Hypoxia

Maternal hypoxemia may lead to fetal hypoxia. Situations where acute maternal hypoxemia may present a challenge for fetal management include acute asthmatic episodes, acute respiratory distress (often associated with sepsis), pulmonary edema with or without preeclampsia, cranial injuries with respiratory failure, amniotic fluid or pulmonary embolism, cardiac decompensation (e.g., pulmonary edema associated with mitral stenosis), pneumonia, irritant inhalation or burns.

Therapy is directed to the primary condition of the mother. Fetal heart rate monitoring is useful in assessing how the fetus is tolerating any reduced oxygen delivery. In the absence of uterine contractions, a hypoxic fetus develops tachycardia and loss of variability; prolonged decelerations are seen

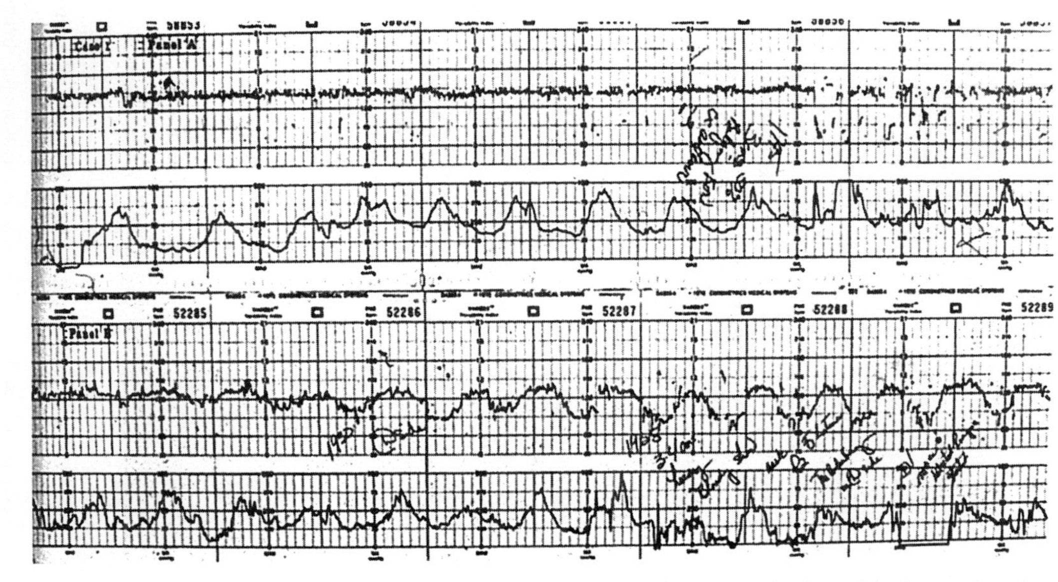

FIG. 22-5 Abruptio placentae. This tracing demonstrates the characteristic contraction pattern (tachysystole: frequent contractions with short or absent relaxation period) and, beginning on the lower panel, persistent late decelerations. In the last half of the lower panel, this patient began actively hemorrhaging. Immediate cesarean delivery revealed a 50-percent abruption.

TABLE 22-1 Candidates for Tocolysis and Corticosteroids with Abruptio Placentae

1. Actively contracting
2. Cervical dilation appropriate for tocolysis (≤4 cm)
3. Gestational age appropriate for tocolysis and corticosteroids (24–34 weeks)
4. No vigorous active bleeding
5. Reassuring fetal heart rate pattern
6. No evidence of significant coagulopathy (fibrinogen >100 mg%, platelet count >100,000/mm^3)
7. No medical contraindications to tocolysis

only preterminally. If contractions are present, late decelerations may be seen. A general goal for optimizing fetal oxygenation is to keep maternal pO_2 above 60 mmHg and O_2 saturation above 95 percent. Levels falling below this, despite supplemental oxygen via rebreathing mask, may require ventilator therapy, the key being to avoid either hyper or hypocarbia. Pregnant women normally hyperventilate. Thus, a pCO_2 of 35 mmHg is normal in pregnancy. Levels significantly below this may be associated with decreased placental perfusion. Accordingly, the goal is to maintain maternal pCO_2 between 35 and 40 mmHg (torr).

While colloid oncotic pressure plays a role in maintaining intravascular volume, intravenous colloid administration should be used with extreme caution in acute situations such as pulmonary edema because supplemental protein may leak into the pulmonary interstitium and further aggravate ventilation-perfusion mismatch. Severe anemia should be corrected with packed red cells, as maximizing oxygen carrying capacity is critical to fetal oxygen delivery.

Delivery is rarely indicated with maternal respiratory failure unless the mother cannot be adequately oxygenated on full ventilatory settings. An uncommon situation which may require delivery, is the mother with severe muscle weakness (e.g., spinal muscular atrophy), where elevation of the diaphragm by the gravid uterus further compromises breathing.

Sickle Cell Crisis

While not truly a hypoxemic event, patients with sickle cell crises have compromised oxygen carrying capacity. Often patients who present with a crisis in the late second or third trimester will have signs of hypoxia on the FHR monitor. Evaluation and management of the fetus is essentially the same as for patients with acute asthmatic episodes or other forms of respiratory failure. Thus, aggressive maternal therapy aimed at maximizing oxygenation and uterine perfusion is important. Intervention for fetal compromise is not usually necessary. Maternal transfusion may be as beneficial for the fetus as for the mother since increasing maternal oxygen carrying capacity improves fetal oxygen transfer. Improvement in the fetal heart rate should be expected as the crisis is resolved.

Anaphylaxis

Anaphylaxis is an acute allergic reaction with systemic manifestations that can include urticaria, respiratory distress, and cardiovascular collapse. The inciting agent may be food or medication. In the setting of either respiratory

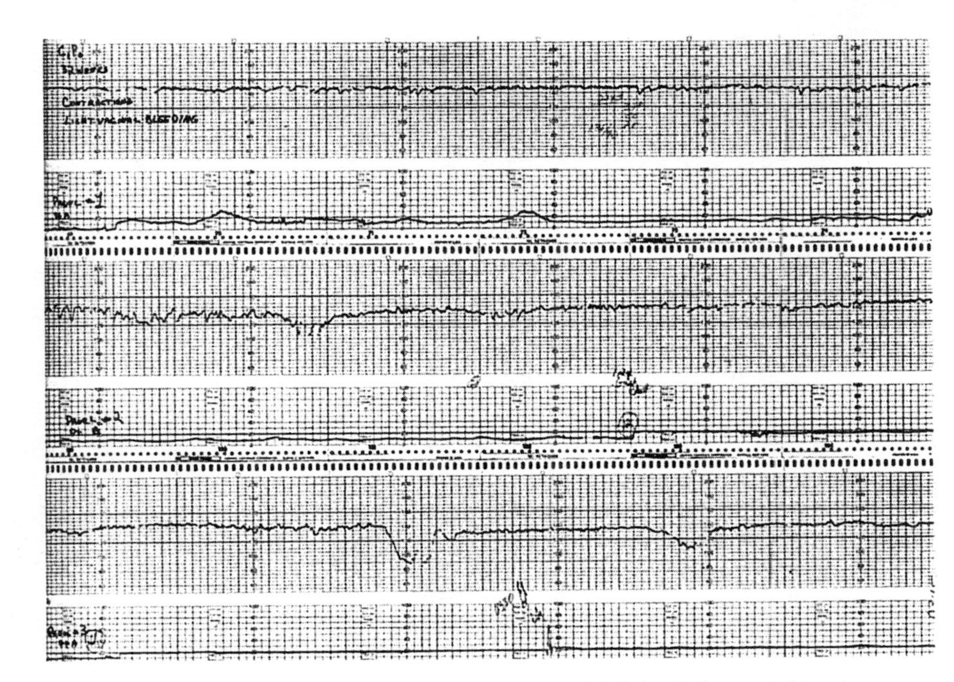

FIG. 22-6 A 32-week patient involved in an automobile collision who sustained mild abdominal trauma. Her uterus was not tender and there was minimal vaginal bleeding. The electronic fetal monitor revealed irregular and infrequent contractions, and on the lower two panels, late decelerations. Immediate cesarean delivery revealed a 30-percent abruption.

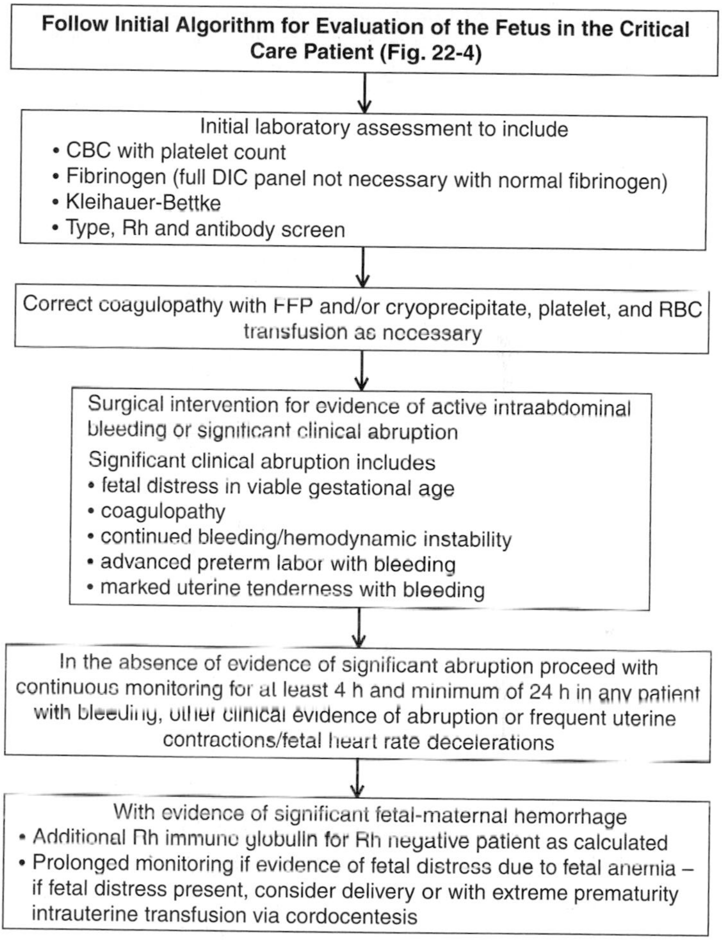

Follow Initial Algorithm for Evaluation of the Fetus in the Critical Care Patient (Fig. 22-4)

↓

Initial laboratory assessment to include
- CBC with platelet count
- Fibrinogen (full DIC panel not necessary with normal fibrinogen)
- Kleihauer-Bettke
- Type, Rh and antibody screen

↓

Correct coagulopathy with FFP and/or cryoprecipitate, platelet, and RBC transfusion as necessary

↓

Surgical intervention for evidence of active intraabdominal bleeding or significant clinical abruption

Significant clinical abruption includes
- fetal distress in viable gestational age
- coagulopathy
- continued bleeding/hemodynamic instability
- advanced preterm labor with bleeding
- marked uterine tenderness with bleeding

↓

In the absence of evidence of significant abruption proceed with continuous monitoring for at least 4 h and minimum of 24 h in any patient with bleeding, other clinical evidence of abruption or frequent uterine contractions/fetal heart rate decelerations

↓

With evidence of significant fetal-maternal hemorrhage
- Additional Rh immune globulin for Rh negative patient as calculated
- Prolonged monitoring if evidence of fetal distress due to fetal anemia – if fetal distress present, consider delivery or with extreme prematurity intrauterine transfusion via cordocentesis

FIG. 22-7 Evaluation of the pregnant patient with blunt abdominal trauma.

compromise or shock, fetal hypoxia should be anticipated. Treatment is similar to that of the nonpregnant patient. Urgent resuscitation includes maintenance of the airway, oxygen administration, epinephrine, diphenhydramine, and intravenous hydration. The fetal heart rate may manifest late decelerations with or without tachycardia. Correction of maternal hypoxia and hypotension should restore placental perfusion and correct fetal hypoxia and the accompanying FHR pattern, although it may require up to 2 hours before the process is complete.

Hypertensive Crisis

Acute hypertensive crisis in pregnancy may occur for reasons similar to those in the nonpregnant patient, such as poorly controlled hypertension, pheochromocytoma, or as a result of severe preeclampsia/ecclampsia (see Chap. 5).

The blood pressure must be lowered to less dangerous levels so as to avoid severe maternal complications such as intracranial hemorrhage. Another benefit of lowering severely elevated blood pressure is the reduced risk of abruptio placentae. However, acute reduction of the blood pressure must be done very carefully, as the fetus may not tolerate too large or rapid a drop in pressure. The goal should be to lower pressure gradually over 30 to 60 minutes, though not to normotensive levels. For example, the patient with an initial blood pressure of 220/130 should be gradually reduced to a pressure of approximately 160 to 170/100 to 105. Medications such as hydralazine, labetalol, or even nitroprusside may be used in small boluses or by continuous, slow intravenous infusion. These drugs allow titration of blood pressure without overshooting, if used appropriately.

In the case of chronic hypertension during early pregnancy, blood pressure should also be controlled with care so as not to overcorrect maternal hypertension. The fetus may demonstrate growth restriction or even hypoxia if maternal blood pressure is overcorrected.

Maternal Acidosis

Though rare, maternal metabolic acidosis in the absence of hypoxemia or shock poses an extraordinary management challenge for the fetal caregiver. Most commonly this is seen with diabetic ketoacidosis, but can also occur with drug- or toxin-induced acidosis (e.g., aspirin overdose). In these cases, the fetus slowly becomes acidotic as buffers, especially HCO_3^-, move slowly across the placenta from the fetal to the maternal intravascular compartment. The ensuing buffer depletion in the fetus gradually results in fetal acidosis, whereby the fetus will demonstrate loss of variability with or without late decelerations on the FHR monitor. Biophysical parameters, including fetal movement, breathing, and tone are reduced or absent. In such situations, correction of maternal acidosis improves the fetal condition; delivery is usually not warranted. A key management point is that fetal acidosis requires several hours, beyond correction of maternal acidosis, to clear (Fig. 22-8), so as to allow the buffer to re-enter the fetal side of the placenta from the maternal system. Continuous fetal heart rate monitoring during correction of maternal acidosis will provide information as to how and when the fetus recovers. Rarely, the fetus may deteriorate before acidosis can be corrected, and can manifest as a preterminal, prolonged deceleration/bradycardia. In this situation, if maternal condition permits and the fetus is of a viable gestational age, emergent cesarean delivery may be required.

In diabetic ketoacidosis and some other nonhypoxic metabolic acidoses, the mother is severely dehydrated, as well. This may result in underperfusion of the placenta; the ensuing fetal hypoxemia may compound the metabolic acidosis. Therefore, it is as important to correct the dehydration with aggressive fluid administration as it is to treat the acidosis (see Chap. 11).

Seizures

Maternal seizures, whether due to ecclampsia, epilepsy, or metabolic disturbances, will usually diminish those aspects of antepartum assessment ascribed to fetal well being, especially with regard to the fetal heart rate. Seizures may alter placental perfusion and fetal oxygenation in several ways. For instance, maternal hypoxia often results from seizure-related apnea, while diversion of blood flow away from the uterus may occur as a result of intense maternal

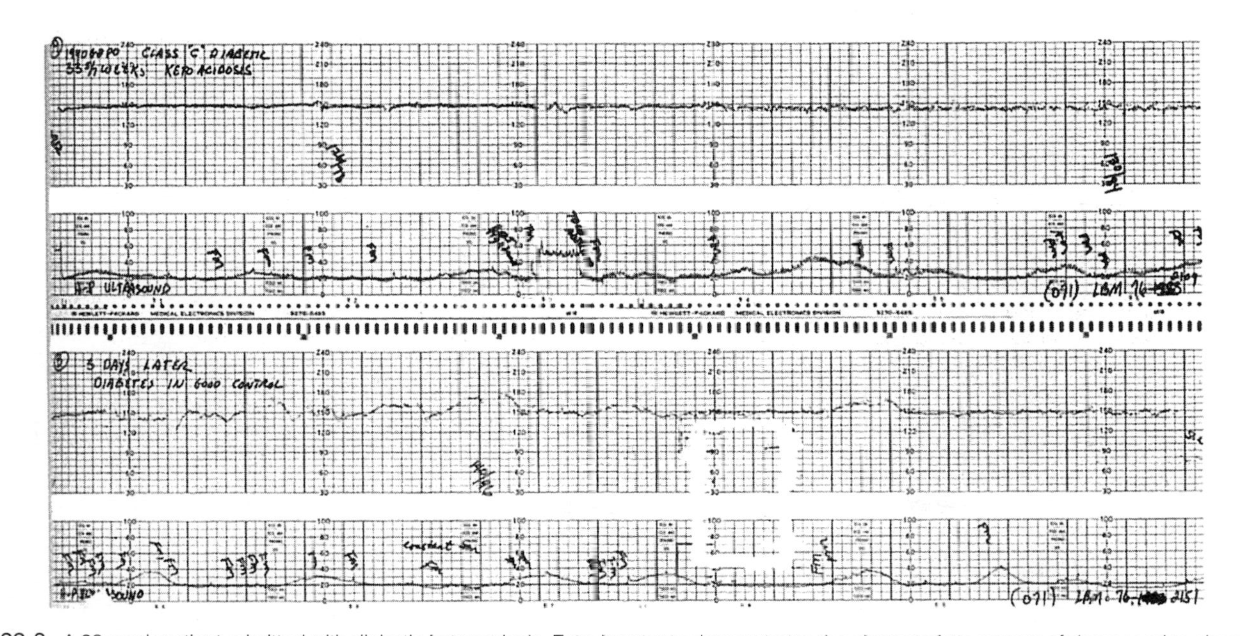

FIG. 22-8 A 33-week patient admitted with diabetic ketoacidosis. Fetal heart rate demonstrates the characteristic pattern of decreased to absent variability (upper panel). After correction of the DKA, the fetal heart rate pattern returned to normal with accelerations and normal variability (lower panel).

muscular activity. Probably as a result of intense uterine ischemia, there often can be tetanic or prolonged uterine contractions during the seizure. Usually, a prolonged deceleration or deep late decelerations occur during the seizure. Once the seizure resolves, however, the deceleration(s) resolve, though a period of tachycardia and reduced FHR variability often occur, lasting up to 2 hours; especially if the FHR preceding these changes is normal and the mother is subsequently well oxygenated and seizure free (Fig. 22-9).

Therapy is directed at the maternal condition. The goal is to maintain the mother's airway and avoid injury. Tilting the mother to her left side will avoid aorto-caval compression. Once the seizure is resolved, treatment is aimed at preventing further seizures and treating the underlying cause, when possible. The choice of medications for treatment of acute seizures or status epilepticus must be made with the fetus in mind. Azodiazepams should be used cautiously if there is a chance that the baby will need to be delivered acutely, especially if the fetus is premature, as these drugs alter thermoregulation and are neurodepressive. In such cases, short-acting barbiturates (e.g., pentobarbital) are reasonable alternatives. Delivery is rarely needed for fetal heart rate changes due to seizure activity; in most situations it is preferable to allow the placenta to resuscitate the fetus, even if delivery is planned (see Chap. 16).

Thyrotoxicosis

Acute thyrotoxicosis and thyroid storm are obstetrical emergencies that pose significant fetal risks. Potential complications include hypoxia, premature labor, preeclampsia, and fetal hyperthyroidism with its attendant problems. The mechanisms of fetal compromise are multifactorial: the maternal hyperdynamic state can divert blood flow away from the uterus and uterine ischemia may lead to fetal growth restriction, fetal hypoxia, and premature contractions. Superimposed preeclampsia, which the thyrotoxic patient is at increased risk of, may further aggravate placental hypoperfusion. Thyroid stimulating immunoglobulin is an IgG antibody that crosses the placenta, potentially causing fetal hyperthyroidism which thereby increases metabolic demands upon the fetus. Thyroid storm provokes even greater hyperdynamism, amplifying the potential for fetal compromise (see Chap. 10). There may also be maternal heart failure and pulmonary edema with superimposed maternal hypoxemia.

The fetal heart rate may be altered in a number of ways, depending on which of the above factors are involved. Tachycardia may be due to either maternal or fetal hyperthyroidism. Late decelerations may occur if placental hypoperfusion is severe. Treatment, as with other situations where correction of the maternal condition will usually improve the fetal condition, does not usually require immediate delivery.

Cardiac Arrest

The presence of an enlarged uterus, especially with a gestational age >24 weeks, can compromise resuscitative efforts for the mother with cardiac arrest. This is primarily due to aorto-caval compression, but is also aggravated by the low resistance utero-placental bed, which draws critically needed blood from the vital organs of the mother. Furthermore, the potential for fetal asphyxia in the case of maternal cardiac arrest is very high.

Cardio-pulmonary resuscitation (CPR) of the pregnant woman involves two additional considerations beyond those employed during CPR upon a nongravid person. The first is to ensure left uterine displacement. Tilting the

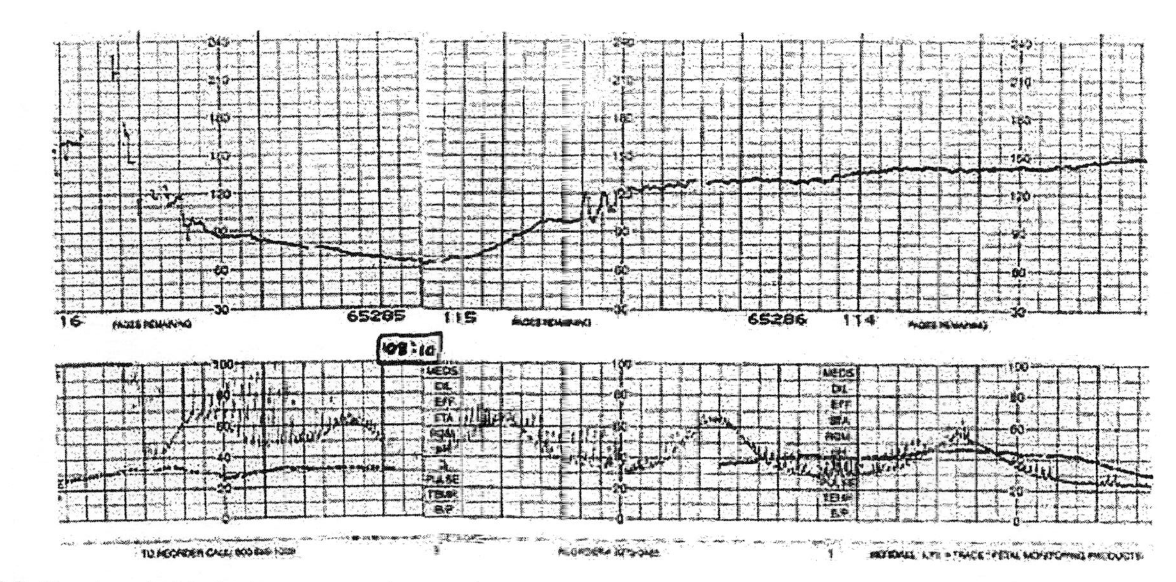

FIG. 22-9 The characteristic fetal heart rate and contraction pattern associated with an acute eclamptic seizure. Note the prolonged deceleration with loss of variability and the tetanic contraction during the seizure, the development of tachycardia and loss of variability following the seizure. This fetus was also being monitored with fetal pulse oximetry: the oxygenation saturation falls to 30 percent during the seizure and returns to normal (50 percent) following its cessation.

maternal trunk may not be the best option as this may compromise the efficiency of chest compression. It is recommended that the patient's backboard be tilted or that an assistant manually displace the uterus to the left. The second consideration relates to the need and timing of delivery. Katz et al. performed a large review of cardiopulmonary arrest in pregnancy. Fetuses delivered within 5 minutes of maternal death all survived and appeared to be neurologically intact. Given this information and the knowledge that pregnancy compromises resuscitation, it is recommended that bedside cesarean delivery be initiated if resuscitation has not restored cardiac function within 4 minutes, so as to accomplish delivery within 5 minutes (see Chap. 17).

Brain Death and Life Support

Prolongation of pregnancy in an effort to reach a viable or near-mature gestation has been reported in mothers who are brain dead but remain on cardiopulmonary life support. In these cases, delivery is required for sepsis, fetal distress, or maternal hypotension. Thus, it is critical to employ continuous FHR monitoring once viability is reached, to optimize utero-placental perfusion with aggressive hemodynamic monitoring and fluid management, and to avoid infection. Tocolysis may be utilized as needed. A bedside setup for immediate cesarean delivery should be available at all times.

SUMMARY

The principles guiding fetal evaluation and management in maternal critical care situations are remarkably similar in most conditions. Correction of the maternal condition and/or stabilization of maternal cardio-respiratory status is always the primary goal. If her condition can be reversed, the goal should be to stabilize the mother without the necessity for premature delivery. If delivery will improve the maternal condition, the mother should, nevertheless, be stabilized prior to delivery. A thorough understanding of the physiologic changes in pregnancy, how they affect maternal evaluation, and how pathologic conditions affect fetal oxygen delivery and utero-placental perfusion are critical components for assessing and managing the fetus of the critical care gravida.

SUGGESTED READING

Behrman RE, Lees MH, Peterson EN, et al.: Distribution of the circulation in the normal and asphyxiated fetal primate. *Am J Obstet Gynecol* 1970;108:956.

Bernstein IM, Watson M, Simmons GM, et al.: Maternal brain death and prolonged fetal survival. *Obstet Gynecol* 1989;74:434.

Boehm FH, Growdon JH: The effect of eclamptic convulsions on the fetal heart rate. *Am J Obstet Gynecol* 1974;120:851.

Connolly AM, Kate VL, Bash KL, et al.: Trauma and pregnancy. *Am J Perinatol* 1997;14:331.

Cruz AC, Spellacy WN, Jarrell M: Fetal heart rate tracing during sickle cell crisis: a cause for transient late decelerations. *Obstet Gynecol* 1979;54:647.

Dias MS: Neurovascular emergencies in pregnancy. In: Pitkin RM, Scott JR (eds), *Clin Obstet Gynecol.* Philadelphia: JB Lippincott 1994; p. 337.

Freeman RK, Garite TJ, Nageotte MP: *Fetal Heart Rate Monitoring,* 3rd edn. Baltimore, MD: Williams & Wilkins, 2003.

Goodwin TM, Breen MT: Pregnancy outcome and fetopmaternal hemorrhage after noncatastrophic trauma. *Am J Obstet Gynecol* 1990;162:665.

Higgins SD, Garite TJ: Late abruptio placenta in trauma patients: implications for monitoring. *Obstet Gynecol* 1984;63:105.

Hurd WW, Miodovni KM, Hertzberg V, et al.: Selective management of abruptio placentae: a prospective study. *Obstet Gynecol* 1983;61:467.

Katz VL, Dotters DJ, Droegemueller W: Perimortem cessarean delivery. *Obstet Gynecol* 1986;68:571.

Kuhlmann RS, Cruikshank DP: Maternal trauma in pregnancy. In: Pitkin RM, Scott JR (eds), *Clin Obstet Gynecol.* Philadelphia: JB Lippincott, 1944; p. 274.

Lees MM, Scott DB, Kerr MG, et al.: The circulating effects of recumbent postural change in late pregnancy. *Clin Sci* 1967;332:453.

LoBue C, Goodlin RC: Treatment of fetal distress during diabetic ketoacidosis. *J Reprod Med* 1978;20:101.

Marx G: Shock in the obstetric patient. *Anesthesiology* 1965;26:423.

Modanlou HD, Freeman RK: Sinusoidal fetal heart rate pattern: its definition and clinical significance. *Am Obstet Gynecol* 1982;142:1033.

Paul RH, Koh KS, Bernstein SG: Changes in fetal heart rate: uterine contraction patterns associated with eclampsia. *Am J Obstet Gynecol* 1978;130:165.

Pearlman MD, Tintinalli JE, Lorenz RP: Blunt trauma during pregnancy. *N Engl J Med* 1990;323:1609.

Rigby FB, Pastorek JG: Pneumonia during pregnancy. *Clin Obstet Gynecol* 1996;1:107.

Rolbin SH, Levinson G, Shnider DM, et al.: Dopamine treatment of spinal hypotension decreases uterine blood flow in the pregnant ewe. *Anesthesiology* 1979;51:36.

Schatz M, Zeiger RS: Asthma and allergy in pregnancy. *Clin Perinatol* 1997;24:407.

Sheldon RE, Peeters LLH, Jones MD Jr, et al.: Redistribution of cardiac output and oxygen delivery in the hypoxic fetal lamb. *Am J Obstet Gynecol* 1979;135:1071.

Sholl JS: Abruptio placentae: clinical management of nonacute cases. *Am J Obstet Gynecol* 1987;156:40.

23 Poisoning in Pregnancy

Steven C. Curry *David J. Watts*

INTRODUCTION

Many emotional, clinical, and ethical issues surface when a physician is confronted with a pregnant patient who suffers from acute or chronic poisoning. Fortunately, with rare exceptions, the proper management of pregnant patients does not differ from the nongravid patient.

Two general principles should be kept in mind when treating pregnant women who are poisoned

1. With rare exception, we save the baby by saving the mother.
2. More harm and damage result from withholding needed therapy from the mother.

Excluding drugs of abuse, the three most common intentional poisonings during pregnancy are those by acetaminophen (APAP), iron, and aspirin. This chapter specifically addresses the perinatal concerns and management of these three poisonings.

ACETAMINOPHEN

Excluding alcohol and drugs of abuse, APAP is the most common drug taken in overdose during pregnancy.

Maternal Concerns

Pathophysiology

Most APAP is metabolized in the liver by being conjugated with sulfate or glucuronide to form nontoxic metabolites that are excreted in the urine (Fig. 23-1). Approximately 7 percent of APAP, however, is metabolized in the liver and kidneys by cytochrome P450 to form a toxic metabolite, *N*-acetyl-*p*-benzoquinoneimine (NAPQI). NAPQI is an extremely reactive molecule that covalently binds to macromolecules, leading to cell injury and death. NAPQI normally undergoes detoxification by combining with glutathione to form a nontoxic mercapturic acid metabolite that is excreted in the urine. With APAP overdose, however, so much NAPQI is formed that glutathione stores become depleted resulting in NAPQI-induced cytotoxicity. Acetaminophen poisoning principally affects the liver and, to a lesser extent, the kidneys.

Toxic Doses and Clinical Course

Patients *acutely* ingesting >140 mg/kg of acetaminophen are at risk for hepatotoxicity. One can predict the risk for developing hepatotoxicity after an *acute, single* ingestion by obtaining a serum APAP concentration at least 4 hours after ingestion. Plotting the resulting level on a standard nomogram estimates the risk for hepatotoxicity (Fig. 23-2). If an antidote is not given within 8 hours and hepatotoxicity develops, it is associated with prolonged prothrombin time and elevation of transaminases (commonly into the thousands). Enzyme values usually peak between 36 and 72 hours after ingestion.

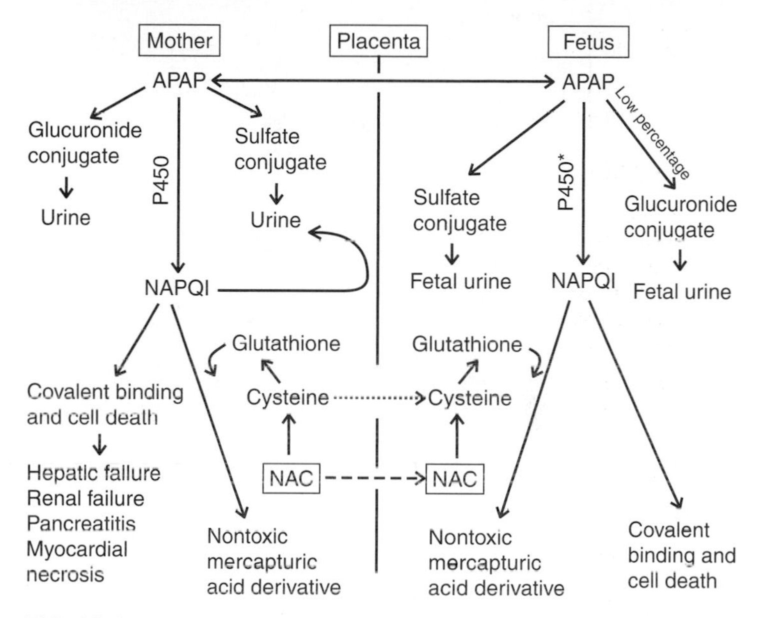

FIG. 23-1 Pathophysiology of acetaminophen poisoning. APAP, acetaminophen; NAC, *N*-acetylcysteine; NAPQI, *N*-acetyl-*p*-benzoquinoneimine; P450* steadily increases after 14 weeks of life.

Jaundice is uncommon. Seriously poisoned patients occasionally suffer from pancreatitis, myocardial necrosis, and heart failure. For reasons that are not understood, persons who take massive overdoses may present in the first few hours (before the onset of liver failure) with coma and severe metabolic acidosis with elevated lactate concentrations.

While nausea and vomiting commonly develop early in APAP poisoning, patients who ingest fatal doses may suffer no symptoms until the onset of symptomatic liver failure, which can occur one to three days later. Therefore, a serum APAP value must be obtained from both symptomatic and asymptomatic patients in order to properly access the severity of the overdose.

Patients who habitually take excessive doses of acetaminophen (usually well in excess of 4 g per day) are more likely to develop renal failure along with hepatotoxicity. Serum APAP concentrations in these patients cannot be correlated with severity of illness or risk of hepatotoxicity.

Treatment

The antidote for APAP poisoning is *N*-acetylcysteine (NAC, Mucomyst) (Fig. 23-3). *N*-Acetylcysteine undergoes conversion to cysteine, which, in turn, is metabolized to glutathione. *N*-Acetylcysteine's main effect is to maintain glutathione stores so that NAPQI can be detoxified. Started within 8 hours of ingestion, NAC prevents serious maternal hepatic and renal toxicity from APAP. To ensure that NAC is started promptly after an acute ingestion, it is generally most prudent to begin NAC therapy immediately and discontinue it only if the serum APAP concentration is found to be in the nontoxic

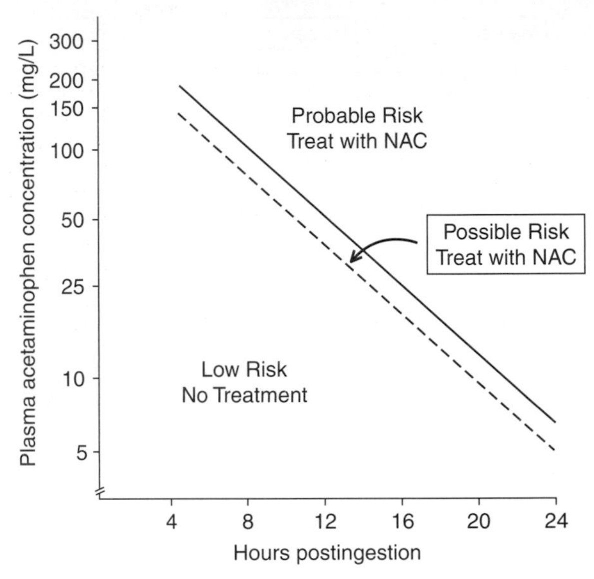

FIG. 23-2 Acetaminophen nomogram. For use only after a single, acute ingestion in a patient who has not recently taken acetaminophen prior to ingestion. A level should not be plotted on the nomogram unless it was obtained at least 4 h after ingestion. If a level falls above the lower line, *N*-acetylcysteine should be continued (if already started) or administered immediately.

range when plotted on the nomogram. Therapy with NAC provides benefit by lessening the severity of hepatic necrosis and increasing chances for survival, even when commenced more than 24 hours after ingestion. Therefore, it is never too late to begin NAC therapy, though efficacy begins to fall the longer the therapy is delayed beyond 8 hours.

A serum APAP concentration (measured at least 4 hours after ingestion) resulting in a value above the lower line of the nomogram necessitates a full course of NAC therapy (e.g., 17 oral doses) be delivered. Although, experienced toxicologists sometimes are confident with slightly shorter courses of therapy in patients who have never exhibited signs of hepatotoxicity, NAC therapy should not be stopped prematurely simply because a repeat serum APAP concentration falls to zero or plots below the lower line on the nomogram.

Patients commonly experience nausea and vomiting following APAP ingestion, sometimes making it difficult to administer oral NAC therapy. In these cases, NAC has been given intravenously. An intravenous formulation is prepared in the pharmacy by aseptically passing sterile inhalable or oral NAC solution through a 0.2-μm filter and diluting it in 5 percent dextrose in water, to create an intravenous solution. An intravenous protocol commonly used in the United States is described in Fig. 23-3.

Occasionally, patients suffer symptomatic histamine release from intravenous NAC and require treatment with antihistamines. On rare occasions,

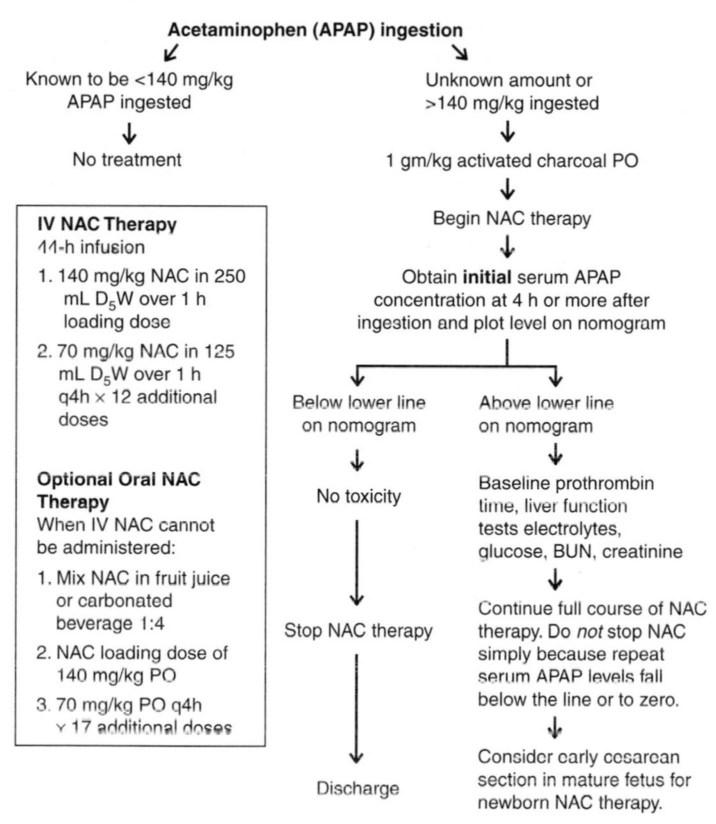

FIG. 23-3 General guidelines for managing acetaminophen poisoning. Oral NAC should be used when IV NAC cannot be prepared by the pharmacy and promptly administered. NAC, *N*-acetylcysteine; APAP, acetaminophen. See text for discussion on role of cesarian section.

patients suffer life-threatening anaphylactoid reactions requiring fluids, epinephrine, antihistamines, and corticosteroids. If the pharmacy cannot timely prepare intravenous NAC, treatment should not be delayed and oral NAC therapy should be started immediately. Treatment for adjunctive complications (e.g., liver failure, renal failure) is entirely supportive and identical to that for other pregnant patients.

Fetal Concerns

Fetal death from APAP overdose has been reported in all trimesters. Maternal NAPQI does not cross the placenta. Maternal APAP, however, does cross and has the potential to produce toxic fetal concentrations. The fetus's ability to produce NAPQI from APAP begins as early as 14 weeks intrauterine life and increases until term. The fetus's ability to detoxify APAP by conjugation with sulfate and glucuronide remains impaired until after birth, possibly shunting more APAP through cytochrome P450. The third trimester fetus, therefore, appears to be at greatest risk for *direct* toxicity from APAP. Nevertheless, fetal loss appears to be most common in the first trimester—not because the fetus is necessarily poisoned, but because maternal illness is more likely to lead to fetal loss at that time.

To our knowledge, medical literature has not reported fetal demise from acetaminophen after an *acute, single* maternal APAP ingestion of less than 140 mg/kg. We are also unaware of APAP-induced fetal demise when the mother habitually ingests excessive amounts of APAP unless maternal toxicity was also present. Finally, we cannot locate reports of fetal demise in mothers who have *acutely* ingested a single toxic APAP dose if NAC therapy was commenced within 8 hours.

NAC does not reliably cross the ovine placenta or perfused living ex vivo human placenta. However, the most recent study addressing this issue reported that serum NAC concentrations in the umbilical cord blood of four infants, whose mothers were treated with oral NAC for APAP toxicity, were equivalent to maternal values (Horowitz et al.). However, an infant would not have had the potential benefit of first-pass effect through its liver that the mother experiences. While the mother's serum NAC concentrations were in the range associated with protection from hepatotoxicity after oral ingestion and first pass through the maternal liver, we do not know whether IV NAC given at doses which would produce levels this low would be protective. In fact, when NAC is given IV at currently used therapeutic doses, serum NAC levels 10 to 100 times higher are achieved. This is one reason why the authors administer IV NAC, rather than oral NAC, to our pregnant patients at our center. Investigators can only speculate whether maternal cysteine, produced from NAC, crosses in amounts large enough to maintain fetal glutathione stores.

At least one authority has recommended consideration for delivery of the mature fetus by cesarean section so that NAC therapy can be administered directly to the baby at risk (i.e., when maternal serum APAP concentrations are toxic). This assumes that the mother is not at undue risk for the procedure because of coagulopathy. Advocates of immediate delivery state that the maternal and fetal risk of late third trimester cesarean section is extremely low in comparison to data from the several case reports describing fetal death from APAP toxicity. Unfortunately, no animal or human studies have examined the benefits of immediate delivery followed by direct newborn NAC therapy. As noted above, literature does not contain reports of fetal demise following acute single APAP ingestions if NAC therapy is begun promptly. Thus, there is support for both positions, and no standard of care to guide clinicians who face this dilemma exists; the decision lies with the treating physician.

IRON

Prenatal vitamins with iron, account for the second most common overdose in pregnant women. Large doses of iron are extremely toxic and may lead to multiorgan system dysfunction and death. Strong evidence indicates that the fetus is protected from elevated maternal iron levels. Iron poisoning is, almost entirely, a situation in which fetal survival depends on saving the mother. Table 23-1 and Fig. 23-4 summarize the pathophysiology of iron toxicity.

TABLE 23-1 Pathophysiology of Iron Poisoning

1. Iron is corrosive to the gastrointestinal tract, producing nausea, vomiting, diarrhea, abdominal pain, gastrointestinal bleeding, and rarely perforations.
2. Systemically absorbed iron causes venodilatation and increased capillary permeability with associated third spacing of fluid.
3. Iron causes cell dysfunction and death by disrupting ATP formation in mitochondria and by catalyzing the formation of oxygen-free radicals that destroy cell membranes. The liver takes the brunt of the injury with potential for fulminant hepatic failure, but in massive iron poisoning, any organ can be affected.
4. Early after ingestion, high serum iron concentrations directly inhibit serine proteases (thrombin) and lengthen the prothrombin time, even in the absence of hepatic failure.

Maternal Concerns

Toxic Doses

To determine how much iron was ingested, the elemental iron content must be calculated. On a milligram basis, ferrous sulfate comprises 20 percent elemental iron; ferrous fumarate 33 percent elemental iron; and ferrous gluconate 12 percent elemental iron. Any patient who ingests more than 20 mg/kg of elemental iron, any patient with symptoms, and/or any patient in whom the amount of ingested iron is not known requires an evaluation.

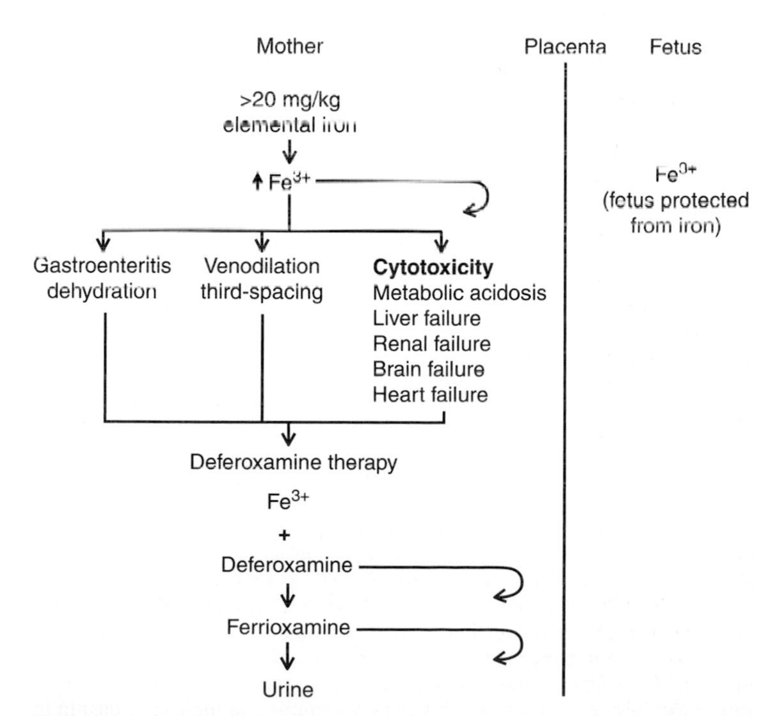

FIG. 23-4 Pathophysiology of iron poisoning and rationale for treatment. See text for conversion of iron salts to elemental iron.

Clinical effects

Traditionally, clinical effects are considered in four stages, although the distinctions between stages are not always clear.

Stage 1 is characterized by abdominal pain, vomiting, and diarrhea, and results from the corrosive effects of iron on the gut. Stage 1 begins 1 to 6 hours after ingestion. Hematemesis is possible, and hypovolemia may result in hypotension and metabolic acidosis. Serum iron levels may be normal or elevated at this stage.

Stage 2 in not always seen, but, when present, lasts for about 2 to 24 hours or so after Stage 1. Stage 2 is characterized by resolution of gastroenteritis, and patients commonly lie in bed quietly. Pallor, metabolic acidosis, and in the face of uncorrected hypovolemia, tachycardia and hypotension may be noted. Physicians may be falsely reassured by the resolution of gastroenteritis in the face of ensuing systemic iron toxicity as tissue iron stores rise. Tachycardia and hypotension are common if hypovolemia has not been corrected. Metabolic acidosis and hypotension result from uncorrected hypovolemia, venodilation, third-spacing of fluid, and the cytotoxic effects of iron. Serum iron concentration may be elevated and liver enzyme values are normal. Prothrombin time may be elevated if serum iron concentrations are high from a direct effect of iron on serum proteases such as thrombin. In severe iron poisoning, the patient may rapidly progress from Stage 1 to Stage 3.

Stage 3 comprises systemic organ damage or failure from the cytotoxic effects of iron. Its onset is observed at any time from ingestion through 48 hours. Stage 3 is characterized by hepatic failure, lethargy/coma/convulsions, renal failure, and, occasionally, heart failure. Hypoglycemia and coagulopathy reflect hepatic damage. In this setting, metabolic acidosis has numerous causes including hepatic failure, low cardiac output, and impaired oxidative phosphorylation. The liver is the major organ affected by the toxicity of iron and typically is the first organ to fail.

Stage 4 is characterized by gastric outlet or small bowel obstruction from gastrointestinal scarring several weeks after the poisoning.

Evaluation and Treatment

Serum Iron Concentrations While most patients who suffer iron poisoning of Stage 2 or greater are thought to have *peak* serum concentrations >350 μg/dL, the actual peak level is seldom observed as a consequence of mistiming. Serum iron levels peak sometime between 2 and 6 hours after ingestion. Normal or mildly elevated serum iron concentrations can be misleading, since they do not always reflect the tissue iron burden, and it is tissue iron that is responsible for systemic toxicity. For example, a normal or low serum iron concentration may represent a decline from previously elevated levels. Therefore, as an isolated finding, a normal serum iron concentration cannot always be used to exclude iron poisoning in the symptomatic patient. The measurement of total iron binding capacity (TIBC) does not assist in the treatment of acute iron poisoning since it is falsely elevated in the face of high serum iron concentrations by some methods and since serum iron concentrations may be quickly changing in their relationship to TIBC.

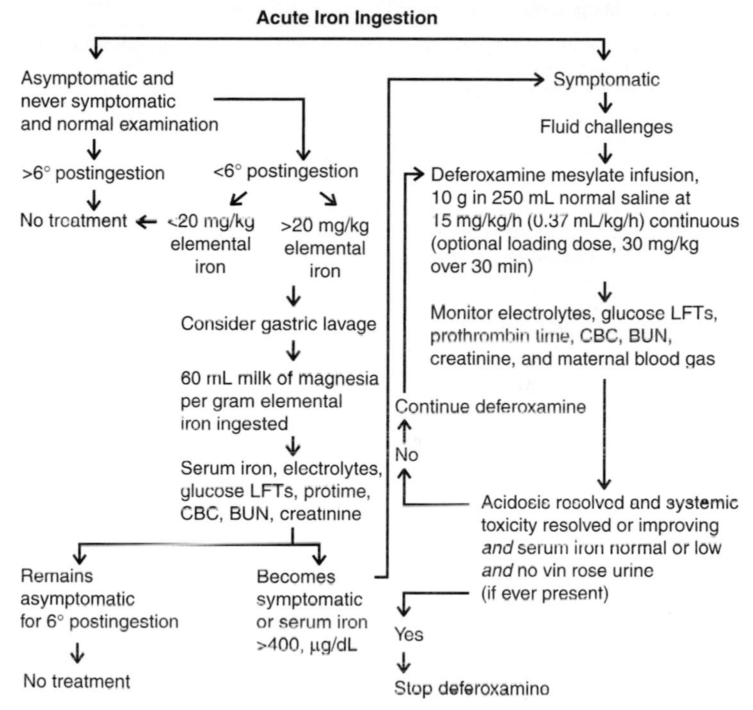

FIG. 23-5 Treatment of acute iron ingestion.

Asymptomatic Patients Generally, patients who remain completely asymptomatic for 6 hours after ingestion and have a normal physical examination do not require treatment for iron poisoning (Fig. 23-5). Asymptomatic patients who ingest >20 mg/kg of elemental iron but are seen within 6 hours might benefit from gastric lavage with saline, but it is not known if this is effective. If vomiting has already occurred, it is not thought that gastric lavage would be of further benefit. We advise *against lavage* with bicarbonate, phosphate, or deferoxamine solutions. A single oral dose of 8 percent magnesium oxide (Milk of Magnesia), 60 mL/g of elemental iron ingested, significantly reduce iron absorption in healthy volunteers.

Symptomatic Patients Patients are considered symptomatic when they present with more than minimal symptoms (e.g., more than one emesis). These patients require treatment with fluids and deferoxamine mesylate, in addition to magnesium oxide (Table 23-2). When a patient has significant clinical symptoms, it is never prudent to wait for results of a serum iron concentration before beginning therapy, including deferoxamine.

Fetal Concerns

The placenta selectively transports maternal transferrin-bound iron only when it is required by the fetus. Animal models of iron poisoning in pregnancy, along

TABLE 23-2 Management: Symptomatic Iron Poisoning

1. With rare exception, all symptomatic patients are hypovolemic. Administering 500–1000 mL fluid challenges (Ringer's lactate or normal saline) to restore fluid volume and ensure urine output of 1–2 mL/kg/h is therapeutic. Patients commonly require maintenance infusions at twice normal rates to keep up with gastrointestinal losses and third spacing.
2. A complete blood count, prothrombin time, electrolytes, serum glucose, liver function studies, arterial blood gases and blood urea nitrogen/creatinine, and serum iron concentration should be obtained. Do not order a total iron binding capacity, as it does not assist in treatment and is frequently falsely elevated in iron poisoning.
3. Deferoxamine mesylate is an iron-chelating agent that is given to remove iron from tissues. Deferoxamine binds with iron to form ferrioxamine, which is excreted in the urine over days or weeks. Ferrioxamine occasionally produces a vin rose color in the urine. This color change is unreliable and inconsistent; it should not be used to determine the need for deferoxamine. Deferoxamine mesylate can be mixed in the crystalloid of choice and should be infused continuously at 15 mg/kg/h after optional loading dose of 30 mg/kg over 30 min (Fig. 23-5)[a].
4. Deferoxamine should be continued until the serum iron concentration is normal or low and systemic toxicity is resolved (e.g., resolved acidosis, liver function studies normal or improving) and if it is present, obvious vinrose-colored urine disappears. Most patients require 12 to 24 h of deferoxamine infusion. Occasionally patients taking very large overdoses require a longer duration of therapy.
5. If renal failure develops, deferoxamine should be continued, but at much lower infusion rates. Assuming that therapeutic deferoxamine levels have been obtained, anuric patients should continue to receive infusions at about 1.5 mg/kg/h, based on the known prolonged half-life in renal failure.
6. General supportive care for attendant complications (e.g., liver failure, gastrointestinal bleeding) is the same as that for any other pregnant patient.

[a]Many statements in the package insert for deferoxamine do not reflect common practice and are misleading or incorrect. Deferoxamine is not contraindicated in pregnancy for the treatment of acute iron poisoning. At 15 mg/kg/h, most patients will receive well over 6 g deferoxamine mesylate per day and this is safe for short-term treatment of iron poisoning. Intramuscular deferoxamine is not recommended.

with human experience, lead to the conclusion that the fetus does not develop elevated iron burdens in the face of maternal iron poisoning (Fig. 23-4). Fetal demise appears to be due, entirely, to maternal illness or death. In addition, deferoxamine and ferrioxamine do not appear to cross the placenta (despite information in the package insert). Fetal outcome depends on the well being of the mother; it is in the interest of both mother and child that significant poisoning be treated promptly with deferoxamine. *Pregnancy or fetal concerns are never reasons to withhold deferoxamine therapy.*

In a review of 61 cases of iron overdose in pregnancy, Tran and colleagues noted that the degree of maternal toxicity was directly related to the risk of fetal loss. Fetal demise appeared to be related to the timing and severity of the maternal illness, rather than to fetal toxicity directly from iron.

SALICYLATE

Sources of salicylate include aspirin (acetylsalicylic acid), oil of wintergreen (methylsalicylate), salicylic acid, and salsalate. All of these compounds are converted to salicylate after absorption. With the exception of aspirin's ability to inhibit platelet function, salicylate is responsible for most of the observed toxic effects.

Salicylate poisoning remains one of the most underestimated and mismanaged poisonings in medicine. This problem is further compounded by pregnancy, when only moderate maternal toxicity may result in fetal demise secondary to the propensity of the drug to concentrate in the fetus. Few intoxications require as much effort on the physician's part for a successful outcome as salicylate toxicity.

Maternal Concerns

Pharmacokinetics and Toxic Doses

Significant salicylate toxicity is said to develop after the acute, single ingestion of at least 150 mg/kg of aspirin (or its equivalent). However, given the fetus's ability to concentrate salicylate, concern arises when an acute, single maternal ingestion exceeds 75 mg/kg. Salicylate levels may not peak until 24 hours after the drug is absorbed. Enteric-coated aspirin may not produce toxic serum concentrations for many hours after ingestion.

Salicylate exists in blood as an equilibrium between the ionized and the nonionized form (Fig. 23-6). The nonionized, nonprotein-bound fraction of salicylate is in equilibrium with tissue stores. This nonionized form easily moves into body compartments because of its lipophilic nature. As serum salicylate levels rise, protein binding becomes saturated, producing a higher free (nonionized) fraction of the drug. As pH falls the nonionized fraction of salicylate increases. Therefore, rises in serum salicylate concentration or falls in blood pH result in an increase in the apparent volume of distribution of salicylate as salicylate moves from blood into tissue. This important concept is critical in understanding both the pathophysiology and the management of salicylate toxicity, since the serum salicylate concentrations can fall while tissue concentrations and severity of toxicity increase.

In salicylate poisoning, most salicylate is eliminated unchanged by the kidneys. Elimination half-lives can be as long as $1\frac{1}{2}$ to 2 days in untreated patients because of saturable elimination kinetics.

Pathophysiology and Clinical Effects

Salicylate produces numerous actions that produce various effects in many organ systems. These diverse clinical manifestations result, in part, because of impaired adenosine triphosphate (ATP) formation from salicylate's actions on cellular metabolism.

Gastrointestinal Irritation Direct corrosive injury to the gut is responsible for abdominal pain, nausea, vomiting, gastrointestinal bleeding, and rare reports of gastric perforation.

Respiratory Alkalosis Salicylate directly stimulates the brain stem to cause hyperventilation. However, the onset of coma or coingestion of sedatives commonly masks hyperventilation, and can even produce hypoventilation and hypercapnia.

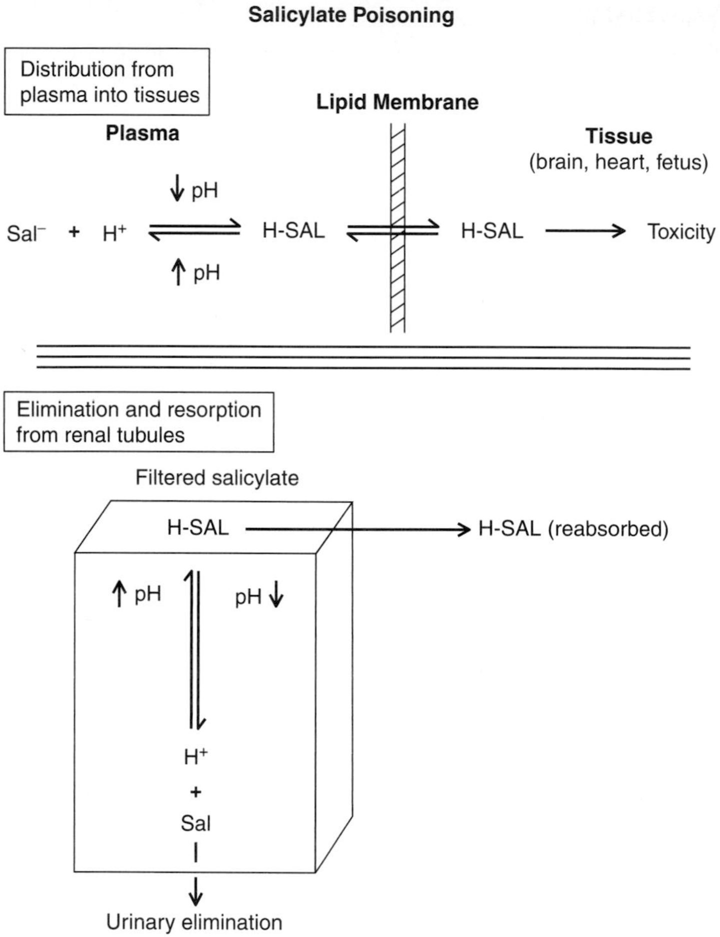

Salicylate Poisoning

Distribution from plasma into tissues

Lipid Membrane

Plasma

Tissue
(brain, heart, fetus)

↓ pH

$Sal^- + H^+ \rightleftharpoons$ H-SAL $\rightleftharpoons$ H-SAL → Toxicity

↑ pH

Elimination and resorption from renal tubules

Filtered salicylate

H-SAL → H-SAL (reabsorbed)

↑ pH ⇅ pH ↓

H^+
+
Sal

↓
Urinary elimination

FIG. 23-6 Salicylate distribution between blood, tissues, and urine. A smaller fraction of salicylate is protein bound at higher concentrations. A fall in pH increases the fraction of unionized salicylate. Therefore, falls in pH or rises in salicylate concentrations result in a greater fraction of the drug that can move into tissues, including the brain and fetus. Alkalinization of the blood helps prevent movement of salicylate into tissue. Alkalinization of urine traps salicylate in an ionized form so it cannot be reabsorbed, enhancing urinary elimination. H-SAL, unionized salicylic acid; SAL^-, ionized salicylate anion.

Metabolic Acidosis Salicylate affects numerous metabolic pathways to inhibit ATP formation. Salicylate inhibits the Krebs' cycle, uncouples oxidative phosphorylation, and enhances lipolysis. All of these actions serve to produce metabolic acidosis. Ketonuria is usually present, and lactate levels are usually normal. The anion gap can be normal or elevated.

Glucose Metabolism Increased glucose demand accompanied by glycogenolysis explains occasional hyperglycemia seen early in poisoning. However, salicylate inhibits gluconeogenesis so when glycogen stores become depleted, hypoglycemia is possible.

Fluid and Electrolytes Dehydration from gastrointestinal losses and hyperventilation is common. Patients may lose 1 to 2 L/h from severe diaphoresis, alone. The average patient with moderate to severe salicylate poisoning has a 6 L fluid deficit. Both hypokalemia and hyperkalemia may be observed. Hypokalemia results from gastrointestinal losses and obligatory urinary excretion of potassium with organic acids (e.g., salicylate). Hyperkalemia usually reflects severe dehydration and prerenal azotemia, sometimes with rhabdomyolysis.

Pulmonary Noncardiogenic (low pressure) pulmonary edema can develop with salicylate poisoning; however, hydrostatic (high pressure) pulmonary edema may also occur in persons with chronic heart disease or salicylate-induced heart failure, or in those whose fluid therapy has not been carefully monitored for fluid balance.

Cardiovascular The metabolic insult to myocardium induced by salicylate results in tachycardia, ventricular arrhythmias, heart failure, hypotension, and sudden death. In the absence of heart disease, metabolic acidosis and neurotoxicity almost always precede severe cardiac dysfunction and shock if the patient has been adequately fluid resuscitated.

Central Nervous System Impaired ATP production produces neurotoxicity which is manifested by hallucinations, agitation, delirium, lethargy, coma, convulsions, malignant cerebral edema, and brain death. Patients who die despite supportive care usually die from cerebral failure.

Coagulation and Platelets Salicylate impairs vitamin K-dependent coagulation factors to prolong prothrombin time in a manner similar to Coumadin. Aspirin (acetylsalicylic acid) also inhibits platelet function, though this is rarely responsible for major morbidity.

Miscellaneous Hyperthermia may be observed, but is the exception. When present, it portends a poor prognosis. Acute tubular necrosis has been reported. Rhabdomyolysis contributes to hyperkalemia, coagulopathy, and renal failure. Tinnitus is common when serum salicylate levels exceed about 25 mg/dL.

Clinical Presentation

Acute Salicylate Poisoning Patients who present shortly after an overdose are usually awake and complain of tinnitus, abdominal pain, nausea, and vomiting. Other abnormalities include tachypnea, respiratory alkalosis with alkalemia, hypovolemia, hypokalemia, and gastrointestinal bleeding.

Progression of the poisoning is characterized by diaphoresis, tachycardia despite correction of hypovolemia, metabolic acidosis and acidemia, progressively severe neurotoxicity, alterations of glucose homeostasis, elevated prothrombin time, pulmonary edema, and cardiotoxicity. The combination of acidemia and neurotoxicity carries a grave prognosis unless aggressive treatment is initiated promptly.

Chronic Salicylate Poisoning Chronic salicylate poisoning is best described as a syndrome resulting from repeated doses of salicylate. Patients are brought in by friends or family because of altered mental status, including lethargy, hallucinations, agitation, seizures, and coma. Occasionally, hypoglycemia contributes to encephalopathy. Prothrombin times are typically elevated, and metabolic acidosis is more common than alkalosis in toxic patients. Pulmonary edema leading to adult respiratory distress syndrome (low pressure) occurs more often than with acute poisoning. As compared to acute salicylate poisoning, serum salicylate concentrations are lower for any given degree of toxicity in chronic poisoning because of larger tissue burdens of salicylate, reflecting a larger volume of distribution.

Evaluation and Treatment

Serum Salicylate Concentrations Interpretation of serum salicylate concentrations can be difficult. Similar levels can have varied effects because of changing tissue burdens of the drug depending on blood pH, protein binding, and other factors. Because of these factors, tissue concentrations of salicylate can actually rise while serum levels are falling, causing the patient's condition to deteriorate while the physician is falsely reassured by falling serum drug concentrations. It is always more important to treat the patient than the serum salicylate concentration.

Furthermore, because of delayed or prolonged absorption, basing treatment and disposition on a single serum salicylate concentration can be misleading and is to be discouraged. We are generally reassured that the mother is out of danger only when serum salicylate concentrations are less than 25 mg/dL and are known to be falling, with the patient exhibiting no laboratory or clinical evidence of toxicity. Because the fetus develops higher serum salicylate concentrations than the mother, it is possible for a mother to have become asymptomatic after an overdose (with low serum salicylate levels) but to have suffered fetal loss or to carry a fetus with significant toxicity.

Hyperbilirubinemia can cause falsely elevated salicylate concentrations when levels are measured using a colorimetric method. In these cases, serum salicylate concentrations should be measured by an immunoassay or by a chromatographic method.

General Principles All patients with salicylate poisoning should be admitted to an intensive care setting, whether in labor and delivery or in a medical intensive care unit. Successful maternal management of acute salicylate poisoning hinges on intensive and attentive medical care (Fig. 23-7). Specifically, frequent attention to fluid balance, electrolyte and acid-base status, bedside examination, and rapid institution of hemodialysis at the earliest signs of central nervous system deterioration are required. As noted below, we also recommend that hemodialysis be performed earlier than in nonpregnant patients, given ability of the fetus to concentrate salicylate.

The rationale behind sodium bicarbonate therapy outlined below has two principal purposes (see Fig. 23-6). Most important, alkalinization of blood helps prevent movement of salicylate out of the serum into target organs. The prime concern is preventing movement of salicylate into the CNS and the fetus. Blood pH should be kept between 7.45 and 7.50. A drop in blood pH from 7.45 to 7.20 can almost double the concentration of nonionized salicylate that is able to move into the brain and fetus. Of lesser importance, alkalinization of urine promotes ionic trapping of salicylate in urine, preventing reabsorption, and enhancing elimination. Urinary salicylate excretion can

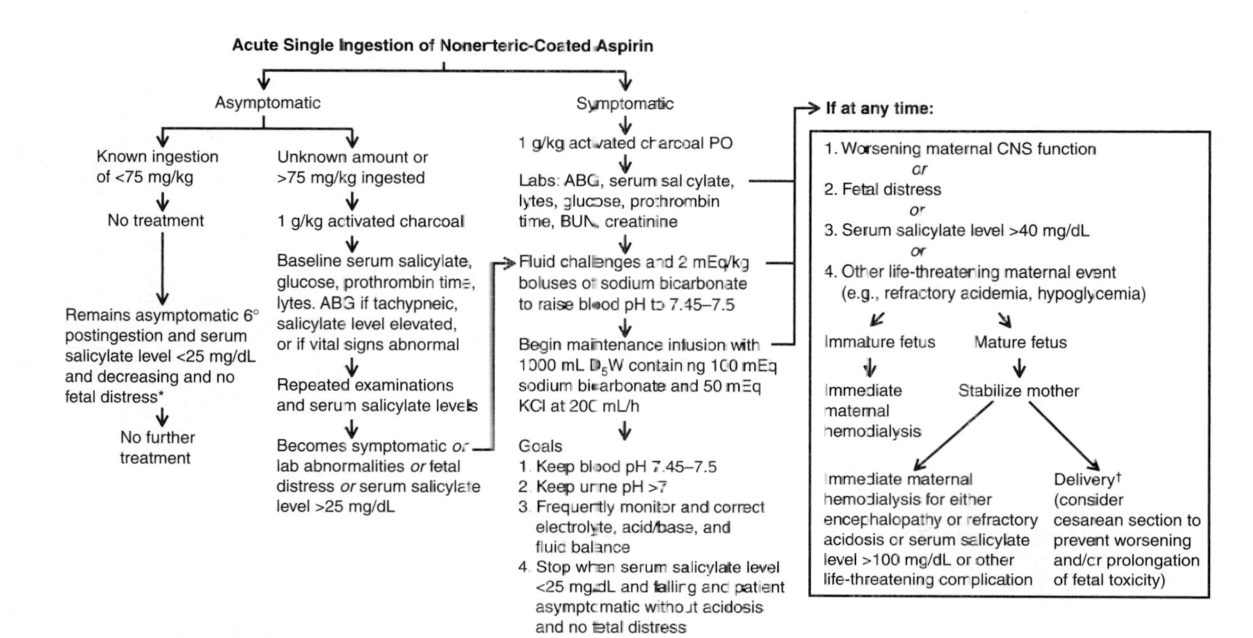

*Enteric-coated aspirin may not produce toxic serum salicylate concentrations until well after 6-h postingestion.

†See text for discussion.

FIG. 23-7 Treatment guidelines for salicylate poisoning

increase 15 times as urine pH increases to pH 8.0, above which there is no additional benefit.

Airway As with many patients, immediate attention to airway and adequate oxygenation are mandatory. If a patient receives narcotics or sedatives, including when used for endotracheal intubation and mechanical ventilation, a drop in an elevated minute ventilation (from salicylate-induced hyperventilation) to normal values can precipitate a rapid decline in blood pH, movement of salicylate into tissues and fetus, and rapid deterioration. Therefore, close attention must be given to maintaining alkalemia with additional doses of IV sodium bicarbonate when sedation or mechanical ventilation is instituted.

Glucose Abnormalities Patients must be monitored for hypoglycemia, especially in the face of any mental status changes. Treatment comprises IV boluses of 50 percent dextrose and infusions of dextrose solutions.

Gastrointestinal Decontamination Most patients suffering from acute salicylate poisoning vomit repeatedly, rendering further attempts at gastric emptying (lavage and ipecac) unnecessary. A single dose of 1 g activated charcoal per kg body weight should be given initially. If salicylate levels continue to rise, repeated doses of 0.25 g activated charcoal per kg body weight, every 4 to 6 hours until levels begin to fall, may be considered if the patient has normal gastrointestinal motility. Phenothiazines are to be discouraged, as they usually are ineffective and lower the seizure threshold.

Fluid and Electrolyte Therapy Most patients are moderately to severely dehydrated and require immediate fluid challenges with normal saline or Ringer's lactate until urine output is 2 to 3 mL/kg/h. Initial sodium bicarbonate boluses of 2 mEq/kg are given, if needed, to raise arterial blood pH from 7.45 to 7.5. A typical patient with moderate to severe salicylate toxicity has a 6-L fluid deficit on presentation.

A recommended *initial* regimen for maintenance fluid therapy *after* fluid resuscitation and establishment of good urine flow is a continuous infusion of 1000 mL of 5 percent dextrose in water to which is added 150 mEq sodium bicarbonate and 50 mEq potassium chloride to run at 200 mL/h. Hypokalemia must be treated aggressively. Urine alkalinity cannot be achieved in the setting of hypokalemia because the kidney will secrete protons rather than potassium ions when reabsorbing sodium. Additionally, for the reasons outlined above, the patient usually presents with a total body potassium debt, and ongoing losses continue as salicylate anions combine with potassium cations in the urine during elimination. Despite intravenous infusions containing 50 mEq/L of KCl, patients almost always require regular additional potassium supplementation. Oral potassium solutions can be used when vomiting has halted.

Fine-Tuning Therapy In moderately to severely ill patients, arterial blood gases, urine pH, electrolytes, and serum glucose should be measured every 1 to 2 hours, at which time fluid balance is also reassessed. Fluid and electrolyte infusions are modified as needed to prevent hypovolemia, fluid overload, normalize electrolytes, ensure adequate urine output, and prevent acidemia and hypoglycemia. Because of fluid losses through hyperventilation, diaphoresis, vomiting, and sometimes, hyperthermia, it is common for moderately to severely ill patients to require more than 500 mL/h of intravenous fluid (e.g., an additional 300 mL/h of lactated Ringer's) to maintain euvolemia and prevent the rises in serum creatinine, sodium, and hematocrit typical of hemoconcentration. Serum salicylate concentrations should be obtained every 1 to 2 hours until it is clear that they are falling, with findings interpreted in the context of the patient's condition. Efforts are directed at preventing drops in arterial pH below 7.45 and at keeping urine pH elevated. Aciduria in the face of alkalemia is treated with further doses of potassium, as long as hyperkalemia is not present. Any deterioration in neurologic function, especially if associated with acidemia, is an indication for immediate hemodialysis.

Noncardiogenic Pulmonary Edema Adult respiratory distress syndrome (ARDS) is more common in chronic toxicity and should be treated with oxygen and continuous positive airway pressure (CPAP) or positive end-expiratory pressure (PEEP), if required. Only cautious use of diuretics is recommended, as these patients are usually volume depleted.

Miscellaneous A 20 mg parenteral dose of vitamin K_1 reverses elevated prothrombin time produced by salicylate over several hours. In an emergency, fresh-frozen plasma rapidly corrects coagulopathy (but not platelet dysfunction). Serial blood hemoglobin values should be followed to determine if gastrointestinal bleeding develops and becomes severe enough to require transfusions. Antacid therapy with proton pump inhibitors or H_2 antagonists are commonly used, but have not been studied in the setting of salicylate poisoning. Serial measurements of serum creatine kinase (CK) activity should be evaluated to rule out rhabdomyolysis, which, if present, will require specific therapy.

Hemodialysis Hemodialysis is effective and life saving in that it removes salicylate and corrects acid base electrolyte abnormalities. It is best performed using high-flux hemodialysis with the largest-surface area cartridge available. Hemodialysis is generally indicated in the following situations:

1. Moderately to severely ill patients with renal insufficiency
2. Onset of significant or worsening neurotoxicity, even if serum salicylate concentrations are falling
3. Other life-threatening complications accompanied by elevated serum salicylate concentrations
4. To ensure fetal survival (see below)

Fetal Concerns

Salicylate crosses the placenta and concentrates in the fetus at higher levels than in the mother, at least in part, by differences in protein binding. Nöschel and colleagues gave 20 mg sodium salicylate per kg maternal body weight IV to pregnant women at the beginning of labor and then measured serum salicylate concentrations in mothers and cord blood at the time of delivery. By 4 hours, the ratio of fetal to maternal serum salicylate values was about 1.5:1. The relative acidemia of the fetus also contributes to a higher relative volume of distribution and, therefore, higher tissue levels for a given serum salicylate concentration. In addition, the fetus has a lower capacity to buffer the acidemic stress imposed by salicylate and, relative to the mother, a reduced capacity to excrete the toxin. Collectively, this places the fetus at greater risk for death and forms the basis for the subsequent recommendation of hemodialysis and/or possible cesarean section.

Premature Fetus

Given that the fetus concentrates salicylate and suffers greater toxicity than the mother, it seems wise to institute hemodialysis for lesser degrees of maternal toxicity than would be done in nonpregnant patients. Unfortunately, there are no studies to guide clinicians in this setting. From our experience, we generally recommend immediate hemodialysis in the face of any signs of fetal distress, in the face of chronic maternal salicylate poisoning (where high tissue levels predominate), or whenever maternal serum salicylate concentrations exceed 40 mg/dL.

Mature Fetus

Using the rationale for premature fetuses, it has been argued that delivery by cesarean section, when safe for the mother, should be considered. However, there are no studies that have addressed this issue, and it is possible that hemodialysis would result in falls in both maternal and fetal salicylate concentrations from the redistribution of salicylate across the placenta. Again, no standard of care exists, and decisions must be made on an individual basis. If cesarean section is not performed, hemodialysis should be instituted.

SUGGESTED READING

Berkovitch M, Uziel Y, Greenberg R, et al.: False-high blood salicylate levels in neonates with hyperbilirubinemia. *Therap Drug Monitor* 2000;22:757–761.

Curry SC, Bond GR, Raschke R, et al.: An ovine model of maternal iron poisoning in pregnancy. *Ann Emerg Med* 1990;19:632–638.

Gray TA, Buckley BM, Vale JA: Hyperlactataemia and metabolic acidosis following paracetamol overdose. *Q J Med* 1987;65:811–821.

Harrison PM, Keays R, Bray GP, et al.: Improved outcome of paracetamol-induced fulminant hepatic failure by late administration of acetylcysteine. *Lancet* 1990;335:1572–1573.

Horowitz RS, Dart RC, Jarvie DR, et al.: Placental transfer of *N*-acetylcysteine following human maternal acetaminophen toxicity. *J Toxicol Clin Toxicol* 1997;35:447–451.

Johnson D, Simone C, Koren G: Transfer of *N*-acetylcysteine by the human placenta. *Vet Hum Toxicol* 1993;35:365.

Levy, G: Salicylate pharmacokinetics in the human neonate. *Basic Therap Aspects Perinatal Pharmacol* 1975:319–330.

Loebstein R, Koren G: Clinical relevance of therapeutic drug monitoring during pregnancy (protein binding changes in fetus). *Therap Drug Monitor* 2002;24:15–22.

Mills KC, Curry SC: Acute iron poisoning. *Emerg Med Clin North Am* 1994;12:397–413.

Riggs BS, Bronstein AC, Kulig K, et al.: Acute acetaminophen overdose during pregnancy. *Obstet Gynecol* 1986;74:247–253.

Rollins DE, von Bahr C, Glaumann H, et al.: Acetaminophen: potentially toxic metabolite formed by human fetal and adult liver microsomes and isolated fetal liver cells. *Science* 1979;205:1414–1416.

Selden BS, Curry SC, Clark RF, et al.: Transplacental transport of *N*-acetylcysteine in an ovine model. *Ann Emerg Med* 1991;20:1069–1972.

Smilkstein MJ, Bronstein AC, Linden C, et al.: Acetaminophen overdose: a 48-hour intravenous *N*-acetylcysteine treatment protocol. *Ann Emerg Med* 1991;20:1058–1063.

Smilkstein MJ, Knapp GL, Lulig KW, et al.: Efficacy of oral *N*-acetylcysteine in the treatment of acetaminophen overdose. Analysis of the national multicenter study (1976–1985). *N Engl J Med* 1988;319:1557–1562.

Tenenbein M: Poisoning in pregnancy, In: Koren G (ed), *Maternal-Fetal Toxicology,* 3rd edn. New York: Marcel Dekker, 2001; pp. 233–256.
Tran T, Wax JR, Philput C, et al.: Intentional iron overdose in pregnancy—management and outcome. *J Emerg Med* 2000;18:225–228.
Wallace KL, Curry SC, LoVecchio F, et al.: Effect of magnesium hydroxide on iron absorption following simulated mild iron overdose in human subjects. *Acad Emerg Med* 1998;5:961–965.

24 Neonatal Resuscitation: Pathophysiology, Organization, and Survival

Keith S. Meredith

INTRODUCTION

For those caring for mothers and their babies, the goal for each pregnancy is to optimize maternal-fetal outcome. Unfortunately, this goal is often challenged by the expected, or, even more challenging, unexpected delivery of a neonate who requires urgent medical attention for a disorder(s) threatening his (her) life. Obstetrical providers are, by training and experience, more skilled in adult than neonatal emergency care. As a consequence, without standards in place that direct personnel, training, and equipment, an obstetrical practitioner may find he (she) is ill prepared to effectively respond to a neonatal emergency. The objective of this chapter is to offer an overview of the pathophysiology, organization, and provision of emergency medical care to the newly born patient for the obstetrical primary care provider.

Each year, an estimated 19 percent of the 5 million neonatal deaths that occur worldwide are the result of birth asphyxia. In the United States, approximately 4 million children are born annually, with a reported perinatal mortality rate of 7.0 for the year 2001. This suggests that every year, among U.S. children who reach 28 weeks gestation, 28,000 die prior to their 28th day of life. A significant portion of those infants who succumb, do so from birth asphyxia. Further, among children reaching term gestation, one to two per 1000 live term births suffer hypoxic ischemic encephalopathy (HIE), (0.3 per 1000 severe HIE). In addition, it is widely accepted that 10 percent of all newborns require some assistance to begin and maintain normal breathing and that 1 percent require aggressive resuscitation. Thus, using the national birth rate data, annually 400,000 newborns need some help during the perinatal period, 40,000 per year require expert assistance to reverse profound cardiorespiratory depression and 1200 per year develop severe HIE. You need only to relate these statistics to your own practice to appreciate the frequency with which you may encounter an infant in need of neonatal resuscitation and at risk for long-term neurodevelopmental sequelae.

This chapter is not meant to replace the information found in references such as the *Textbook of Neonatal Resuscitation*. Instead, the reader will be guided through an approach of creating an environment conducive to facilitating optimal neonatal emergency care. This will include a brief discussion of the pathophysiology of brain injury, a description of the organization of neonatal resuscitation teams and equipment, and a review of resuscitation guidelines. Readers interested in more detail will find additional resources in the selected list of suggested readings. All obstetrical clinicians will find completing Neonatal Resuscitation Program (NRP) certification useful and are encouraged to do so.

PATHOPHYSIOLOGY OF HYPOXIC ISCHEMIC ENCEPHALOPATHY

The onset of an aberration in fetal well being marked by concerning changes in vital signs, like fetal heart rate, is a common herald of a potentially deteriorating fetus. Clinicians respond to this with measures designed to improve oxygen and energy substrate (glucose) delivery to the fetus. Ominous changes in fetal heart rate and the clinician's response to it highlight, in great measure, one of the most concerning disturbances in homeostasis occurring to the unborn child—ischemia and hypoxemia. The result of worsening oxygen and energy delivery to the fetus is the onset of a series of changes in fetal status that must be reversed to avoid an untoward neurodevelopmental outcome. The scope of this chapter is not intended to cover prepartum management, but the same sequence of events can continue into the immediate postpartum period prompting the need for infant management. A brief review of the fetal response to hypoxia is useful (Fig. 24-1).

Studies in newly born animals describe the importance of both low oxygen states and decreased cerebral flow in the development of perinatal depression

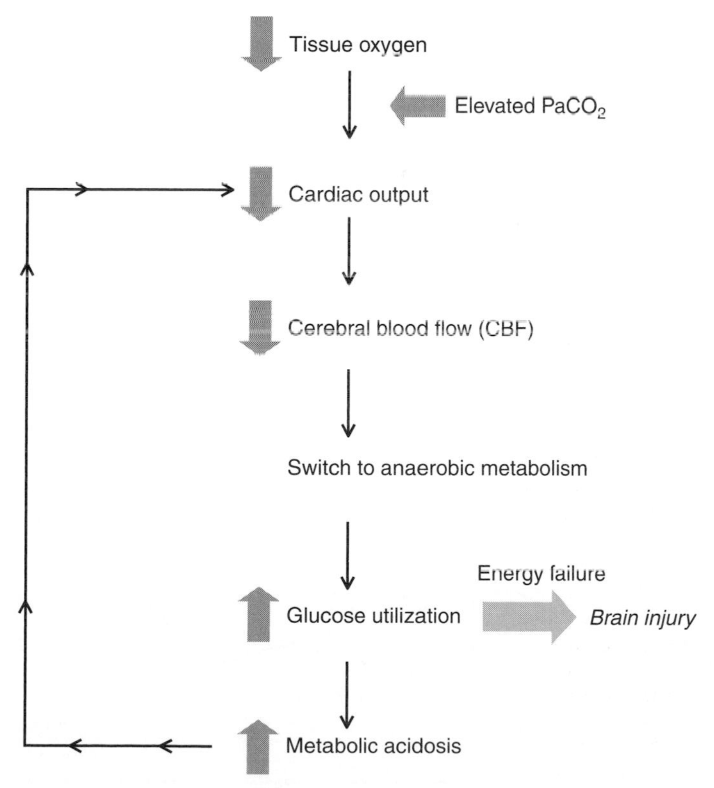

FIG. 24-1 Schematic, relative to time, of physiological events resulting in neonatal birth depression and leading to brain injury.

and, if uninhibited, HIE. The addition of absent breathing and resulting respiratory acidosis common to clinical events distinguishes the human experience from animal research. However, from limited studies in nonhuman primates, we know that complete asphyxia results in a series of fetal responses. Initially, there is an increase in muscular activity with tachypnea followed by a period of muscular quiet and apnea (primary apnea). The apnea lasts for about 1 minute, is followed by a few minutes of gasping respirations, and simple stimulation of the baby is usually adequate to restore normal breathing. During this time the fetal heart rate is below the allowed threshold, 100 beats per minute. After 4–5 minutes without resolution, secondary apnea with progressive fetal bradycardia occurs. This is unresponsive to simple stimulation. Fetal arterial blood pressure, and as a consequence, cardiac output and cerebral blood flow have also been decreasing coincident with the lowered heart rate (Fig. 24-1).

As tissues receive less and less oxygen from the combination of low fetal oxygen content and decreased cardiac output (low heart rate not compensated for by an increase in stroke volume), glycolytic pathways switch from aerobic to anaerobic. This results in increasing metabolic acidosis followed by primary energy failure from inefficient glucose utilization (recall that under aerobic conditions a unit of glucose produces 16 times more high-energy phosphate ATP than under anaerobic conditions). This further inhibits the effectiveness of myocardial contractility and a positive feedback back loop develops with disastrous consequences (Fig. 24-2). As this sequence of events

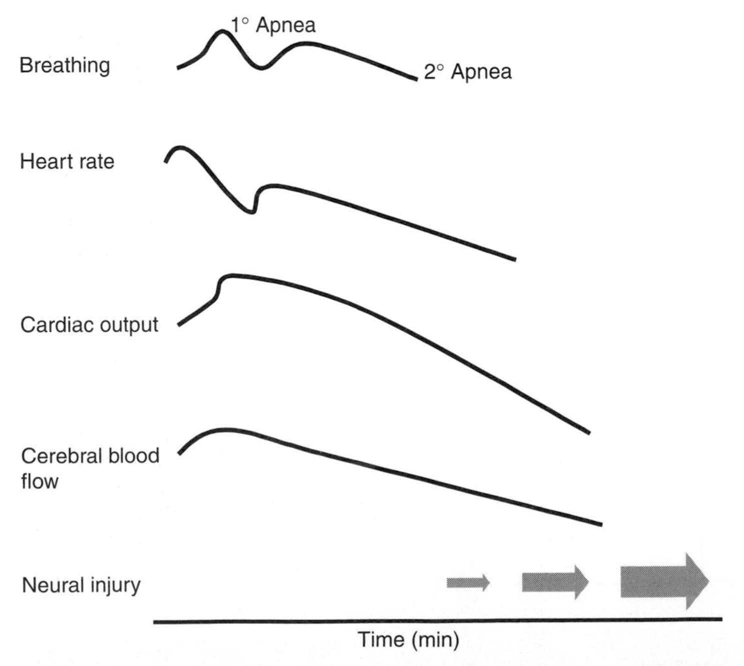

FIG. 24-2 Pathophysiological events leading to brain injury and positive feedback loop.

TABLE 24-1 Organization of Neonatal Resuscitation

Identification of peripartum risk factors for fetal/neonatal depression
• Antepartum
• Intrapartum
Personnel
• Team identification
• Team training
• Intra-team communication
Equipment
• Inventory
• Maintenance

continues, the fetus or newborn infant develops a deepening derangement in vital functions and the opportunities for recovery without sequelae rapidly diminish. The key ingredients to this are depression of fetal oxygenation, impaired cardiac output, altered central nervous system and myocardial energy stores, and neural cell death. Resuscitative efforts designed to mitigate this process as it develops are discussed below. The essentials needed to develop and implement the resource capabilities required to assure state-of-the-art neonatal resuscitation are shown in Table 24-1, and will form the blueprint for the remainder of this discussion.

ORGANIZATION

Identification of Peripartum Risk Factors

Anticipating the specific clinical circumstances leading to the need for neonatal resuscitation in the delivery room is very helpful. Not enough can be said for the value of time to prepare for a sick newborn. In addition, while the basics of resuscitation do not vary from one patient to the next, certain clinical situations will require the resuscitation team to be prepared to provide specific medical care beyond the usual. For example, the needs of an uncomplicated 28-week premature infant delivered for worsening maternal preeclampsia will be quite different from a term infant with particulate meconium stained amniotic fluid, or a 36-week-old child with nonimmune hydrops fetalis. Table 24-2 shows many of the more common ante- and intrapartum conditions likely to result in the initiation of neonatal resuscitation. Some of the additional requirements of children presenting under these circumstances are shown in Tables 24-3 and 24-4. An unusual example of this is the EXIT procedure (ex utero intrapartum treatment). This operating room procedure is used when a prenatal diagnosis is made of a fetus with airway anatomy likely to make endotracheal tube intubation difficult. The delivered infant's umbilical cord blood flow is not interrupted until airway access is secured. This allows the intubation to proceed without immediate concern for asphyxia. In addition, if a tracheotomy is anticipated, the provision of anesthetic to the maternal circulation can provide the fetus with pain relief adequate for the procedure to be performed. Thus, advance preparation will optimize even the most complex and dire delivery room events.

Team Identification

In order to function properly, each member of the resuscitation team (and back up members in the event of simultaneous resuscitations, e.g., multiple gestation) should be identified for each shift. All team members should

TABLE 24-2 Clinical Conditions Commonly Leading to Neonatal Resuscitation

Antepartum
Maternal conditions
Age <16 or >35 years
Substance abuse (recreational or prescribed)[a]
Chronic illness
Endocrine[a]
Cardiac
Autoimmune[a]
Pulmonary
Renal
Central nervous system
Oligohydramnios[a]
Polyhydramnios[a]
Premature rupture of membranes
Multiple gestation
Medications
Beta blockers[a]
Magnesium sulfate[a]
Anesthesia/analgesia[a]
Diabetes
No prenatal care[a]
Fetal conditions
Decreased fetal movement
Fetal malformation[a]
Anemia
Isoimmunization
Infection
Intrauterine growth retardation
Macrosomia
Intrapartum
Maternal conditions
Vaginal breech
Vacuum extraction
Forceps delivery
Prolonged rupture of membranes
Chorioamnionitis
Medications
Anesthesia/analgesia[a]
Placenta previa[a]
Abruptio placentae[a]
Vasa previa[a]
Umbilical cord prolapse
Meconium stained amniotic fluid[a]
Neonatal conditions
Preterm birth
Non-reassuring fetal heart rate pattern
Congenital diaphragmatic hernia[a]
Esophageal atresia[a]
Omphalocele/gastroschisis[a]
Congenital hydrops fetalis[a]
Suspected airway compromise[a]
Campomelic dysplasia
Severe micrognathia

[a]Conditions which usually require additional peripartum neonatal management measures (see Table 24-3).

TABLE 24-3 Maternal Conditions Requiring Additional Neonatal Resuscitative Measures

Maternal condition	Neonatal issues
Substance abuse	Avoid naloxone
Endocrine	
Grave's disease	Thyrotoxicosis–propranolol, PTU
Diabetes	Hypoglycemia–glucose, glucagon
Autoimmune (systemic lupus erythematosus)	Neonatal third-degree heart block—pace maker
Multiple gestation	More babies than resuscitators
Oligohydramnios	Airway obstruction—tracheal suction
Polyhydramnios	Presence of anomalies—anomaly specific
Medications	
Beta blockers	Hypoglycemia—glucose
Magnesium sulfate	Respiratory depression/hypotonia
Anesthesia/analgesia	Respiratory depression/drug specific
No prenatal care	Hepatitis B or C exposure, etc.
Placental abnormality (previa, abruption, vasa previa)	Hypovolemia—volume replacement
Meconium stained amniotic fluid	Meconium aspiration syndrome—selective tracheal suctioning, management of syndrome

respond to high-risk deliveries and to urgent calls from the delivery room. In addition, it is standard of care for the team to attend all cesarean deliveries. A recommended team composition and delineation of responsibilities are listed in Table 24-5. Note the considerable overlap of duties. The nature of a neonatal delivery room emergency requires that all team members are capable of performing multiple tasks, as the circumstance requires. Indeed, a child who needs a thoracentesis for a spontaneous pneumothorax or large pleural effusion will need the most skilled practitioner to perform this procedure. Usually, this clinician is the one managing the airway. He (she) will have to relinquish that responsibility to another to be free to emergently evacuate the chest of air or fluid. Team flexibility is a requirement rather than a luxury.

TABLE 24-4 Fetal Conditions Requiring Additional Neonatal Resuscitative Measures

Fetal condition	Neonatal management or problem
Congenital diaphragmatic hernia	Lung hypoplasia, bowel in thorax—orogastric tube placement
Esophageal atresia	Excessive oral secretions—secretion drainage
Omphalocele/gastroschisis	Heat/fluid loss—sterile moist inclusive cover, avoid vascular compromise to gut
Congenital hydrops fetalis	Large pleural, pericardial, peritoneal effusions—emergent fluid drainage
Suspected airway compromise	Difficult endotracheal intubation—EXIT procedure, ENT or pediatric surgery

TABLE 24-5 Resuscitation Team Composition and Duties (Suggested)

Team member	Responsibility
Neonatologist Pediatrician Neonatal nurse practitioner	• Obtain perinatal history • Lead resuscitation • Endotracheal intubation • Manage airway (bagging, suctioning, etc.) • Order/administer medications • Perform chest compressions • Obtain vascular access
Neonatal nurse Obstetrical nurse	• Evaluate neonatal heart rate—air entry • Documentation • Administer medications • Apply patient identification • Perform chest compressions • Obtain intravenous access • Apply monitoring equipment
Respiratory care practitioner Additional personnel	• Endotracheal intubation • Manage airway (bagging, suctioning, etc.) • Evaluate air entry—heart rate • Administer surfactant replacement • Perform chest compressions • Documentation • Apply patient identification • Apply monitoring equipment

Team Training

In addition to completing and maintaining NRP certification, each team member should be responsible for participating in periodic *mock codes*. These training exercises are extremely valuable for evaluating the team member knowledge of resuscitation procedures, adequacy of communication systems and response times, and for identifying general logistical problems unique to each institution (reliability of elevators, distance to operating rooms and delivery rooms, location of personnel and adequacy of equipment, etc.). After each mock and real code, a debriefing to evaluate team performance is strongly recommended. This activity creates the methodology to systematically identify and correct deficiencies noted during the code.

Communication

Critical to successfully completing a neonatal resuscitation is getting the resuscitation team to the delivery. This may seem a trite comment to make, and, therefore, one not worth making. However, once the delivering department of a hospital comes to rely upon a designated team of individuals to provide a service, no one else is likely to provide it. A simple and effective communication means becomes the backbone of the team's function, notifying members of the timing and location of the anticipated need. This is accomplished by facilities in many ways.

Some utilize broadcast paging. This method allows multiple so-called *Code Pagers* to be accessed with a single pager number entry. This minimizes the time required for contacting multiple parties but is vulnerable to pager battery life and black out areas. Others employ overhead paging that disturbs uninvolved patients and staff, is vulnerable to ambient noise interference and areas not served with speakers, and can be confusing. Many institutions use both of the above. Recent technological communication advances have increasingly permitted direct voice communication between staff members. This is accomplished both by localized FM transmitted telephone communications (zone phones), direct voice-to-voice technologies (modified walkie-talkies), or by digital cellular telephones with web-based direct connection to on-call clinicians. The latter permits user to call one telephone number and access the communication device of the clinician(s) on-call using a web-based system that also permits the entry of backup providers. While dependent upon battery life and signal adequacy, direct voice-to-voice communication allows clinicians to share critical case-specific information while simultaneously proceeding to the location required (i.e., time waiting for someone to return their page is mitigated).

Once alerted, the team should be familiarized with the details of the case to allow them to adequately prepare for any needs particular to each circumstance (Tables 24-3 and 24-4). Again, adequate preparation should not be undervalued.

EQUIPMENT

Inventory and Maintenance

A list of standard equipments needed for neonatal resuscitation is presented in Table 24-6. Medications for resuscitation, their doses and indications are listed in Table 24-7. These items should be placed in the same order and in

TABLE 24-6 Equipment and Supplies for Neonatal Resuscitation

Suction equipment
Bulb suction syringe
DeLee mucous trap with No. 10 French catheter
Wall or mechanical suction
Suction catheters, No. 5, 8, 10 French
Bag and mask ventilation equipment
Infant resuscitation bag with pressure gauge/release valve
Face masks, newborn and premature sizes (cushioned rim preferred)
Oral airways, newborn and premature sizes
Oxygen with flow meter and tubing
Intubation equipment
Laryngoscope and straight blades, No. 0 (premature) and No. 1 (term)
Extra light bulbs (unless fiberoptic) and batteries
Endotracheal tubes, sizes 2.5, 3.0, 3.5, 4.0 mm o.d.
Stylet (optional)
Scissors
Gloves
Vascular access equipment
Umbilical vessel catheters, 3.5 and 5.0 Fr.
Umbilical vessel catheterization kit
24 and 26 g peripheral intravenous catheters
Thoracentesis equipment
18 and 20 g intravenous catheters
20 and 30 mL syringes
Three-way stopcock

TABLE 24-7 Medications for Neonatal Resuscitation

Medication	How supplied	Dose and indication
Epinephrine	1:10,000; 3 or 10 mL ampules	0.1–0.3 mL/kg, IV or IT: bradycardia not responsive to stimulation or adequate ventilation
Normal saline Ringer's lactate	250 mL bag	10 mL/kg IV: push or over 10–30 min if hypovolemia suspected
Sodium bicarbonate	4.2% (0.5 mEq/mL); 10 mL ampule	1–3 mEq/kg: after adequate ventilation established, if persistently poor perfusion noted and hypovolemia not suspected
Dextrose	10% 250 mL bag	2 mL/kg: once resuscitation completed and poor perfusion persists (not responsive to other measures)
Naloxone HCl (neonatal Narcan)	0.02 mg/mL; 2 mL ampule	0.5 mL/kg: for respiratory depression with known recent maternal narcotic treatment[a]

[a]Do not use in newborns whose mother has known narcotic addiction.

the same place at all resuscitation stations. The identification of individuals responsible for ensuring that each equipment and medication store is adequately stocked is critical. Confirmation of adequate supplies should be accomplished in each shift and after each resuscitation. Documentation of this confirmation is strongly encouraged. Inadequate supplies noted during a resuscitation are inexcusable.

RESUSCITATION

Since the preparation has been accomplished and the clinician is now armed with a fundamental understanding of the pathophysiology of perinatal asphyxia and has advanced warning about the clinical scenario of each case, he (she) is prepared to provide emergency care to a recently delivered depressed newborn. Figure 24-3 depicts the general considerations of performing essential tasks. It is imperative not to underestimate the importance of a patent airway and adequate gas exchange. The overwhelming proportion of newborns requiring the institution of life-sustaining support in the delivery room will respond to proper oxygenation and ventilation alone. No amount of external cardiac compressions or intravenous/intratracheal epinephrine will adequately restore the heart rate and perfusion if appropriate gas exchange cannot be achieved. Medications for resuscitation, their doses and indications, are shown in Table 24-7. The interested reader is again encouraged to complete NRP certification.

SURVIVAL

Tables 24-8 and 24-9 show survival and outcome data for in excess of 11,000 infants born recently in the United States. The first of the two (Table 24-8)

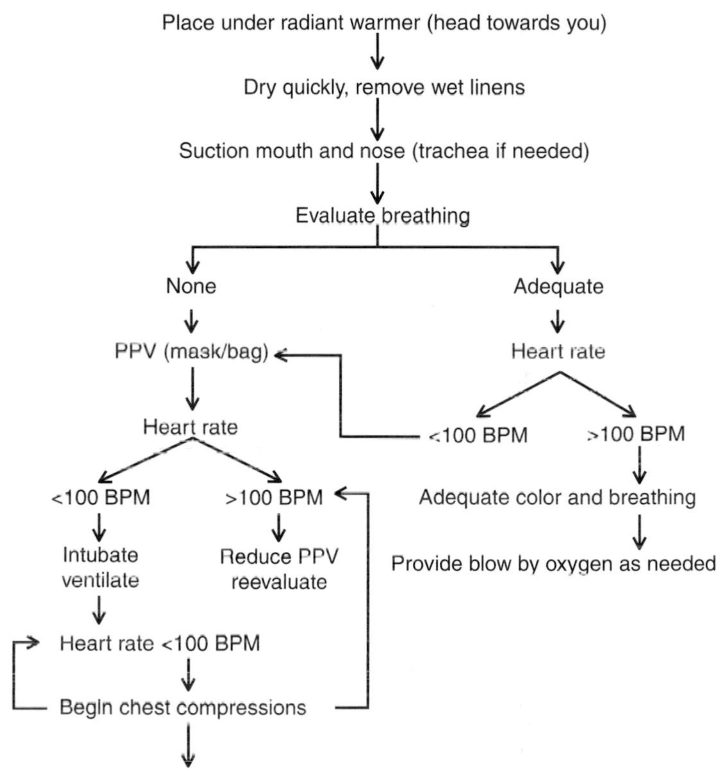

If after 30–60 s of chest compressions after adequate ventilation has been assured and heart rate remains <100 BPM, begin pharmacological management (see Table 24-7), and consider other pathophysiology (see Tables 24-3 and 24-4).

FIG. 24-3 Algorithm for neonatal resuscitation.

shows pure survival by both birth weight and estimated gestational age (EGA). The second (Table 24-9) demonstrates survival without two significant disorders that are predictive of impaired long-term neurological development (severe intraventricular hemorrhage and retinopathy of prematurity). This format is particularly useful to the obstetrical clinician since at the bedside, gestational age is more often used to discuss pregnancy status than is birth weight. If both birth weight and gestational age are known, then the tables are especially valuable. The obvious advantages of reaching birth weight over 1000 g and EGA at (or) above 29 weeks is evident. At these levels, good survival exceeds 90 percent. Intentional resuscitation of infants below 24 weeks gestation remains the subject of significant controversy. Families considering this option should be heavily counseled about the poor survival rates below 24 weeks and the poor long-term neurodevelopmental outcome of those that do survive.

TABLE 24-8 Percent Survival by Estimated Gestational Age (EGA) and Birth Weight[a]

	EGA (weeks)											
Birth weight (g)	23	24	25	26	27	28	29	30	31	32	33	Total
250–500	13	33	48	33								30
501–750	32	56	73	75	85	84						64
751–1000		69	74	88	89	91	95	99	93	100		87
1001–1250				87	93	99	97	99	96	99	100	96
1251–1500					91	95	97	99	99	100	99	98
1501–1750							98	98	99	99	99	99
1751–2000								97	100	99	99	99
2001–2250									97	99	100	99
2251–2500										100	99	99
>2500											99	99
Total	28	55	71	83	89	94	97	98	98	99	99	93

[a]The outcomes of 11,252 neonates born at, cared for, and discharged from 98 different hospitals in 26 different states from 1998 to 2000. These numbers are an estimate. The likelihood of a good outcome is influenced by many variables only two of which are estimated gestation age and birth weight.

Source: Pediatrix-Obstetrix Outcomes Data: Survival by estimated gestational age (EGA) and birth weight. NATAL U Clinical Research Center (http://www.natalu.com/clinical_research_center.asp?log=1) 2000, Pediatrix Medical Group, Inc. Used with permission.

TABLE 24-9 Percent Survival without Severe Intraventricular Hemorrhage or Retinopathy of the Premature by Estimated Gestational Age (EGA) and Birth Weight[a]

	EGA (weeks)											
Birth weight (g)	23	24	25	26	27	28	29	30	31	32	33	Total
250–500	5	20	30	20								18
501–750	17	34	51	63	78	65						46
751–1000		39	53	72	83	85	90	96	90			75
1001–1250				71	85	93	95	97	95	99	100	92
1251–1500					82	89	95	97	97	98	98	96
1501–1750							98	95	98	98	98	98
1751–2000								95	98	99	99	98
2001–2250									96	99	99	98
2251–2500										100	99	99
>2500											98	96
Total	14	33	50	68	82	88	94	96	97	99	99	89

[a]The outcomes of 11,252 neonates born at, cared for, and discharged from 98 different hospitals in 26 different states from 1998 to 2000. These numbers are an estimate. The likelihood of a good outcome is influenced by many variables only two of which are estimated gestation age and birth weight.

Source: Pediatrix-Obstetrix Outcomes Data: Survival without severe IVH or ROP by estimated gestational age (EGA) and birth weight. NATAL U Clinical Research Center (http://www.natalu.com/clinical_research_center.asp?log=1) 2000, Pediatrix Medical Group, Inc. Used with permission.

SUMMARY

The most important resuscitation elements are understanding the capabilities and limitations of the facility, followed by temperature support, the provision of adequate ventilation and oxygenation, and reestablishing cardiovascular stability. Once these important technical aspects of perinatal resuscitation are understood and the organization and management of obstetrical and pediatric emergency services are in place, what remains are the ethical and legal concerns regarding the provision of life-sustaining support. The obstetrical provider is encouraged to seek out additional information regarding national- and institution-specific survival and morbidity data and state-specific statutes that govern perinatal care.

SUGGESTED READING

American Heart Association/American Academy of Pediatrics. *Textbook of Neonatal Resuscitation*, 4th edn. Dallas: American Heart Association National Center, 2000.

MacDorman MF, et al.: Annual summary of vital statistics—2001. *Pediatrics* 2002;110:1037.

Mychaliska GB, et al.: Operating on placental support: the ex utero intrapartum treatment procedure. *J Pediatr Surg* 1997;32:227.

Thacker SB, Stroup DF, Peterson HB: Efficacy and safety of intrapartum electronic fetal monitoring: an update. *Obstet Gynecol* 1995;86:613.

World Health Report. Geneva, Switzerland: World Health Organization, 1995.

25 Fluid and Electrolyte Therapy in The Critically Ill Obstetric Patient

Cornelia Graves

INTRODUCTION

The ultimate goal of fluid and electrolyte therapy is to maintain a balance between the intracellular and extracellular compartments. This, easier said than done, means that fluid replacement and electrolyte balance become an afterthought of therapy instead of a goal. Many disease states in pregnancy can change the intracellular and extracellular compartments. Preeclampsia is a prime example of how changes in the dynamics of the intracellular and extracellular compartments can affect overall fluid physiology. Common therapies used during pregnancy such as terbutaline or magnesium can change electrolyte balance. The purpose of this chapter is to explain basic fluid and electrolyte balance and to provide guidelines for initiating the therapy.

Fluid Compartments

The human body is composed mostly of water. Approximately, 50 percent of total body weight in an average female is body water. [TBW (total body water) = 1/2 wt (kg)]. Given that, total blood volume increases by 50 percent during pregnancy with only 20 percent of that increase attributed to an increase in red cell mass, one can extrapolate that 60 to 65 percent of the total body weight in pregnancy can be attributed to TBW. The intracellular fluid compartment (ICF) contains 66 percent of TBW. The extracellular compartment is composed of 34 percent TBW. The extracellular fluid compartment (ECF) is composed of both intravascular and the interstitial components. Most of the extracellular fluid compartment is interstitial (26 percent), plasma composes 8 percent (Fig. 25-1). Other examples of ECF include cerebrospinal fluid, synovial fluid, and secretions from the gastrointestinal tract. The fluid compartments are separated by semi-permeable membranes. Water and smaller molecules may pass through the membranes; larger colloid substances and proteins are confined to the intravascular space. Hydrostatic pressure assists in maintaining an overall fluid balance as water moves by osmosis, from the area with the lowest concentration of plasma proteins (interstitial compartment) to the area with the highest concentration of plasma proteins (blood).

Osmotic Activity

Osmotic activity is the expression of the concentration of solute or the density of solute particles in a fluid. In the ECF, osmotic activity can be defined as the sum of the individual osmotic activities of each solute in the fluid. Plasma osmolality can be calculated using the following formula:

$$2 \times [\text{Na}] + \frac{\text{glucose}}{18} + \frac{\text{BUN}}{28}$$

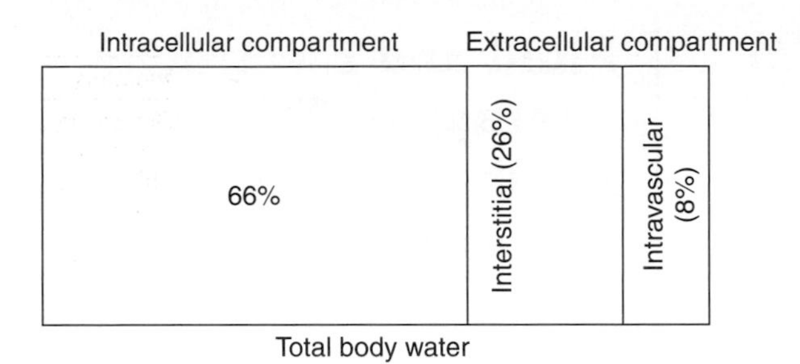

FIG. 25-1 A breakdown of the human body fluid compartments.

Colloid osmotic pressure (COP) is produced by serum albumin (60 to 80 percent) with fibrinogen and the globulins accounting for the remainder. Normal COP is decreased in pregnancy. While COP can be measured with electronic equipment, the equation in Table 25-1 below can estimate COP by using total protein (TP) in g/dL (Table 25-1).

Evaluation of Volume Status

In the obstetrical patient, depletion of intravascular volume can occur in two ways: overall fluid loss, e.g., vomiting, diarrhea, perspiration, or by shifting of the intravascular volume to the interstitial space. Overall fluid loss may be manifested by a clinical examination that reveals orthostasis, poor skin turgor, dry mucous membranes, and a thready pulse. These clinical findings respond to rehydration (Table 25-2).

Shifting of intravascular fluid occurs in disease states such as preeclampsia. Evaluation of volume status in this subset of patients may be much more difficult. In critically ill patients, the evaluation of volume status can be obtained by the judicious use of central pressure catheters (Table 25-3). The central venous pressure (CVP) may be used to evaluate long-term trends in fluid status; however, in patients with cardiac disease or preeclampsia, the CVP may not reflect left ventricular filling. For acute management of the disease states previously mentioned, a pulmonary artery catheter can be more useful in guiding therapy. The left ventricular end-diastolic pressure is best reflected by the pulmonary artery occlusion (wedge) pressure (PAOP). Numerous formulas have been used to evaluate the effect of volume replacement on ventricular filling pressures; we present the 7-3 rule as a handy guideline (Table 25-3).

TABLE 25-1 Colloid Osmotic Pressure[a]

	Normal pregnant (mmHg)	Preeclampsia (mmHg)
Antepartum COP	22	18
Postpartum COP	17	14

[a]Calculation of COP: COP = 2.1 (TP) + 0.16 (TP^2) + 0.009 (TP^3) mmHg.
Nonpregnant COP: 25–28 mmHg.

TABLE 25-2 Signs of Hypovolemia

Clinical	Laboratory
Pulse: Weak, thready, and >120 bpm	Urine specific gravity >1.025
Orthostatic vital signs	Hemoconcentration
Dry mucous membranes	Urine Na > 10 meq/L
Poor skin turgor	BUN/creatinine > 20
Prolonged capillary refill	

INTRAVENOUS FLUID THERAPY

The majority of intravenous fluid therapy is directed at expanding the plasma component of the ECF. Some of the most common questions asked are: which fluid should I use, how much should I use, and when should I use it? The goal of this section is to review the pharmacology of the available colloid and crystalloid therapies and discuss their pros and cons.

Crystalloids

As sodium is the major cation and determinant of osmotic pressure in the ECF, it is not surprising that most crystalloid preparations contain mixtures of sodium chloride and other physiologically active solutes. As crystalloid fluids are designed to expand the interstitial space, only about 20 percent remain in the vascular space. Indications for the use of crystalloid include extracellular losses, as in dehydration, acute hemorrhage, and acute volume replacement.

Normal saline, 0.9 percent, is isotonic to normal body fluid, and, therefore, does not alter osmotic movement of water across the cell membrane. It is the most common fluid used for acute volume expansion. There are variations of this fluid such as one-half normal saline, 0.45 percent; however, these hypotonic fluids have no place in acute volume expansion. Infusing normal saline may produce a hyperchloremic metabolic acidosis; however, this occurrence is rare.

Ringer's lactate is an isotonic fluid that may be used interchangeably with normal saline in the treatment of hypovolemia or shock. Ringer's lactate is a balanced electrolyte solution that substitutes potassium and calcium for some of the sodium. Lactate is added as a buffer. The concern that acidosis may be worsened by the installation of Ringer's lactate during shock is unfounded; however, it is recommended that extreme caution should be taken while using the fluid in patients with diabetes or renal failure.

Hypertonic sodium-containing solutions (600 to 2400 mOsm/L) may be used in patients in whom a large volume load is contraindicated. Some studies have noted that the infusion of a hypertonic solution may reduce interstitial

TABLE 25-3 The Effect of Volume Replacement on Ventricular Filling Pressures

Measure hemodynamic parameters
Fluid bolus of 200–500 mL of isotonic fluid
Measure PAOP 30 min after fluid challenge
PAOP increase > 7 mmHg → no more fluid
PAOP increase 2–7 mmHg (over baseline) → wait 10 min
If PAOP still > 3 mmHg → stop
If PAOP ≤ 3 mmHg → continue fluid administration

edema as well as create a positive inotropic effect. Care should be taken to use a slow infusion rate and to monitor sodium regularly to avoid hypernatremia.

Plasmalyte is a highly buffered fluid that has a pH equivalent to plasma. Although theoretically its adjusted pH may be preferential to saline or Ringer's lactate, there are no definitive studies that show a great difference in its effects on vascular volume.

Dextrose-containing Solutions

Dextrose, 5 percent in water, is isotonic; but unlike normal saline, it penetrates the cell leaving behind the infused water. It provides a carbohydrate source during brief periods of fasting. One liter of a 5 percent solution contains approximately 170 kcal and a 10 percent solution contains 340 kcal. When dextrose is added to normal saline or to Ringer's lactate, it raises the osmolality of the fluid to roughly twice that of plasma. This can promote significant changes in serum osmolality when large volumes of fluid are infused.

Colloid

Colloids are large molecular weight substances that do not pass readily across capillary walls. The rationale for the use of colloids is to expand the vascular volume and to decrease the amount of fluid that leaves the intravascular space (see Chap. 2).

Human Serum Albumin

Albumin, which is synthesized in the liver, is the major oncotic protein of plasma. Responsible for about 80 percent of the colloid osmotic pressure of plasma, it also serves as the major transport protein for drugs and ions. The preparation is available as 5% (50 g/L) and 25 percent solution (250 g/L) in isotonic saline. The 5 percent solution has a colloid osmotic pressure (COP) of 20 mmHg which is equivalent to plasma (COP); the 25 percent solution has a COP of 70 mmHg. An infusion of 100 mL of 25 percent albumin will expand the plasma volume to about 500 mL. The effect of the albumin infusion persists for 24 to 36 hours. Contrary to popular belief, albumin will eventually pass into the interstitial space. This may produce delayed pulmonary edema in patients at risk. Caution should also be exercised when using large volumes since dilutional coagulopathy can occur.

Hydroxyethyl Starch (Hespan)

Hetastarch is a synthetic colloid that closely resembles glycogen. It was introduced as a less expensive alternative to albumin. A 6 percent solution has a COP of 30 mmHg, and the acute volume expansion is equivalent to that of albumin. Hetastarch has a longer half-life than albumin with 50 percent of the osmotic effect persisting for 24 hours. Coagulopathies are less common than with albumin. The clinician should be aware that serum amylase may be elevated in patients receiving hetastarch as amylase is used to cleave polymers in order to facilitate renal excretion. This elevation usually persists three to five days after use.

Dextran

The dextrans are another group of synthetic colloids that are polysaccharides derived from the juice of sugar beets. The available preparations are dextran-40 (mean molecular weight—40,000) and dextran-70 (mean molecular weight—70,000). Dextran-40 is available as a 10 percent solution with a COP of 40 mmHg. The acute volume expansion from dextran-40 is about twice the infused volume. However, more than 50 percent is cleared after six hours. While an effective artificial colloid, significant side effects limit its use. Dextrans may inhibit platelet aggregation, decrease platelet factor 3, and produce an anticoagulation effect. Anaphylactic reactions can occur in up to 1 percent of patients. Dextrans coat the surface of red blood cells and interfere with the ability to cross match blood. Dextran-induced renal failure or an osmotic diuresis may interfere with the overall fluid status (Tables 25-4 and 25-5).

Crystalloid or Colloid

Much debate has raged over the use of cystalloid versus colloid solution. Colloids are much more expensive and associated with an increased risk of side effects. Champions of colloid use maintain that the cost and the side effects are outweighed by the benefit of colloid use. Proponents of crystalloid use point out that the infusion of crystalloid increases intravascular volume and that the shift in interstitial fluid is a result of the underlying pathological process. Pulmonary edema may occur with both types of fluid, although the edema associated with colloid use may be delayed. While judicious use of colloid may be useful in some clinical situations, it is the opinion of the author that crystalloid resuscitation is preferred in the obstetrical population.

ELECTROLYTE BALANCE AND ABNORMALITIES

As the major cation of the ECF and the major determinant of osmolality, sodium maintains the concentration and volume of the ECF. Normal sodium ranges from 135 to 145 mg/dL in most labs. Sodium maintains irritability and conduction in nerve and muscle tissue and assists in the regulation of acid-base balance. Since most diets have an excess of sodium, the kidney maintains normal levels through excretion of sodium and retention of free water.

Hypernatremia

Hypernatremia is defined as a sodium level greater than 145 mEq/L. It is a relative state of free water deficit and an increase in the solute concentration in all body fluids. The three major hypernatremic states result from loss of water, hypotonic fluid loss, and sodium retention.

Water Loss

Pure water loss usually occurs with increased insensible loss through the skin. Thermal burn injury is associated with the greatest risk of insensible water loss. Diabetes insipidus, which results in massive amounts of dilute urine output, can be seen in patients with severe preeclampsia. Figure 25-2 offers a simple algorithm for the treatment of hypernatremia due to this cause.

Hypotonic Fluid Loss

Hypotonic fluid loss is the most common cause of hypernatremia. It is usually caused by dehydration due to gastroenteritis or an osmotic diuresis. Signs of ECF depletion may be present. Oliguria will be present unless the osmotic diuresis has been induced. Treatment is outlined in Fig. 25-3.

TABLE 25-4 Common Intravenous Fluids

Solution	Na^+ (mEq/L)	K^+ (mEq/L)	Cl^- (mEq/L)	Mg^{2+} (mEq/L)	Ca^{2+} (mEq/L)	Lactate (mEq/L)	Other	Approx pH	Osmolality (mOsm/kg)
0.9 NaCl	154		154					4.2	308
Lactated Ringer's	130	4.0	109		3.0	28		6.5	273
Hypertonic saline									
3%	513		513					5.0	
5%	855		855					5.6	
Plasmalyte	140	5.0	98	3.0			Acetate (27 mEq/L) Gluconate (23 mEq/L)	7.4	295
D_5W							Dextrose (5 g/dL)	5.0	278
Albumin 5%	145		145						
Hespan	154		154				Hetastarch (6 g/L)	5.5	
Dextran-70	154		154						

TABLE 25-5 Intravenous Fluids: A Comparison

Solution	Pros	Cons
Isotonic saline	Slightly hypertonic to . plasma. Minimizes fluid shifts	May produce hyperchloremic metabolic acidosis
Lactate Ringer's	Relatively isotonic to plasma	Use with caution in patients with renal or adrenal disease. May interact with drugs due to calcium binding
Hypertonic saline	Less volume required. May reduce the interstitial edema	May cause hypernatremia. Rapid correction of sodium may increase risks of cerebral edema
Plasmalyte	Isotonic to plasma	Theorectically, magnesium may interfere with compensatory vasoconstriction
Dextrose	Provides substrate and caloric intake	Osmotic load. Can fuel production of lactic acid especially in the CNS
Albumin	May help maintain colloid osmotic pressure and decrease interstitial edema	Coagulopathy. Allergic reactions
Hespan	Equivalent to 5% albumin	Cleared entirely by the kidneys. May increase serum amylase
Dextran	Volume expansion with small amounts	Reduction of Factor VIII, promotes fibrinolysis, anaphylactic reactions in 1% of pts. May interfere with the ability to cross match blood. Can cause acute renal failure

Sodium Retention

Sodium retention is an uncommon phenomenon. It is usually seen only when hypertonic saline- or bicarbonate-containing solutions are being infused.

Hyponatremia

Hyponatremia is defined as a serum sodium level of 135 mEq/L or less. Three major categories of hyponatremia exist: isotonic (pseudohyponatremia), hypertonic, and hypotonic. Severe hyponatremia (less than 120 mEq/L) is a serious life-threatening condition. Mortality rate may exceed 50 percent; however, rapid correction of sodium may produce central pontine myelinolysis and cerebral edema which can be fatal.

Isotonic

Isotonic hyponatremia is characterized by a low serum sodium level but a normal plasma osmolality. Common causes include hyperproteinemic states and hyperlipidemic states. The management requires evaluation and

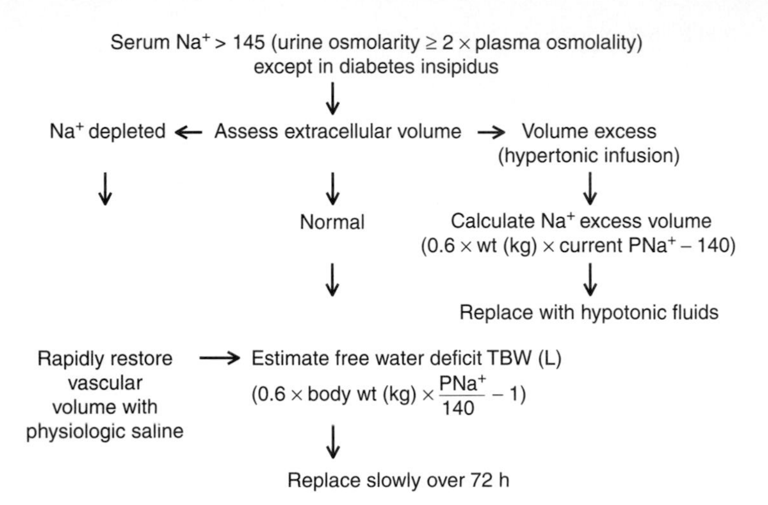

*Management of diabetes insipidus, vasopressin may be necessary 5–10 units aqueous dDAVP, sub q every 4–6°

FIG. 25-2 Hypernatremia.

correction of the underlying cause. The following correction factors may be used to assist in correcting the sodium concentration:

$$\text{Plasma triglycerides (g/L)} \times 0.002 = \text{mEq/L decrease in plasma Na}^+$$

$$\text{Plasma [protein] greater than 8 g/dL} \times 0.025 = \text{mEq/L decrease in plasma Na}^+$$

Hypertonic

Hypertonic hyponatremia is diagnosed by a low serum sodium and a plasma osmolality of greater than 290 mOsm/kg H_2O. The most common cause of this disorder is hyperglycemia seen in association with diabetic ketoacidosis (see Chap. 11). Correction of hyponatremia requires addressing the underlying disorder and replacing the free water deficit (Fig. 25-3).

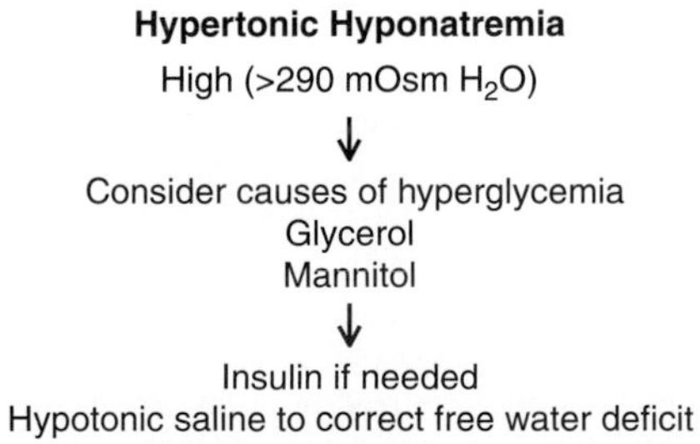

Hypertonic Hyponatremia

High (>290 mOsm H_2O)

↓

Consider causes of hyperglycemia
Glycerol
Mannitol

↓

Insulin if needed
Hypotonic saline to correct free water deficit

FIG. 25-3 Hypertonic hyponatremia.

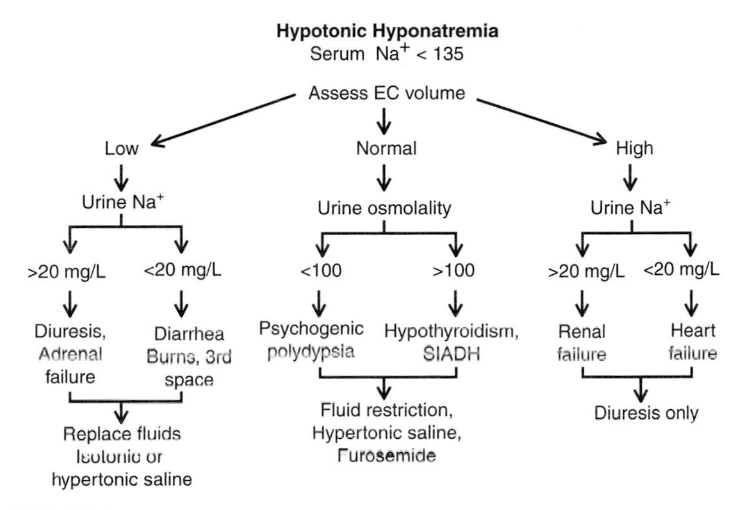

FIG. 25-4 Hypotonic hyponatremia.

Hypotonic

Hypotonic hyponatremia is characterized by a low serum sodium and plasma osmolality. It can be divided into three subtypes: isovolemic, hypervolemic, and hypovolemic. The clinician should address three major concerns. The patient's neurological status, volume status, and adrenal function.

Isovolemic hyponatremia is characterized by a small gain in free water. This may be related to inappropriate secretion of antidiuretic hormone or in rare instances psychogenic polydipsia. Numerous drugs, including oxytocin, have been implicated in this disorder and they are listed as follows:

- Morphine
- Nonsteroidal anti-inflammatory drugs
- Carbamazepine
- Oxytocin

Hypovolemic hyponatremia is characterized by the loss of fluid that is isotonic to plasma combined with volume replacement using a hypotonic fluid. This results in a net sodium loss. The most common causes of this disorder are diuretics, adrenal insufficiency, or diarrhea. A urine sodium can help to identify the etiology (i.e., renal or extrarenal) of the hyponatremia.

Hypervolemic hyponatremia occurs in patients in which there is excess water and sodium gain. Edema is common in this population. Causes include heart, renal, and liver failure. The evaluation and management of hypotonic hyponatremia is presented in Fig. 25-4.

Potassium

Potassium is the major intracellular cation. The normal plasma potassium concentration is 3.5 to 5.0 mmol/L. Renal excretion is the major route of elimination of dietary or other sources of excess potassium. The clinician should keep in mind that serum potassium may be falsely elevated in the

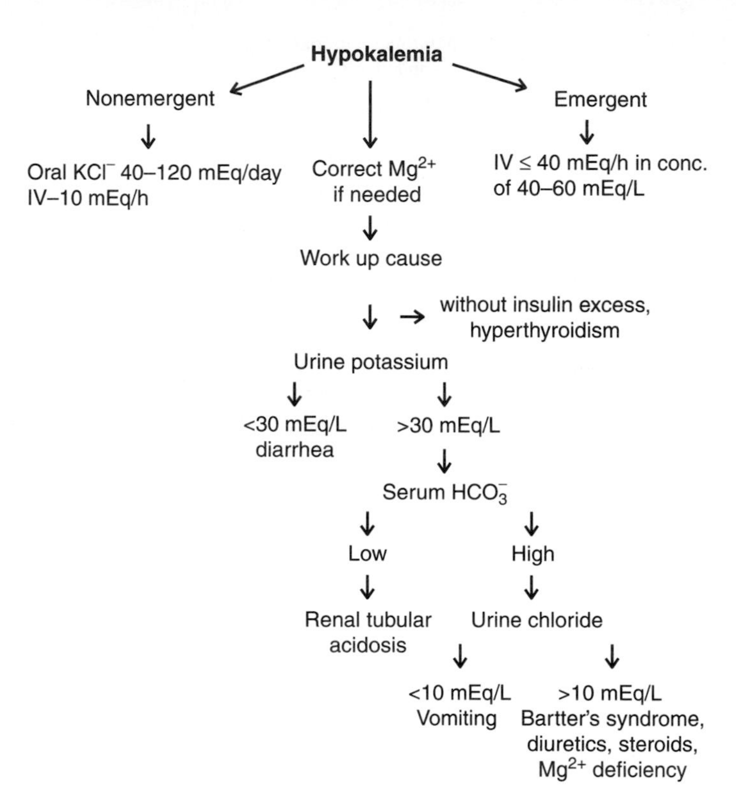

FIG. 25-5 Hypokalemia.

presence of hemolysis or factitiously decreased when processing of a lab sample is delayed.

Hypokalemia

Hypokalemia is defined as a serum potassium concentration below 3.5 mEq/L. The causes of hypokalemia may be classified as transcellular shift, as in the use of beta agonist (i.e., terbutaline), or from depletion. The major causes of the latter are renal loss, most commonly caused by diuretic therapy, or extrarenal, usually seen with excessive diarrhea. A number of drugs listed below are also associated with hypokalemia. Treatment is outlined in Fig. 25-5.

- Laxatives
- Gentamycin-cephalexin combo
- Prostaglandin F2 alpha
- Steroids
- Furosemide

- Penicillins
- Lithium
- Beta agonists

Hyperkalemia

Hyperkalemia is defined as a serum potassium above 5.5 mEq/L. It is caused by the release of potassium into the extracelluar fluid such as in myonecrosis, or by reduced renal excretion.

Hyperkalemia can be associated with fatal cardiac arrythmias; therefore, it should be treated much more aggressively than hypokalemia (Fig. 25-6).

Magnesium

Magnesium is not uniformly distributed in the body fluid compartments. Over half of the total body stores are located in the bone and less than 1 percent are distributed in plasma. This distribution creates a problem in diagnosing disturbances in magnesium balance. Magnesium levels are frequently overlooked in the critically ill patient and are not often replaced. For these reasons, magnesium may be the most common electrolyte

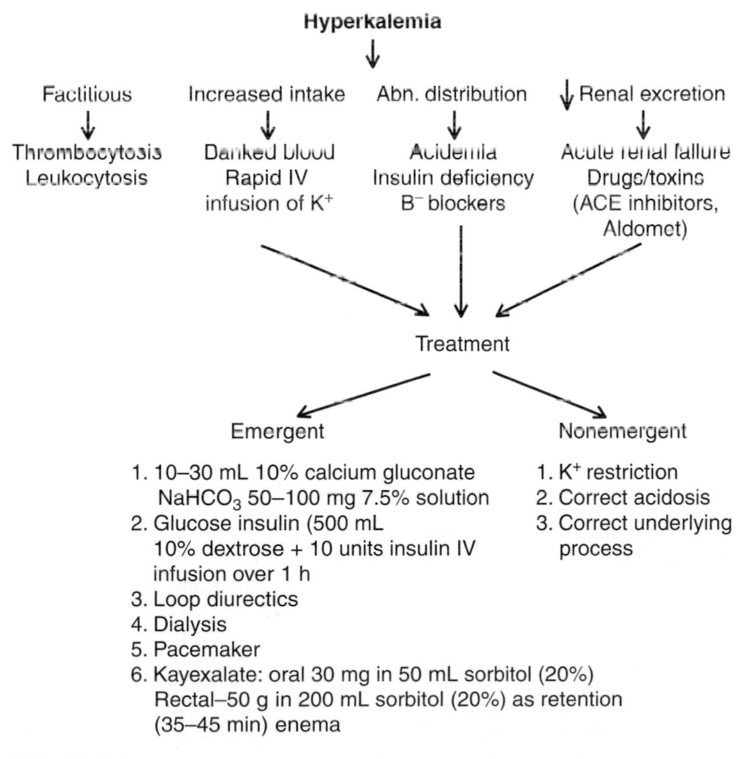

FIG. 25-6 Hyperkalemia.

TABLE 25-6 Magnesium Disorders

Hypomagnesemia
Oral magnesium oxide 500–2000 mg/day
$MgSO_4$ 1 mEq/kg for first 24 h; and 0.5 mEq/kg/c over 3 days
Severe, symptomatic[a]
2 g $MgSO_4$ over 1–2 min, follow with 5 g $MgSO_4$ over next 6 h
Continue 5 g $MgSO_4$ every 12 h (continuous infusion) for next 5 days
Hypermagnesemia
Discontinue magnesium infusion
20 mg 10% calcium gluconate over 5–10 min (if symptomatic)[b]
Infusion of D5.45NS with IV furosemide (40–80 mg IV every 1–2 h to enhance excretion)
Consider dialysis

[a]Care should be taken in patients with renal disease.
[b]May substitute calcium chloride.

abnormality in critically ill patients. In obstetrics, the use of magnesium for tocolysis and for neuroprophylaxis can further complicate the picture. The most common cause of magnesium depletion in our population is the use of diuretics.

The use of amnioglycosides can also lower magnesium levels. Alcoholism is a rare cause of magnesium depletion in obstetrical patients. Low levels of magnesium may potentiate cardiac arrythmias.

Hypermagnesamia is almost always associated with renal insufficiency, with excess magnesium intake, or in cases of diabetic ketoacidosis. Infusion of magnesium in patients with preeclampsia or other diseases that may be associated with renal insufficiency should be done with care. Hypotension can be seen with magnesium levels of 3.0 to 5.0 mEq/L. A level greater than 12 mEq/L can be associated with respiratory depression. Levels greater than 14 mEq/L can be associated with cardiac arrest. Treatment protocols are outlined in Table 25-6.

Calcium and Phosphorus Balance

There are three fractions of calcium in the blood. About 50 percent of calcium is bound to serum proteins—with albumin accounting for 80 percent of protein binding. Five to ten percent of calcium is bound to anions like bicarbonate. The remainder of calcium is present as the free or "ionized" form of calcium. The interpretation of calcium levels must be adjusted for change in serum albumin. A correction factor, that increases the total calcium by 0.8 mg/dL for each 1 mg/dL decrease in albumin, should be used. Obtaining an ionized calcium may avoid using the above correction factor; however, changes in pH or other factors may also alter calcium levels.

Hypocalcemia

The most common cause in an acute care setting is magnesium depletion. Other causes such as hypoparathyroidism are usually not a concern in an acute setting. Massive transfusion, panacreatitis, and burns are other causes of decreased calcium level in this patient population.

TABLE 25-7 Treatment of Calcium Disorders

Hypercalcemia	Saline + forced diuresis (furosemide, 40–80 mg IV every 2 h) Calcitonin 4 u/kg IM or subq every 12 h Mithracin 25 mcg/kg IV every 2–3 days* Dialysis
Hypocalemia	
Severe	Calcium gluconate 10 mL of 10% solution over 10 min
Symptomatic	Calcium chloride 10 mL of 10% solution in 50 mL D_5W over 30 min Correct Mg^{2+} and K^+ deficits Treat hyperphospatemia if needed
Nonemergent asymptomatic	Calcium gluconate or calcium lactate 2–4 g/day in divided doses every 6 h Supplemental vitamin D

*Pregnancy category X.

The clinical manifestations include neuromuscular excitability, which may vary, cardiovascular excitability including decreased myocardial contractility, and a prolonged QT interval. Treatment includes the infusion of calcium chloride or gluconate.

Hypercalcemia

Hypercalcemia should be treated when the serum calcium level approaches 13 mg/dL or higher. Causes of hypercalcemia include malignancy and hyperparathryoidism. Mental status changes are the most common clinical symptoms and warrant immediate therapy. The aim of the therapy is to facilitate the excretion of calcium in the urine (Table 25-7).

Phosphorous

Like magnesium and potassium, phosphorous is predominately an intracellular ion. While phosphorous levels may show diurnal variation, severe hypophosphotemia (serum level below 0.5 mg/dL) is uncommon. The most common causes of hypophosphotemia in the obstetrical population are recovery from diabetic ketoacidosis, aluminum antacid use, or respiratory alkalosis. Phosphate deficiency reduces cardiac contractility, shifts the oxygen dissociation to the left, and may contribute to skeletal muscle weakness. Intravenous replacement is recommended (Table 25-8).

Hyperphosphatemia is seen in the face of renal failure or tissue destruction, such as rhabdomyolysis. Management is directed at correcting the underlying problem. Aluminum-containing antacids may also be administered (Table 25-8).

SUMMARY

Caring for the critically ill obstetrical patient requires a coordinated effort involving the maternal-fetal medicine specialist, internist, neonatologist, and other members of the critical care team. Meticulous attention to fluid and electrolyte balance will enable the clinician to restore the altered physiology that results from the underlying pathological process.

TABLE 25-8 Treatment of Phosphate Disorders

Hyperphosphatemia
Restrict PO_4 intake <200 mg/day
Saline infusion
Oral phosphate binders (aluminum hydroxide antacids)
Correct hypocalcemia
Dialysis
Hypophosphatemia
Profound depletion <1 mg/dL
Potassium or sodium phosphate (2.4–5.0 mg/kg/6 h)
Follow serum PO_4^-, Ca^{2+}, Mg^{2+}, K^+ every 12 h
Depletion
Neutra-phos (250 mg/tablet); 2 tabs every 8–12 h
Phospho-soda (129 mg/mL); give 5 mL every 8–12 h

SUGGESTED READING

Berl T, Robertson GL: Pathophysiology of water metabolism. In: Brenner BM (ed), *Brenners and Rectors, The Kidney,* 6th edn. Philadelphia: W.B. Saunders, 2000; p. 866–924.

Halperin ML, Kamel KS: Potassium. *Lancet* 1998;352:135.

Hand H: The use of intravenous therapy. *Nursing Standard* 2001;15:47–55.

Layen JA, Kerby PR: Fluids and electrolytes in the critically ill. In: Civetta JM, Taylor RW, Kirby RR (eds), *Critical Care*. Philadelphia: JB Lippincott, 1996.

Marino PL: *The ICU Book,* 2nd edn. Malvern: Lee & Febiger, 1994.

Miller RD: *Anesthesia,* 5th edn. Churchill Livingston, New York, 2000.

Verbalis JG: Adaptation to acute and chronic hyponatremia: Implications for symptomatology, diagnosis and therapy. *Semin Nephrol*, 1998;18:3.

26 Human Immunodeficiency Virus in Pregnancy

Linda R. Chambliss Robert Myers

INTRODUCTION

Despite all we have learned about the HIV virus, HIV infection continues to ravage the world, particularly in underdeveloped nations. The United Nations estimates that over 35 million people are infected with the HIV infection and 16,000 new infections occur each day. The care of HIV-infected pregnant women is more complex today than ever. Pregnant women who are infected with the HIV virus present a challenge to even the most experienced clinician. Drug therapies have increased exponentially since the epidemic was first recognized. Obstetricians caring for HIV-infected women should only manage them in concert with clinicians who are fluent with the most current recommendation regarding drug therapies. HIV-infected patients should be managed by a team experienced in the medical, obstetrical, and psychosocial needs of these women.

It is important to remember that HIV seropositivity is not synonymous with AIDS. This is especially true today, as current HIV drug regimens have allowed many HIV seropositive patients to survive free from an AIDS defining condition for years.

The HIV epidemic is increasingly affecting women, especially women from minority groups. The vast majority of these women are of reproductive age. During the initial period of the epidemic, most obstetricians had no experience treating an HIV positive pregnant woman but with the dramatic increase in HIV infections in women, more and more obstetricians can expect to have an HIV positive pregnant woman among their patients. Women account for almost a third of the cases of AIDS reported in the United States.

However, the good news is that the majority of HIV positive patients who receive appropriate antiretroviral therapy can expect a much longer survival than those infected early in the epidemic. Likewise, the use of antiretroviral drugs during pregnancy has drastically reduced the risk of perinatal transmission of HIV.

PATHOGENESIS

HIV is an RNA retrovirus. There are two types of HIV virus, HIV-1 and HIV-2. In the United States, HIV-1 causes the vast majority of infections. The virus is composed of viral particles surrounded by a lipid membrane. The RNA retrovirus recognizes certain cell receptors and adheres to the cell wall. After adhering, the viral particles enter the host cell's cytoplasm. Once inside, the RNA virus is capable of using an enzyme called reverse transcriptase to make DNA using the viral RNA. The viral DNA enters the cell's nucleus where it can begin to direct cell function. The viral DNA uses the host cell to make viral products including more viral RNA. Billions of new virions are made each day. When CD4 lymphocytes are infected, the consequence is impaired function and a shortened half-life. As the number of CD4 lymphocytes falls over time, the patient becomes increasingly susceptible to HIV-related opportunistic complications. Viral production lasts for the life of the cell. New RNA viruses can be shed into the body continuing the cycle in other target cells. Many different types of cells and tissues are susceptible to HIV infection. These include B-lymphocytes, macrophages, the cervix, brain, myocardium, kidney, retina, colon, and liver among others. Since both T and B cells are affected, the HIV infection impacts both humoral and cellular immunity.

PRIMARY HIV INFECTION

Primary HIV infection can be asymptomatic, mildly symptomatic with a flu-like presentation, or severely symptomatic. Symptomatic primary HIV infection is called the acute retroviral syndrome. Antibody to HIV may not be present at the time of the acute retroviral syndrome, but HIV RNA (viral load) will be high. Symptoms usually occur from within 5 to 30 days after the infection. The two most common symptoms are fatigue and fever. Other common symptoms include rash, headache, pharyngitis, weight loss, lymphadenopathy, night sweats, and diarrhea. The patient may have neutropenia, thrombocytopenia, anemia, or lymphopenia. The syndrome resembles mononucleosis. The diagnosis is often not considered. Patients recover and become asymptomatic but will develop AIDS within 10 to 12 years if HIV is not diagnosed and treated. However, the course of HIV infection can vary depending upon the host's immune system, comorbid conditions, and the virulence of the virus. Some patients will show evidence of advanced immune deficiency much earlier and on rare occasions a patient may have a fulminant course, rapidly progressing to AIDS. The list of signs and symptoms predictive of progression to AIDS are as follows:

- Oral candidiasis
- Constitutional symptoms (weight loss, diarrhea, fever, sweats)
- CD4 lymphocyte count <200/mL^3
- CD4 lymphocytes <25% of total lymphocytes
- Anemia (nonpregnant)
- Thrombocytopenia

A very small percentage (<5 percent) of patients who become infected never develop an AIDS-defining condition.

TESTING FOR HIV INFECTION

It is wise to have a liberal policy with regard to offering any patient HIV testing and to offer HIV testing to *all* pregnant women. The list of patients who should be offered testing are as follows:

- Patients who are pregnant
- Patients who request HIV testing
- Patients with a sexually transmitted disease
- Patients with clinical/laboratory findings suggestive of HIV infection
- Patients with cervical dysplasia or evidence of human papillomavirus
- Patients age 15–44 years admitted to hospitals with HIV seropositive rates >1% or where AIDS patients account for >1/1000 discharges
- Patients who engage in intravenous drug use or who have partners that do
- Patients who have sex with men who have sex with other men
- Patients with active tuberculosis
- Patients from "endemic areas"
- Patients with an occupational exposure to blood or body fluids

- Donors of semen, blood, or other organs
- Those transfused between 1978 and 1985

Patients may not admit to risk behaviors or may be unaware of their partners' risk behaviors. A patient may have seroconverted since a previously negative test. Testing pregnant patients becomes imperative since perinatal transmission rates drop from approximately 25 percent in the untreated HIV positive mother to less than 1 percent in a mother effectively treated with antiretroviral drugs.

HIV testing consists of both a screening HIV test (ELISA) and a confirmatory test (Western blot) if the ELISA is reactive. Both tests detect antibodies to HIV-1 proteins. As with all testing, both false positive and false negative results occur. The incidence of these is related to the prevalence of the disease in the population. An ELISA is reported as either nonreactive or reactive. A nonreactive test does not require additional testing unless a patient continues to have risk behaviors, in which case testing should be reconsidered in 6 to 12 months. However, there are several conditions that can result in a false positive ELISA. The list of conditions that may cause a false positive ELISA are as follows:

- Autoimmune disease
- Antibodies against class II HLA antigens
- Positive rapid plasma reagin (RPR)
- Recent vaccination, especially influenza
- Recent viral infections
- Liver disease including alcoholic or primary biliary cirrhosis
- Sclerosing cholangitis
- Chronic renal failure
- Lymphoma or hematological malignancies

There are also conditions that can result in a false negative ELISA. The list of conditions that may cause a false negative ELISA are as follows:

- Seroconversion (patient has not yet made antibodies)
- Seroreversion (occurs in end stage disease)
- An atypical host response
- Agammaglobulinemia
- Infection with certain strains of HIV-2 virus
- Lab or clerical error

A positive ELISA makes it necessary to perform a confirmatory Western blot. A Western blot can be reported as negative, indeterminate, or positive. A reactive ELISA and a negative Western blot suggests a false positive ELISA. The patient is considered *not infected* and no further testing is required. An indeterminate Western blot means that the patient has antibodies to one or two bands on the Western blot. It may be the result of recent infection and therefore, on-going seroconversion, or may be a false positive. Approximately, 4 to 20 percent of Western blots are reported as indeterminate. Indeterminate Western blots appear to be more common during pregnancy. On the Western blot, anti-gp 160/120 antibodies appear first followed by anti-p24 antibody and anti-gp41 soon after. If the Western blot is indeterminate, measurement of HIV RNA viral load may help determine if the patient is HIV infected or not. The HIV RNA is not a diagnostic test, but may be helpful to determine if a Western blot is indicative of seroconversion. Alternatively, another option

TABLE 26-1 Interpretation of HIV Serological Testing

Test	Result	Interpretation	Further testing
ELISA	Nonreactive	Not HIV infected	Not necessary Retest 6–12 months if same risk factors
ELISA	Reactive	Possible HIV infection	Western blot
Western blot	Negative	Not HIV infected	Not necessary Retest 6–12 months if same risk factors
Western blot	Indeterminate Reacts to bands gp41 + gp 120/160 or p24 + gp160	Seroconversion or false positive	RNA viral load or IFA or Repeat Western blot in 1 month
Western blot	Positive	HIV infection	See Table 26-3

is the use of an immunoflourescent assay (IFA), as a confirmatory test. If that is negative, the patient should be considered negative. A patient is considered HIV infected if both the ELISA and the Western blot are positive. The Western blot has a 2 percent rate of false positives. Most patients will have positive HIV antibody test within three months of infection. A minority may not seroconvert until six months or later after the infection.

Other methods of testing are available but rarely used. In addition to blood, HIV tests can be performed on saliva, vaginal secretions, and urine. HIV testing of vaginal secretions can be helpful in cases of sexual assault. These tests are either serological or culture. These tests are not better than standard screening but may be helpful in difficult cases. Table 26-1 summarizes how to interpret serological testing.

INTERPRETING VIRAL LOADS AND CD4 COUNTS

The single best indicator of disease activity is the *quantitative* viral load. The viral load can be measured by one of two ways, the b-deoxyribonucleic acid assay (bDNA) or the reverse transcription polymerase chain reaction assay (PCR). A viral load is considered to be undetectable at 50 copies/mL or less. Viral loads can be artifactually increased after viral infections or vaccinations. Therefore, a viral load should not be drawn until at least four and preferably six weeks after an infection or a vaccination to avoid misinterpreting a spurious increase. When the viral load has become undetectable, there can still be *viral blips* or small increases in the viral load that are usually 400 copies/mL or less. These blips do not appear to be clinically significant. The viral load should be undetectable within the first six months after starting treatment. If it is not, treatment compliance should be evaluated and HIV resistance testing obtained. The viral load should be repeated monthly in pregnancy until the virus is undetectable and then every two to three months thereafter.

The CD4 (helper T lymphocyte) cell count is also an important measure of disease activity. Certain complications tend to occur below given CD4 counts. As a rule, CD4 counts should be repeated before any therapeutic decision is made. The trend of CD4 counts is probably more helpful than a single measurement. Multiple factors can depress the CD4 count and should be considered in the evaluation of a patient. In an asymptomatic non-pregnant patient, antiretroviral treatment should start when the CD4 count is between 200 and 350/mm^3. A CD4 count of <200/mm^3 constitutes AIDS. If the patient is stable, the count should be followed every three months. The list of factors that should be considered in the evaluation of the CD4 count are as follows:

- Pregnancy
- Recent steroid use
- Antibiotics
- Diurnal variation (lowest at 12 p.m. and highest at 8 p.m.)
- Major surgery
- Intra/interassay variation
- Infections
- Seasonal/monthly variation

RESISTANCE TESTING

The HIV virus can easily mutate because of the enormous amount of virus that is replicated on a daily basis, and the high rate of error in the reverse transcriptase enzyme. Mutations lead to drug resistance. Resistance testing is recommended when the viral load fails to become undetectable after six months of treatment or when patients have previously been exposed to antiretrovirals and therapy is being restarted. Some have suggested that all pregnant patients have resistance testing regardless of whether they are antiretroviral naïve or not. The resistance testing is done in one of two ways: genotypic or phenotypic. Genotype testing uses point mutations in the viral genome structure to predict which therapies the virus would be sensitive to. Phenotype testing has been likened to *culture and sensitivity* and predicts viral susceptibility based on the ability of the virus to grow in various concentrations of antiretrovirals. Results are reported as the amount of drug needed to reduce viral production by 50 percent. Genotype testing is generally more widely available, less expensive, and faster to obtain. The interpretation of both tests is complex and each test has its limitations. Testing has not been shown, in randomized trials, to be of consistent value in predicting how patients respond to various drugs. Some point mutations may mean increased resistance to a given drug, but enhanced sensitivity to another. Only clinicians with significant expertise in treating HIV patients should interpret the result. The tests are more helpful in deciding which drugs should not be used rather than deciding which drugs should be used. Table 26-2 compares the two types of testing.

TABLE 26-2 Genotype Versus Phenotype Testing

Genotype	Phenotype
Uses point mutations or structural changes in viral genome to predict drug sensitivity	Uses ability of virus to grow in varying concentrations drug(s) to predict sensitivity
Cheaper	More expensive
More widely available	Less widely available
Faster	Slower (requires virus to grow in culture)
Low specificity	Low specificity
More sensitive than phenotype testing	

IMMUNE SYSTEM CHANGES IN PREGNANCY

There are a variety of pregnancy-related changes in the immune system. The peripheral white blood cell count rises during gestation and also rises again in labor. In labor, the WBC count can approach $30,000/mm^3$. The increased white count is primarily due to increased segmented neutrophils. Cell-mediated immunity appears to change so as to allow tolerance for the foreign fetus. T-helper cell and natural killer cells decrease. There is increased maternal morbidity and mortality associated with a number of viral infections including varicella, malaria, and cytomegalovirus. Some women with autoimmune diseases, which are thought to be cell mediated, improve. There is improved antibody-mediated immunity. T-helper 2 cells increase. However, levels of IgM, IgG, and IgA all decrease.

PREGNANCY AND HIV INFECTION

Early, in the HIV epidemic, there were concerns that pregnancy would hasten the progression of HIV infection since there are changes in cell-mediated immunity in pregnancy. However, in controlled studies of HIV positive pregnant women who were compared to asymptomatic HIV positive nonpregnant women, pregnancy had no effect on disease progression. Pregnancy does not make HIV infection worse.

The care of HIV positive women requires a multidisciplinary team consisting of experts in HIV/AIDS care and obstetricians and pediatricians who are knowledgeable about HIV infection in pregnancy and vertical transmission. The team should also include nurses, nutritionists, and social service support. The initial evaluation of a pregnant woman with HIV infection is given in Table 26-3.

ANTIRETROVIRAL THERAPY

The decision to initiate antiretroviral therapy in pregnant women may not be an easy one, but antiretroviral therapy clearly reduces the risk of vertical transmission. The clinician and the patient need to consider a number of factors. There is no perfect combination of drugs nor a standard regimen that can be given to all patients. As with any therapeutic decision, there are risks and benefits of antiretroviral therapy. The benefits are a longer disease-free interval due to preservation of immune function and less risk of transmission of the virus to others. Antiretrovirals have toxicities, both short term and long term for which we have incomplete understanding. The patient must adhere to complex medication schedules making compliance difficult. Noncompliance can quickly result in viral resistance making future therapy much more difficult and generally less effective. Additionally, one must consider the possible fetal effects of drugs administered during pregnancy. Table 26-4 lists several considerations that need to be addressed before initiating antiretroviral therapy.

There are four major classes of antiretroviral drugs: nucleoside reverse transcriptase inhibitors, non-nucleoside reverse transcriptase inhibitors, protease inhibitors, and nucleotide reverse transcriptase inhibitors. Table 26-5 outlines the available drugs and their class. Doses may need to be altered in certain circumstances depending upon the combinations used. Dosing regimens are complex and should only be undertaken in consultation with an expert in HIV therapy.

The original study, demonstrating the efficacy of antiretroviral therapy in decreasing the risk of vertical transmission, utilized zidovudine monotherapy.

TABLE 26-3 Initial Assessment of an HIV-Infected Pregnant Woman

History:
Complete prior medical and surgical history with attention to prior AIDS defining diagnosis(es)
Current and past medications, especially prior antiretroviral use
Immunization status
Prior or current sexually transmitted disease including dysplasia
Substance abuse history including alcohol use and smoking
Mental health history: depression, domestic violence, and dementia
Availability of support systems
Postpartum contraception plans

Physical exam:
Weight
Vital signs (particularly temperature and respiratory rate)
Skin: abscesses, dermatitis, rashes, vesicles, violaceous macules, evidence of prior SQ or IV injection drug use
Lymph nodes: lymphadenopathy
HEENT: dentition, funduscopic exam and visual fields, oral thrush or ulcers
Pulmonary: breath sounds, cough, sputum, dyspnea
Cardiac: cardiomegaly, murmurs, rubs
Abdomen: hepatosplenomegaly, fundal height, fetal heart tones
Genitourinary: vaginal discharge, genital lesions
Neurological: mental status, confusion, ability to concentrate, memory deficits, focal neurological deficits or neuropathy, weakness
Psychiatric: affect, mood, evidence of psychosis, support systems

Laboratory:
Appropriate prenatal labs, baseline assessment of hematological, renal, and liver function, hepatitis B and C serology, CMV and toxoplasmosis titers, CD4 count, HIV-1 RNA viral load, possible resistance testing (especially if prior antiretroviral use), TB skin test

Radiological:
Ultrasound to determine gestational age and evaluate fetal anatomy

Miscellaneous:
Nutritional assessment
Reduction of transmission (abstinence or safe sex practices, and prohibition against breastfeeding)

Many experts feel that zidovudine should be a component of any antiretroviral regimen used in pregnancy. Some women who receive antiretroviral therapy during pregnancy, but who otherwise do not meet current guidelines for antiretroviral therapy, may elect to discontinue treatment after delivery.

In addition, pregnant women should receive antimicrobial prophylaxis to prevent opportunistic infections according to the guidelines published by the U.S. Public Health Service.

PREVENTION OF VERTICAL TRANSMISSION

The cornerstone of preventing vertical transmission of the HIV virus is to recognize which pregnant women are infected and use antiretroviral therapy to reduce their viral load. Antiretroviral therapy should be initiated after the first trimester. The infant should be treated for the first six weeks of life. Reducing viral load is far and away the most important factor in reducing vertical transmission. However, there are other measures that may help as well.

TABLE 26-4 Considerations in Starting Antiretroviral therapy

- Does the patient meet criteria for treatment?
  - Patients with acute retroviral syndrome
  - Patients within 6 months of seroconversion
  - Patients with symptomatic HIV infection or AIDS
  - Patients who are asymptomatic, but otherwise meet criteria
  - CD4 count <200–350/mm^3
  - Rapidly declining CD4 count
  - HIV RNA viral load >55,000 (controversial)
  - Is the patient willing to continue long-term treatment?
- Does the patient understand the importance of compliance?
- Does the patient have the resources to continue treatment?
  - Funds to pay for treatment, stable living situation, absence of psychosis, severe depression, dementia, substance abuse
- What is known about the medication in pregnancy?

Table 26-6 outlines these measures. About 70 percent of perinatal transmission occurs at delivery and 30 percent occurs in utero. About two-thirds of the in utero transmissions are thought to occur within the last 14 days before delivery. If the patient has a viral load of >1000 copies/mL, the American College of Obstetricians and Gynecologists recommends that she be offered an elective cesarean section at 38 weeks before the onset of labor to reduce her chances of vertical transmission. The estimated gestational age should be based on as much clinical data as is available, but amniocentesis to document fetal lung maturity presents an unknown risk of transmitting HIV infection to the fetus and is *not* recommended. Cesarean section offers a reduction in vertical transmission, especially if the mother has a high viral load. However, the benefits of cesarean section are not as pronounced once labor has started or if ruptured membranes are present. The decision about the route of delivery should be individualized. Cesarean sections are not without risk, particularly if the mother's viral load is high. The higher the maternal viral load, the greater the risk of postpartum infectious morbidity.

Unfortunately, about 15 percent of HIV positive women do not receive prenatal care and have not had antenatal antiretroviral therapy. The list of drugs that are recommended by the Public Health Task Force for treating HIV positive women in labor who have not had antepartum antiretroviral therapy is as follows:

- Zidovudine
- Nevirapine
- Zidovudine-lamivudine
- Nevirapine and Zidovudine

OTHER CONSIDERATIONS IN PREGNANCY

HIV affects humoral immunity and B cell function. As a result, HIV-infected patients may produce a range of antibodies including antiphospholipid antibodies. These are not associated with an increased risk of thrombosis.

Protease inhibitors have been associated with carbohydrate intolerance in pregnancy. However, the development of gestational diabetes is not a contraindication to their continued use. Gestational diabetes should be managed in a conventional manner.

If an HIV-infected patient requires an antepartum transfusion, she should receive CMV negative blood even if she has prior evidence of CMV infection

TABLE 26-5 Antiretroviral Therapy

Generic	Trade name	Side effects
	Nucleoside reverse transcriptase inhibitors	
Zidovudine (AZT)	Retrovir	Anemia, nausea, headaches
Didanosine (ddI)	Videx	Pancreatitis especially in alcoholics Peripheral neuropathy Avoid using with d4T in pregnancy
Dideoxycytidine (ddc)	Hivid	Peripheral neuropathy
Stavudine (d4T)	Zerit	Peripheral neuropathy Avoid using with ddI in pregnancy
Lamivudine	Epivir	Rare hepatic dysfunction
Abacavir	Ziagen	Hypersensivity reaction Can be fatal if continued
Emtricitabine	Emtriva	Headache, diarrhea, nausea, rash
	Non-nucleoside reverse transcriptase inhibitors	
Nevirapine	Viramune	Rash, increased LFTs, hepatitis
Delavirdine	Rescriptor	Rash, headaches
Efavirenz	Sustiva	Avoid in pregnancy
	Protease inhibitors	
Indinavir	Crixivan	Renal stones, hepatic dysfunction, diarrhea, hyperbilirubinemia, lipodystrophies, diabetes, drug interactions
Amprenavir	Agenerase	GI intolerance
Lopinavir	Kaletra	GI complaints, pancreatitis, hyperlipidemia, lipodystrophy, hyperglycemia
Saquinavir	Invirase, Fortovase	
Nelfinavir	Viacept	Diarrhea, hepatic dysfunction, drug interactions, lipodystrophies, diabetes
Ritonavir	Norvir	Perioral paresthesia, diarrhea, liver dysfunction, hyperglycemia, drug interaction, diabetes, lipodystrophies
Atazanavir	Reyatax	Hyperbilirubinemia
	Nucleotide reverse transcriptase inhibitors	
Tenofovir	Viread	Major side effects not well known at this time
	Entry inhibitors	
Enfuvirtide (T-20)	Fuzeon	Injection site reactions

TABLE 26-6 Measures to Reduce the Risk of Vertical Transmission

Keep the mother's viral load at 50 copies or less (undetectable)
- Cesarean section for women with viral loads of 1000 or more at 38 weeks of gestation
- Maximize the chance of a term delivery
  - Reduce maternal smoking (preterm premature rupture of membranes)
  - Reduce maternal substance use including drugs or alcohol
  - Treat maternal infections
- Treat vitamin A deficiency
- Avoid invasive fetal procedures
  - Chorionic villus sampling, amniocentesis, percutaneous fetal blood sampling
- Avoid scalp electrodes, fetal scalp sampling, artificial rupture of membranes, operative vaginal delvieries
- Avoid episiotomies
- Wash the infant in an antimicrobial bath as soon as possible and immediately *before* administering parenteral medication or obtaining blood
- Avoid breastfeeding

because of the possibility of infecting the fetus. Although primary CMV infection presents a greater risk to intrauterine infection, secondary CMV infection can also cause morbidity. If she receives a postpartum transfusion, her CMV status should be determined if possible and she should receive CMV negative blood if she is CMV negative.

Breastfeeding is associated with a risk of HIV transmission to the infant. It is estimated that breastfeeding increases the risk of transmission by about 15 percent. Women in the developed world should not breast-feed.

The combination of stavudine and didanosine should be avoided in pregnancy, as there have been reports of fatal lactic acidosis when they have been used together.

SAFETY PRECAUTIONS FOR THE LABOR AND DELIVERY TEAM

Caring for obstetrical patients presents a risk of exposure to body fluids for health care workers (HCW). The Centers for Disease Control and Prevention established universal precautions in 1987. Table 26-7 lists these universal precautions. At least one blood exposure can be documented in over 30 percent

TABLE 26-7 Body Fluids and Universal Precautions

Universal precautions necessary	Universal precautions not necessary *unless* contaminated with blood
Blood	Breast milk
Semen	Urine
Vaginal secretions	Sputum
Tissue	Sweat
Fluids	Vomitus
Amniotic	Feces
Peritoneal	Nasal secretions
Pericardial	Tears
Pleural	Saliva
Synovial	
Cerebrospinal	

of surgical procedures, most (75 percent) of which may have been preventable. Suggestions to reduce exposure with needles or sharp instruments are as follows:

- Observe universal precautions
- Do not recap needles
- Wear double gloves
- Place sharps boxes near where sharps are used
- Announce all sharp instruments prior to passing them
- Pass sharp instruments in an emesis basin
- Use instruments to load needles
- "One wound, one surgeon"
- Check hourly for disruptions of protective barriers

The overall risk of HIV transmission to an HCW depends upon the type of exposure, the volume of the blood, the patient's viral load, and possibly, the immune response of the HCW. The risk of HIV infection with a percutaneous exposure is 0.3 percent while the risk with a mucous membrane exposure is much less, about 0.09 percent. There appears to be minimal risk with exposure to intact skin. The risks are higher with large bore needles, deep intramuscular injections, larger volumes of blood, and higher viral loads. The risks after exposure to other body fluids have not been well defined.

If exposure occurs, the contact area should be washed immediately with soap and water. Other solutions such as betadine are not superior. Eyes should be flushed with sterile normal saline. The exposed HCW should be evaluated as soon as possible for postexposure prophylaxis.

Figures 26-1 and 26-2 provide the current CDC recommendations for postexposure prophylaxis (PEP) in an HCW. It is always important to seek expert opinion after HCW exposure, particularly in special circumstances such as pregnancy in the HCW or exposure with a drug-resistant virus. Animal studies have shown that early initiation of PEP and a small inoculum of blood are the most predictive of successful PEP.

SUMMARY

The care of HIV-infected pregnant women is challenging and constantly evolving as new therapies arise. Unfortunately, since this epidemic continues, many obstetricians can expect to care for an HIV-infected patient at some point. Fortunately new therapies, especially the protease inhibitors, have markedly reduced the risk of perinatal transmission and have significantly increased the life expectancy of HIV-infected women. It is crucial for obstetricians to continue to alert patients to the risks of HIV, to screen all pregnant women for the infection, and to consult with experts in HIV therapy to appropriately manage antiretroviral therapy and HIV-related complications.

APPENDIX: AIDS DEFINING CONDITIONS (CENTERS FOR DISEASE CONTROL AND PREVENTION)

- *Candida* infection of esophagus, trachea, bronchi, or lungs
- Invasive cervical cancer[a]
- Coccidiomycosis, extrapulmonary
- Cryptococcosis, extrapulmonary

[a]Must be HIV seropositive.

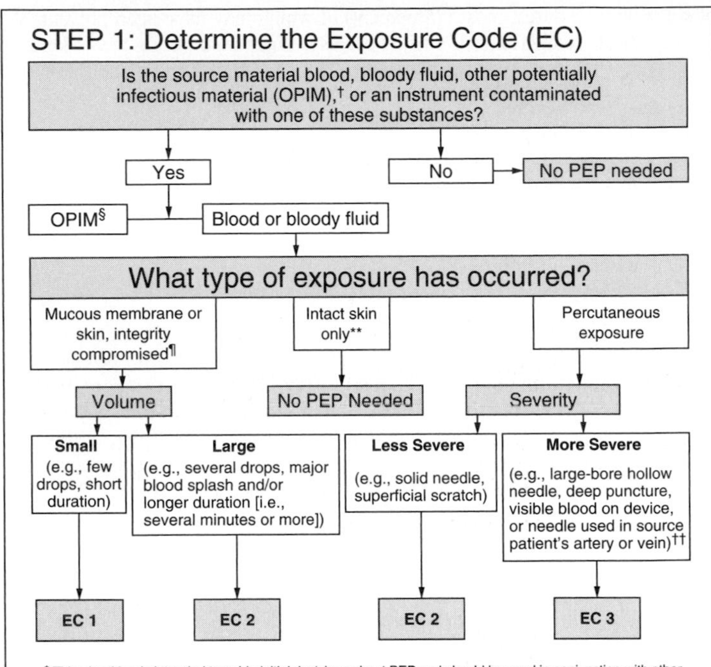

* This algorithm is intended to guide initial decisions about PEP and should be used in conjunction with other guidance provided in this report.

† Semen or vaginal secretions; cerebrospinal, synovial, pleural, peritoneal, pericardial, or amniotic fluids; or tissue.

§ Exposures to OPIM must be evaluated on a case-by-case basis. In general, these body substances are considered a low risk for transmission in health-care settings. Any unprotected contact to concentrated HIV in a research laboratory or production facility is considered an occupational exposure that requires clinical evaluation to determine the need for PEP.

¶ Skin integrity is considered compromised if there is evidence of chapped skin, dermatitis, abrasion, or open wound.

** Contact with intact skin is not normally considered a risk for HIV transmission. However, if the exposure was to blood, and the circumstance suggests a higher volume exposure (e.g., an extensive area of skin was exposed or there was prolonged contact with blood), the risk for HIV transmission should be considered.

†† The combination of these severity factors (e.g., large-bore hollow needle and deep puncture) contribute to an elevated risk for transmission if the source person is HIV-positive.

FIG. 26-1 Determining the need for HIV postexposure prophylaxis (PEP) after an occupational exposure (Step 1).

- Cryptosporidiosis with diarrhea >1 month
- Cytomegalovirus of any organ except the liver, spleen, or lymph nodes
- Herpes simplex with mucocutaneous ulcer >1 month or bronchitis, pneumonitis, or esophagitis
- HIV dementia: disabling cognitive and/or motor function interfering with occupation or activities of daily living
- HIV wasting: involuntary weight loss >10% of baseline plus chronic diarrhea (2 stools/day >30 days) or chronic weakness and enigmatic fever >30 days
- Isosporiasis with diarrhea >1 month
- Kaposi sarcoma if <60 years or >60 years and HIV+
- Lymphoma of the brain if <60 years or >60 years and HIV+
- Lymphoma, non-Hodgkin's of B cell or unknown immunotype or immunoblastic sarcoma

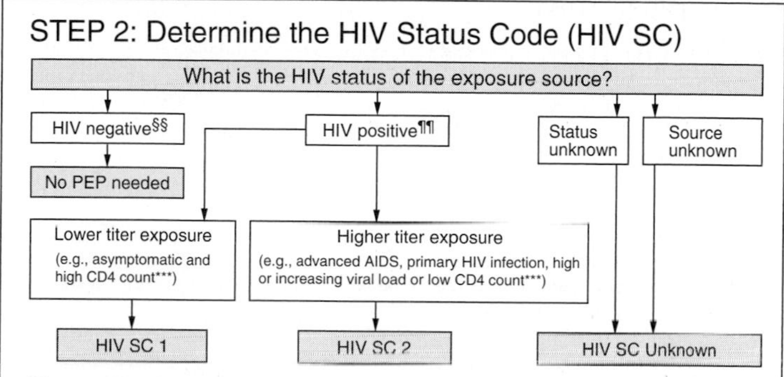

§§ A source is considered negative for HIV infection if there is laboratory documentation of a negative HIV antibody, HIV polymerase chain reaction (PCR), or HIV p24 antigen test result from a specimen collected at or near the time of exposure and there is no clinical evidence of recent retroviral-like illness.

¶¶ A source is considered infected with HIV (HIV positive) if there has been a positive laboratory result for HIV antibody, HIV PCR, or HIV p24 antigen or physician-diagnosed AIDS.

*** Examples are used as surrogates to estimate the HIV titer in an exposure source for purposes of considering PEP regimens and do not reflect all clinical situations that may be observed. Although a high HIV titer (HIV SC 2) in an exposure source has been associated with an increased risk for transmission, the possibility of transmission from a source with a low HIV titer also must be considered.

STEP 3: Determine the PEP Recommendation

EC	HIV SC	PEP recommendation
1	1	**PEP may not be warranted.** Exposure type does not pose a known risk for HIV transmission. Whether the risk for drug toxicity outweighs the benefit of PEP should be decided by the exposed HCW and treating clinician.
1	2	**Consider basic regimen.**††† Exposure type poses a negligible risk for HIV transmission. A high HIV titer in the source may justify consideration of PEP. Whether the risk for drug toxicity outweighs the benefit of PEP should be decided by the exposed HCW and treating clinician.
2	1	**Recommend basic regimen.** Most HIV exposures are in this category; no increased risk for HIV transmission has been observed but use of PEP is appropriate.
2	2	**Recommend expanded regimen.**§§§ Exposure type represents an increased HIV transmission risk.
3	1 or 2	**Recommend expanded regimen.** Exposure type represents an increased HIV transmission risk.
Unknown		If the source or, in the case of an unknown source, the setting where the exposure occurred suggests a possible risk for HIV exposure and the EC is 2 or 3, consider PEP basic regimen.

†††Basic regimen is four weeks of zidovudine, 600 mg per day in two or three divided doses, and lamivudine, 150 mg twice daily.

§§§Expanded regimen is the basic regimen plus either indinavir, 800 mg every 8 hours, or nelfinavir, 750 mg three times a day.

FIG. 26-2 Determining the need for HIV postexposure prophylaxis (PEP) after an occupational exposure (Steps 2 and 3).

- *Mycobacterium avium* or *Mycobacterium kansasii*, disseminated
- *Mycobacterium tuberculosis*, disseminated[a]
- *Mycobacterium tuberculosis*, pulmonary[a]
- Nocardiosis
- *Pnemocystis carinii*, pneumonia
- Recurrent pneumonia[a]
- Recurrent, nontyphoid *Salmonella* septicemia[a]
- Extraintestinal strongyloidosis
- Toxoplasmosis of any internal organ

[a]Must be HIV seropositive.

SUGGESTED READING

American College of Obstetricians and Gynecologists. Scheduled cesarean delivery and the prevention of vertical transmission of HIV infection. ACOG Committee Opinion No. 219. Washington, DC: American College of Obstetricians and Gynecologists, 1999.

Antiretroviral Treatment for Adult HIV Infection in 2002: Updated Recommendations of the International AIDS Society—USA Panel. *JAMA* 2002;288:222–235.

Bartlett J, Gallant J: *Medical Management of HIV Infection.* Baltimore: Johns Hopkins University Press, 2001–2002.

Gabbe S, Niebyl J, Simpson JL: *Obstetrics: Normal and Problem Pregnancies*, 4th edn. New York: Churchill Livingston, 2002.

HIV/AIDS Medical Practice Guidelines. The National Institute of Health. Available at: http://aidsinfo.nih.gov/guidelines.

HIV in pregnancy. Minkoff H, guest editor in *Clinical Obstetrics and Gynecology*, Vol. 44, No. 2, June 2001.

Knowledge, Action, and Health: A Woman's Guide to HIV Treatments. Los Angeles: Women Alive, 1997.

Minkoff H: HIV infection in pregnancy. *Obstet Gynecol* 2003;101:797–810.

Public Health Service Guidelines for the Management of Health-Care Worker Exposures to HIV and Recommendations for Postexposure Prophylaxis. *MMWR* May 15, 1998.

Signs D: HIV infection. In: Tan J (ed), *Expert Guide to Infectious Disease*. Philadelphia: American College of Physicians, 2002.

Sweet R, Gibbs R: *HIV/AIDS in Infectious Diseases of the Female Genital Tract*, 4th edn. Philadelphia: Lippincott, Williams & Wilkins, 2002.

Watts H, Brunham R: Sexually transmitted diseases including HIV infection in pregnancy. In: Holmes K, Sparling P, Mardh P, et al. (eds). *Sexually Transmitted Diseases*, 3rd edn, 1999.

27 Systemic Lupus Erythematosus in the Pregnant Patient

Bob Silver

INTRODUCTION

Systemic lupus erythematosus (SLE) is a multisystemic chronic inflammatory disease that affects patients in many different ways over a varying course of time. The disease is typically characterized by periods of remission and relapse, although the causes of exacerbation remain uncertain. SLE, like most autoimmune diseases, has a clear predilection for women. Indeed, women are affected seven times more frequently than men. The disorder may be diagnosed between the ages of 15 and 50 years, although it is most often detected in women in their 20s. Therefore, SLE is the most commonly encountered autoimmune disease in pregnancy. Although no specific gene mutation for SLE has been identified, the disease likely has a genetic component. Approximately 10 percent of affected patients have a relative with SLE and monozygotic twin studies demonstrate that 50 percent of affected twins are concordant for the disease.

The symptoms of SLE are extremely heterogeneous which can make the diagnosis difficult. The disease may affect joints, skin, kidneys, lung, nervous system, and other organs. The most common presenting complaints are extreme fatigue, arthralgias, fever, and rash (Table 27-1).

In 1982, the American Rheumatism Association (ARA) revised previously set criteria for the diagnosis of SLE (Table 27-2). According to the ARA, a person must have had at least 4 of the 11 specific criteria in order to carry the diagnosis of SLE. However, many patients have less than four clinical or laboratory features of SLE and do not meet strict diagnostic criteria. These patients should not be considered to have SLE, but are often referred to as having lupus-like disease. Such individuals may benefit from therapies for SLE and some will ultimately develop the clinical syndrome.

LUPUS IN PREGNANCY

The Effect of Pregnancy on SLE

Fertility

Typically, patients with SLE do not have impaired infertility. However, patients on high dose steroids may become amenorrheic or anovulatory. Women with end stage lupus nephritis requiring dialysis are also frequently amenorrheic. In addition, depending on the cumulative dose of medication and the age of the patient, 10 to 60 percent of patients who have been treated with cyclophosphamide become permanently amenorrheic. Patients with mild-moderate disease have fertility rates comparable to the general population and should be counseled appropriately about contraception unless they desire to become pregnant.

TABLE 27-1 Frequency of Clinical Symptoms in Patients with SLE

Clinical symptom	Frequency (%)
Fatigue	80–100
Fever	80–100
Arthritis	95
Myalgia	70
Weight loss	60
Photosensitivity	60
Malar rash	50
Nephritis	50
Pleurisy	50
Lymphadenopathy	50
Pericarditis	30
Neuropsychiatric	20

Maternal Complications

Lupus Flares

There is an association between estrogen and SLE, as evidenced by the female predilection for the disorder. Thus, conditions such as pregnancy that are associated with high estrogen levels have the potential to exacerbate SLE. The incidence of flares during pregnancy ranges between 15 and 63 percent. Several retrospective, uncontrolled studies performed prior to 1985 suggest that pregnancy exacerbates lupus flares. Table 27-3 reviews multiple studies on the frequency of lupus flares during pregnancy. It is difficult to interpret available data because control groups were often unmatched, and the SLE cohorts among studies vary greatly regarding patient characteristics, severity of disease, and the definition of lupus flares. Furthermore, normal physiologic changes of pregnancy such as palmar erythema, facial blushing, proteinuria, and alopecia can be misinterpreted as lupus flares.

Doria and colleagues recently investigated the relationship of steroid hormone levels in pregnancy to SLE activity. The group prospectively studied 17 women with lupus during pregnancy and matched them to eight

TABLE 27-2 American Rheumatic Association Criteria for the Diagnosis and Classification of SLE

Malar rash
Discoid rash
Photosensitivity
Oral ulcers
Arthritis
Serositis
Nephritis (proteinuria ≥ 500 mg/day or cellular casts)
Neurologic disorder (seizures, psychosis, stroke)
Hematologic disorder (hemolytic anemia, thrombocytopenia, leukopenia, lymphopenia)
Immunologic disorder (anti-dsDNA, anti-Sm, positive LE, false positive RPR)
Antinuclear antibodies

Note: Patient must have four of the following criteria either serially or simultaneously

TABLE 27-3 Studies on the Frequency of Lupus Flares During Pregnancy

Author	Pregnancies (*n*)	Results
Lockshin (1984)	33	No difference
Lockshin (1989)	80	No difference
Mintz (1986)	102	No difference
Urowitz (1993)	79	No difference
Nossent (1990)	39	Increased
Wong (1991)	29	Increased
Petri (1991)	40	Increased
Ruiz-Irastorza (1996)	78	Increased

healthy pregnant controls. They reported that women with SLE had significantly lower serum levels of estradiol and progesterone than controls. Furthermore, the highest levels of estrogen and progesterone occurred in the third trimester, when patients with SLE had both the lowest disease activity and serum immunoglobulin levels. These data challenge previous work that supports the association between increased levels of steroid hormones and lupus activity, and raise the question of whether or not estrogens and progesterones suppress humoral immune responses and therefore disease activity.

Regardless of whether or not the rate of SLE flares increase during pregnancy, flares are common and may occur in any trimester, or in the postpartum period. In general lupus flares during pregnancy are mild and easily treated. Furthermore, it has been demonstrated that active disease at the time of conception, active nephritis, a systemic lupus erythematosus disease activity index (SLEDAI) score of five or more, and abruptly stopping hydroxychloroquine therapy are significant risk factors for lupus flares. Approximately, 50 percent of patients with active disease at the time of conception experience flares during pregnancy compared to 20 percent of patients who are in remission when they conceive. Conversely, patients who have been in remission for six months prior to conception have a lower risk of lupus flares and do better than those with active disease.

Preexisting Renal Disease

Approximately, 50 percent of patients with lupus will develop renal disease. Lupus nephritis is a result of immune complex deposition, complement activation, and inflammation in the kidney. Several reports have emphasized the potential for a permanent decrease in renal function after pregnancy in women with lupus nephritis. On the other hand, more recent series indicate excellent outcome for most women with mild renal disease. Burkett reviewed several retrospective reports including 242 pregnancies in 156 women with lupus nephritis. He demonstrated that 59 percent of patients had no change in their renal function, 30 percent experienced transient renal impairment, and 7 percent had permanent renal insufficiency.

It is clear that there is a strong correlation between renal insufficiency prior to conception and the risk of deterioration during and after pregnancy. Women with a serum creatinine level greater than 1.5 mg/dL have a significantly increased risk of deterioration in renal function. Conversely, patients with serum creatinine levels less than 1.5 mg/dL can be reassured that pregnancy will not

TABLE 27-4 Laboratory Tests that may be Used to Distinguish Preeclampsia from a Lupus Flare

Test	Preeclampsia	SLE
Decreased complement levels	+	+++
Increased anti-dsDNA	–	+++
Antithrombin III defiency	++	+/–
Microangiopathic hemolytic anemia	++	–
Coombs postitve hemolytic anemia	–	++
Thrombocytopenia	++	++
Leukopenia	–	++
Hematuria	+	+++
Cellular casts	–	+++
Increased serum creatinine	+/–	++
Hypocalcuria	++	+/–
Increased liver transaminases	++	+/–

increase the rate of deterioration of renal function. The specific type of renal disease as demonstrated by histologic studies does not appear to influence pregnancy outcome or postnatal renal function.

Preeclampsia

Preeclampsia is among the most common pregnancy complications in patients with SLE. The incidence ranges between 20 and 35 percent. The cause of the increased incidence of preeclampsia in women with SLE is not clear, but may be due to unrecognized renal disease that is likely present in many patients with SLE. Renal disease, hypertension, and antiphospholipid syndrome all increase a patient's risk for developing preeclampsia. In the prospective study of Lockshin et al., 8 of 11 (72 percent) patients with lupus nephritis developed preeclampsia compared to 12 of 53 (22 percent) women who did not have nephritis.

In some cases, it is difficult to distinguish preeclampsia from a lupus flare manifesting as lupus nephritis. Both disorders may be characterized by increased proteinuria, hypertension, and fetal growth restriction. Table 27-4 lists several features that may aid in the distinction of preeclampsia from nephritis. Despite these parameters, it is often difficult to distinguish between the two, and in some cases a renal biopsy may be required to differentiate between the conditions. For example, confirmation of lupus nephritis may prevent unnecessary iatrogenic preterm birth in an attempt to treat preeclampsia. Although there is a theoretical increased risk of complications from the procedure, it has been performed safely during pregnancy. Preeclampsia and lupus nephrits may also coexist and a definitive diagnosis cannot always be made.

Fetal Complications

Pregnancy Loss

Patients with SLE have, an overall increased risk of pregnancy loss. The rate of first trimester spontaneous miscarriage is as high as 35 percent. The risk of fetal death is also increased and approaches 22 percent in some series. Several factors have been associated with pregnancy loss in women with SLE including antiphospholipid syndrome (see below), renal disease, active disease during pregnancy, and a history of fetal loss. However, in the absence of these, SLE patients have similar pregnancy loss rates to the general population.

Preterm Delivery

There is a higher incidence of preterm birth in patients with lupus than in healthy women. Preterm delivery <37 weeks has been reported in as few as 3 percent and as many as 73 percent of SLE pregnancies (median 30 percent). The variation in preterm birth in these studies may be due, in part, to the tendency of some obstetricians to intentionally deliver patients with SLE in order to avoid increased fetal morbidity. However, a well-designed cohort study by Johnson et al. including careful obstetric detail, reported a 50 percent rate of preterm birth in patients with SLE. Preterm delivery typically occurs because of preeclampsia, fetal growth impairment, abnormal fetal testing, and preterm premature rupture of membranes. Increased disease activity, chronic hypertension, and antiphospholipid antibodies are all associated with an increased risk for preterm delivery.

Neonatal Lupus Erythematosus

Neonatal lupus erythematosus (NLE) is a rare condition that occurs in approximately 1:20,000 live births. The disease is characterized by neonatal or fetal heart block, skin lesions, or less commonly, anemia, thrombocytopenia, and hepatitis. Approximately, 50 percent of fetuses with NLE have skin lesions, 50 percent have heart block, and 10 percent have both. NLE is an immune-mediated disease and is a result of transplacental passage of maternal autoantibodies. Most cases are associated with antibodies to the cytoplasmic ribonucleo-proteins SSA (Ro), more specifically the 5 anti-SS2-kDa epitope of SSA. SSB (La) antibodies are also detected in 50 to 75 percent of these women. However, NLE is rarely associated with isolated antibodies to SSB.

Typical skin lesions associated with NLE are erythematous, scaling plaques usually seen on the scalp or face of the infant. The lesions appear within the first weeks after delivery and last only for a few months. Skin biopsies of the lesions show changes typical of cutaneous lupus in adults. The hematologic abnormalities of NLE also resolve within a few months, coinciding with the disappearance of maternal autoantibodies.

Cardiac lesions associated with NLE are heart block and endocardial fibroelastosis. The anti-SSA (most specifically anti-SSA-52), binds to myocardial tissue. Histologic analysis of affected fetal hearts demonstrates mononuclear cell infiltration, fibrin deposition, calcification of the conduction system (specifically the AV and SA nodes), and diffuse fibroelastosis throughout the myocardium. It is hypothesized that the earliest effect of the antibody-mediated disease is global pancarditis with subsequent fibrosis of the conduction system. Congenital heart block is usually detected as fetal bradycardia with a rate between 60 and 80 beats per minute between 16 and 25 weeks gestation. Fetal echocardiography demonstrates a structurally normal heart with AV dissociation. In some cases, fetal hydrops develops in utero.

The presence of autoantibodies alone is insufficient to cause NLE. This is demonstrated by the fact that approximately 30 percent of patients with SLE have anti-SSA antibodies, and 15 to 20 percent of patients have anti-SSB autoantibodies. However, prospective studies indicate that the incidence of congenital heart block in infants born to women with SLE is only 2 percent. Also, the recurrence risk ranges between 5 and 25 percent and there are reports of twins who are discordant for NLE. Thus, anti-SSA alone does not always lead to NLE. It is also important to recognize that maternal SLE is not a prerequisite for NLE. In fact, up to 50 percent of cases occur in the offspring of healthy women with circulating autoantibodies. Some, but not all of these women eventually develop connective-tissue disorders.

The clinical course of NLE is highly variable. Cuteaneous and hematologic abnormalities resolve by six months of age. However, heart block is a permanent condition that is associated with significant morbidity and mortality. Approximately, one-third of fetuses affected with heart block die within three years of age, and the remaining two-thirds require permanent pacemakers.

Whether treatment of heart block detected in utero is beneficial is not clear. Many clinicians advocate the use of flourinated corticosteroids since they cross the placenta. The rationale for steroid treatment is based on the fact that the cardiac histology of fetuses with CHB demonstrates diffuse inflammation, IgG, fibrin, and complement deposition. Slight improvement in myocardial function has been reported by some investigators. However, others note that once diagnosed, heart block is complete and irreversible. Furthermore, there are significant maternal and fetal risks to treatment with flourinated corticosteroids including osteoporosis, glucose intolerance, fetal growth restriction, and developmental delay. Therefore, the efficacy, of steroid therapy in the treatment of congenital heart block diagnosed in utero, needs to be addressed in prospective studies.

The Management of Pregnancies Complicated by SLE

Table 27-5 summarizes the management of a patient with SLE during pregnancy. Ideally, women with SLE should have preconceptual counseling to discuss both medical and obstetric risks including lupus flares, preeclampsia, fetal growth restriction, pregnancy loss, and preterm delivery. Patients should also be made aware of the risk of NLE and the clinical implications of the disease. All patients with SLE should have an assessment of their renal function in the form of a serum creatinine level and a 24-hour urine analysis for protein and creatinine clearance. In addition, a hematocrit and platelet count should be determined to exclude hematologic abnormalities associated with SLE. Finally, all patients should be tested for antiphospholipid antibodies (see below). A number of studies have demonstrated that active lupus at the time of conception is associated with a higher risk of lupus flares, preeclampsia, and fetal loss. Thus, the optimal timing of conception in SLE patients is after a patient has been in remission for six months. In addition, nonsteroidal anti-inflammatory drugs (NSAIDs) and cytotoxic agents should be stopped prior to conception (see below).

During pregnancy, patients with the disease should be co-managed by an obstetrician and a rheumatologist. Obstetric visits should be as frequent as every two weeks during the first and second trimesters, and weekly during the third. Blood pressure, urinalysis, and symptoms of a lupus flare should be assessed at each visit. Serial ultrasounds should be preformed to screen for fetal growth restriction. Nonstress testing and evaluation of the amniotic fluid should begin at 32 weeks gestation.

Routine testing for ANA titers and complement levels do not improve obstetric outcome and are unnecessary. Some physicians advocate routine testing for anti-SSA and SSB antibodies in all patients with SLE. However, these tests are not cost effective since one would neither advise a patient against a pregnancy, nor institute a specific treatment if the serum titers were positive. Cesarean

TABLE 27-5 Management Protocol for Patients with Systemic Lupus Erythematosus

I. Priorities

A. Avoid medications that are harmful to the fetus
B. Prompt detection of preeclampsia and uteroplacental insufficiency
C. Discern between lupus exacerbations and preeclampsia
D. Appropriate detection and treatment of lupus flares

II. Management

A. Preconception counseling

1. Discuss potential pregnancy complications including preeclampsia, preterm labor, miscarriage, fetal death, fetal growth restriction, and neonatal lupus.
2. Clinically evaluate lupus activity. Delay pregnancy until remission.
3. Evaluate patient for nephritis, hematologic abnormalities, and antiphospholipid antibodies.
4. Discontinue NSAIDs and cytotoxic agents.

B. Antenatal care

1. Frequent visits to assess SLE status and to screen for hypertension.
2. Serial ultrasounds to evaluate interval fetal growth.
3. Antenatal surveillance at 32 weeks or earlier if indicated.

C. Treatment of SLE exacerbations

1. Mild to moderate exacerbations
   a. If the patient is taking glucocorticoids, increase the dose to at least 20–30 mg/day.
   b. If the patient is not taking glucocorticoids, start 15–20 mg prednisone/day.
2. Severe exacerbations without renal or CNS manifestations
   a. Rheumatology consult and consider hospitalization.
   b. Glucorticoid treatment 1.0–1.5 mg/kg. Expect clinical improvement in 5–10 days.
   c. Taper the glucocorticoids once the patient demonstrates clinical improvement.
   d. If the patient cannot be tapered off high doses of glucorticoids, consider starting cyclosporine or azathioprine.
3. Severe exacerbations with renal or CNS involvement
   a. Hospitalization and rheumatology consult.
   b. Initiate intravenous glucocorticoid treatment, 10–30 mg/kg/day of methylprednisolone for 3–6 days.
   c. Maintain patient on 1.0–1.5 mg/kg of oral prednisone.
   d. When the patient responds, taper the glucocorticoid.
   e. For unresponsive patients, consider starting cyclophosphamide or plasmapheresis.

delivery should be reserved for the usual obstetric indications. In cases of fetal heart block, vaginal delivery may still be safely accomplished with the use of a fetal pulse oximeter in labor to assess fetal oxygen status.

Medications

The medical management of SLE includes four categories of drugs: NSAIDs, antimalarials, corticosteroids, and cytotoxic agents (Table 27-6).

TABLE 27-6 Medications Used for the Treatment of SLE in Pregnancy

Medication	Pregnancy category	Recommendations
NSAIDs	B	Avoid, especially in the third trimester.
Hydroxychloroquine	C	Limited data available on the use of hydroxychloroquine in pregnancy. Teratogenicity based on studies of chloroquine. Stopping hydroxychloroquine is associated with an increased risk of SLE flares. Therefore, recommend continuing if needed to control SLE.
Glucocorticoids	B	Avoid fluorinated glucocorticoids because they cross the placenta. High doses associated with significant maternal side effects and subsequent fetal side effects. Avoid empiric treatment.
Cyclosporine A	C	Extensive experience with the use of cyclosporine in pregnant renal transplant patients. Not an animal teratogen. Appears safe in humans. Long term follow up studies are limited.
Azathioprine	D	Teratogenic in animals. Appears safe in humans
Cyclophosphamide	D	Associated with cleft palate and skeletal abnormalities. Avoid if possible. May be needed in severe cases of proliferative nephritis.
Methotrexate	X	Avoid. The drug is embryolethal. Also associated with multiple types of congenital anomalies.

Nonsteroidal Anti-inflammatory Drugs

NSAIDs are the most common anti-inflammatory agents used in the treatment of SLE. Unfortunately, their use during pregnancy is associated with significant fetal morbidity. NSAIDs readily cross the placenta and can block prostaglandin synthesis in fetal tissue. The use of NSAIDs during pregnancy is associated with premature closure of the ductus, fetal pulmonary hypertension, necrotizing enterocolitis, and fetal renal insufficiency. There was speculation that selective COX-II inhibitors might cause fewer fetal side-effects than nonselective inhibitors. However, untoward fetal effects occur even with selective COX-II inhibitors. Aspirin crosses the placenta and may adversely affect fetal platelet function. The use of aspirin in the third trimester is associated with intracranial fetal hemorrhage. Aspirin should be avoided in pregnancy.

Glucocorticoids

Glucocorticoids are the first line of treatment for SLE in pregnancy. They are not considered to be human teratogens. Hydrocortisone, prednisone, and prednisilone are the steroids of choice since these agents are inactivated by 11-beta hydroxysteroid in the placenta, allowing less then 10 percent of active drugs to reach the fetus. The incidence of fetal adrenal suppression after maternal gucocorticoid use is extremely low.

There are severe maternal side effects from glucocorticoid use including osteoporosis, glucose intolerance, sodium and water retention, infection, hypertension, and avascular necrosis. There is also an increased risk of obstetric complications such as gestational diabetes, preeclampsia, preterm premature ruptured membranes, and fetal growth restriction. Typically, the benefits of glucocorticoid use for controlling lupus flares in pregnancy outweigh the risks. However, patients should be maintained on the lowest possible dose and weaned off if symptoms permit. Patients receiving chronic steroids (20 mg or more of prednisone for a duration of ≥3 weeks during the last six months) should receive stress doses in labor.

Antimalarials

Chloroquine has been associated with congenital anomalies raising concern for the safety of using antimalarial medications during pregnancy. However, hydroxychloroquine is not associated with an increased risk for fetal malformations and is considered *safe* during pregnancy. In fact, a recent prospective study by Cortes-Hernandez and colleagues demonstrated that stopping hydroxychloroquine treatment during pregnancy was associated with a significant increase in the risk of lupus flares. Therefore, if a patient requires this medication to control her disease, stopping the drug is ill adversed.

Cytotoxic Agents

Cyclosporine is a pregnancy category C drug. There is abundant data obtained from transplant patients regarding the use of cyclosporine in pregnancy. The use of this medication appears to be safe, but long-term follow-up studies are limited. Azathioprine does not appear to be a teratogen in humans. However, its use in pregnancy has been associated with fetal growth restriction. In severe cases of SLE in pregnancy requiring chronic high doses of glucocorticoids, either cyclosporine or azathioprine may be added to help control symptoms and to lower the dose of steroids used. Cyclophosphamide is an alkylating agent and is the drug of choice in nonpregnant patients for the treatment of proliferative lupus nephritis. However, this drug is known to cross the placenta and is associated with fetal cleft palate and skeletal abnormalities. It should be used only with extreme caution in pregnancy. Methotrexate, an antimetabolite, is sometimes used in SLE patients. It is embryolethal in early pregnancy and is also a known human teratogen when used later in gestation. It is pregnancy category X and is absolutely contraindicated in the treatment of pregnant women with SLE.

Treatment of Lupus Flares

Lupus flares in pregnancy are usually mild, and most commonly are manifested by skin lesions or joint pain. However, patients may present with severe nephritis, stroke, seizures, or psychosis as a result of a lupus exacerbation. Treatment of lupus flares depends on the severity of the patient's symptoms, and with few exceptions can be controlled with NSAIDs, hydroxychloroquine, and glucocorticoids.

Lupus Nephritis

Patients with severe nephritis may present with acute renal insufficiency. As discussed above, the differential diagnosis includes preeclampsia and in transplant patients, acute rejection. Interestingly, there are only rare case reports of recurrent lupus nephritis in transplanted kidneys. Therefore, acute renal insufficiency in transplant patients is likely due to transplant rejection or preeclampsia. However, the distinction between rejection, nephritis, and preeclampsia is often difficult and may require a renal biopsy.

Patients frequently respond well to glucocorticoids. However, patients with proliferative nephritis may require cyclophosphamide. A recent study comparing low dose to high dose cyclophosphomide for the treatment of proliferative nephritis demonstrated that low doses were as effective as high doses and associated with fewer maternal side effects. Patients who do not respond to medical therapy, and who have serum creatinine levels >3.5 mg/dL should be started on dialysis in order to optimize pregnancy outcome.

Neuropsychiatric SLE

There are many different central nervous system manifestations of SLE, making the treatment of neuropsychiatric SLE complex. These include peripheral neuropathy, headaches, seizures, chorea, stroke, mood disorders, and psychosis. It is also essential to exclude other causes of neurologic symptoms such as metabolic abnormalities, infection, and intracranial lesions. Infection is especially common in SLE patients with chronic steroid use. Thus, a complete evaluation for infection including cerebral spinal fluid analysis is required. In addition, brain imaging and EEG are often helpful in excluding other causes of neurologic abnormalities.

Unfortunately, there are no randomized-controlled studies regarding the appropriate treatment of lupus cerebritis. As such, treatment is empiric. Patients presenting with recurrent psychosis, mood changes, or delirium do not readily respond to mood stabilizing medications, but instead typically respond to high dose steroids. Cyclophosphamide may be added, if needed, to help lower the dose of steroids required to control symptoms. Patients with mild neuropsychiatric symptoms (infrequent seizures, mild depression, headaches, peripheral neuropathy) and no other manifestations of systemic disease may be treated symptomatically. Lupus patients presenting with a thrombotic stroke often also have antiphospholipid antibodies. The primary treatment for these women is anticoagulation with heparin.

In general, with the exception of methotrexate, cyclophosphamide, and NSAIDs, the benefits of medical therapy for the treatment of severe lupus flares far exceed the risks. Although these medications should be used prudently, there are circumstances wherein they are indicated in pregnancy.

LUPUS AND ANTIPHOSPHOLIPID SYNDROME

The antiphospholipid syndrome (APS) is an autoimmune disorder defined by distinct clinical and laboratory features including the presence of antiphospholipid antibodies (aPL) (Table 27-7). aPL are a heterogeneous group of autoantibodies that bind phospholipids, proteins, or a phospholipid-protein complex. Approximately, 30 percent of patients with SLE also have antiphospholipid antibodies. Individuals with SLE and APS are considered to have secondary APS, while those with APS and no other connective tissue disorders have primary APS.

Although several aPL have been described, lupus anticoagulant and anticardiolipin antibodies are the two best characterized, and are recommended for clinical use. Lupus anticoagulant is a misnomer because patients may not have SLE and they are hypercoagulable as opposed to anticoagulated. It is also an unusual name for an antibody. Lupus anticoagulant is detected in plasma using one of several phospholipid-dependent clotting tests (e.g., activated partial thromboplastin time or dilute Russel viper venom time). If the autoantibody is present, it will interfere with clotting, thus prolonging the clotting time. Confirmatory tests are then performed to exclude other reasons for prolongation of clotting assays (such as clotting factor deficiency). Clinicians may order a *lupus anticoagulant screen* in a *blue top tube* which is reported as either present or absent.

Anticardiolipin antibodies are detected in a more traditional fashion via immunoassay. Results are reported in a semiquantitative manner and the assay is standardized using standard sera obtained from the Antiphospholipid Standardization Laboratory in Atlanta, GA. Medium-high titers of the IgG isotype are most strongly associated with the clinical features of APS. Low-positive

TABLE 27-7 Criteria for the Classification of the Antiphospholipid Syndrome

Clinical criteria

(1) Vascular thrombosis: One or more episodes of arterial, venous, or small vessel thrombosis in any tissue or organ confirmed by imaging, Doppler studies, or histopathology. Superficial venous thromboses are excluded.

(2) Pregnancy morbidity:

- (a) One or more unexplained deaths of a morphologic normal fetus at or beyond the 10th week of gestation, with normal morphology documented by ultrasound or direct examination of the fetus OR
- (b) One or more premature births of a morphologically normal neonate prior to 34 weeks gestation because of severe preeclampsia, eclampsia, or severe placental insufficiency OR
- (c) Three or more unexplained consecutive spontaneous miscarriages prior to the 10th week of gestation, with maternal anatomic or hormonal abnormalities, and paternal and maternal chromosome causes excluded.

Laboratory criteria

(1) Anticardiolipin of IgG and/or IgM isotype in blood present in medium to high titer on two or more occasions at least six weeks apart. Titers must be measured by a standard enzyme-linked immunoabsorbent assay for beta2 glycoprotein I-dependent anticardiolipin antibodies.

(2) Lupus anticoagulant present in plasma on two or more occasions at least six weeks apart, detected according to the guidelines of the International Society on Thrombosis and Hemostasis.

Note: Definite antiphospholipid syndrome is present if a patient meets at least one of the clinical criteria and one of the laboratory criteria.

results and isolated IgM or IgA antibodies are common, nonspecific, and are of questionable clinical relevance. They are not considered diagnostic criteria for APS.

Several other autoantibodies have been associated with APS. Some are aPL such as the false positive serologic test for syphilis and antiphosphatidylserine antibodies. Others are antibodies against proteins such as anti-beta$_2$-glycoprotein-I. Although these antibodies may eventually prove to be clinically useful, they are not recommended for routine testing in the absence of further study.

APS is associated with significant medical problems including arterial and venous thrombosis, recurrent pregnancy loss, and autoimmune thrombocytopenia. Pregnancies resulting in live births are often complicated by obstetric disorders associated with uteroplacental insufficiency such as preeclampsia, fetal growth restriction, and abnormal antenatal testing. Preeclampsia has been reported in one-fourth to one-half of women with well-characterized APS. It often is severe and occurs prior to 34 weeks gestation. Although women with APS are at increased risk for preeclampsia, most women with preeclampsia do not have APS. This is not surprising given the relative frequency of preeclampsia compared to APS.

In utero fetal growth restriction is also associated with antiphospholipid antibodies, occurring in 15 to 30 percent of women with APS. It appears that fetal growth restriction is more likely in patients with higher levels of IgG anticardiolipin antibodies. Abnormal fetal heart rate tracings indicative of uteroplacental insufficiency are also more common in APS patients. In a large cohort study of women with APS, 50 percent of patients had abnormal antenatal testing which ultimately prompted obstetric intervention and delivery. Placental insufficiency, manifested by abnormal fetal heart rate tracings, may occur as early as the second trimester.

The increased incidence of preeclampsia, fetal growth restriction, and abnormal fetal heart rate tracings all contribute to iatrogenic preterm birth in women with APS. Preterm birth occurs in up to one-third of women with APS. Delivery prior to 34 weeks is most likely in women with strict clinical and laboratory criteria for APS.

Treatment for APS

Initially, high dose prednisone (40 mg daily or greater) in combination with low dose aspirin was the accepted treatment for antiphospholipid syndrome in pregnancy. This regimen resulted in a 60 to 70 percent successful pregnancy rate. Subsequently, the use of heparin in the treatment of antipshospholipid syndrome was proposed. Several case series demonstrated a success rate comparable to that of high dose prednisone. A small randomized trial comparing heparin and prednisone demonstrated that heparin and prednisone are equally efficacious. However, patients treated with prednisone had a higher rate of adverse obstetric events including preeclampsia, preterm premature rupture of membranes, and preterm labor. These results have been confirmed by other randomized studies. Thus, heparin is the treatment of choice for APS in pregnancy. Intravenous immune globulin has been used as adjunctive therapy in patients refractory to heparin. It is not recommended for use as primary therapy due to cost and a lack of improved efficacy compared to heparin alone.

Heparin is also potentially useful for the treatment of APS during pregnancy due to an increased risk of thrombosis, even in women without history of thromboembolism. Patients without a prior history of thrombosis should be treated with thromboprophylactic doses of heparin (10,000 to 20,000 units of unfractionated heparin daily). Patients with a history of thrombosis should receive a dose of heparin that will provide full anticoagulation. The goal of therapy is to maintain the activated partial thromboplastin time (aPTT) 1.5 to 2.5 times the normal value. Patients with no history of thrombosis should continue anticoagulation therapy until six weeks postpartum. Individuals with APS and prior thromboses should be anticoagulated for life. Heparin may be exchanged for sodium warfarin in the postpartum period. Despite initial concerns about transfer through breast milk, it is safe to take warfarin while breastfeeding.

It is important to remember that the lupus anticoagulant causes a prolongation of the activated partial thromboplastin time. Therefore, this test cannot be used to monitor anticoagulation in patients who test positive for the lupus anticoagulant. Rather, antifactor Xa levels can be followed. To achieve full anticoagulation using unfractionated heparin, antifactor Xa levels should fall between 0.4 and 0.7 U/mL.

Side effects of heparin are uncommon but potentially serious and include bleeding, osteopenia, and thrombocytopenia. Heparin-induced osteoporosis with fractures occurs in 1 to 2 percent of women treated during pregnancy with unfractionated heparin. Patients should therefore be encouraged to engage in weight bearing exercise and take calcium supplements. In addition, heparin causes an immune mediated thrombocytopenia in approximately 5 percent of patients. Thrombocytopenia is detected within 21 days after the initiation of therapy. Accordingly, platelet counts should be checked serially through the initial three weeks of heparin therapy.

Low molecular weight heparin (LMWH) has been used with increasing frequency in pregnancy. Initially it was thought that LMWH might cross the placenta and cause fetal hemorrhage. However, several studies have shown that this does not occur and LMWH is safe in pregnancy. In order to achieve full anticoagulation, the recommended dose of enoxaparin is 1 mg/kg, administered subcutaneously in two equal doses 12 hours apart. However, due to the increased plasma volume and renal blood flow in the pregnant patient, the pharmacokinetics of enoxaparin is altered by pregnancy. It is necessary to monitor antifactor Xa levels in order to ensure adequate dosing. The target antifactor Xa level for full anticoagulation using LMWH is 0.5 to 1.1 U/mL. LMWH appears to have less risk for osteopenia and thrombocytopenia than unfractionated heparin. However, it is more expensive and has a longer half life, making it less convenient for intrapartum anticoagulation. Table 27-8 summarizes the management of pregnant women with APS.

Catastrophic APS

A majority of patients with APS experience single large vessel thrombotic events. In patients with recurrent thrombosis, the subsequent event typically occurs months to years after the initial episode. In 1992, Asherson et al. described a small subset of patients with APS who presented with what has been described as *catastrophic APS*. Unlike the majority of patients with APS, those with catastrophic APS suffer microvascular thromboses in multiple organs, most commonly the kidneys, lungs, and gastrointestinal tract. The heart, brain, liver, and adrenal glands are less frequently involved. Catastrophic APS has a 50 to 65 percent mortality rate.

TABLE 27-8 Management Protocol for Patients with Antiphospholipid Syndrome

I. Goals of therapy
A. Embryonic and fetal survival B. Prompt detection of uteroplacental insufficiency and preeclampsia C. Prevention of thrombosis
II. Management
1. Preconception counseling a. Review pregnancy risks such as miscarriage, fetal death, preeclampsia, fetal growth restriction, unteroplacental insufficiency, and preterm birth. b. Evaluate the accuracy of the diagnosis. Confirm the presence of antiphospholipid antibodies if necessary.
2. Antenatal care a. When a live embryo is detected, start subcutaneous unfractionated heparin 10,000–20,000 units/day in divided doses or the equivalent dose of low molecular weight heparin (prophylactic). Higher doses (therapeutic) should be used in patients with prior thrombosis. b. Calcium supplementation and weight bearing exercise. c. Frequent assessment for the development of preeclampsia. d. Serial ultrasounds to evaluate interval fetal growth. e. Fetal surveillance starting at 32 weeks or earlier if complications arise. f. If a patient has a history of a thromboembolic event, or suffers an acute episode during pregnancy, start therapeutic doses of heparin to maintain the PTT 1.5–2.5 times normal, or low molecular weight heparin, 1 mg/kg twice a day. g. If using low molecular weight heparin, anti factor Xa levels should be checked every trimester in order to maintain levels of 0.5–1.1 U/mL.

In a retrospective review of 50 patients with catastrophic APS, Asherson found that 78 percent presented with renal involvement which typically resulted in concurrent malignant hypertension. Renal biopsies in these patients demonstrated frank microangiopathy and occasional renal infarctions. Sixty-six percent of patients demonstrated pulmonary involvement. The most common presenting symptom was severe dyspnea. Approximately, half of patients with pulmonary involvement developed ARDS and 25 percent had pulmonary embolism. In this series, 56 percent of patients had central nervous system involvement. Symptoms were highly variable and included confusion, drowsiness, stupor, seizures, and infarction of either large or small vessels. Half of the patients had myocardial involvement and 38 percent had gastrointestinal involvement. The most common symptom of patients with gastrointestinal involvement is severe abdominal pain. Occlusion of the mesenteric vessels (both arterial and venous) was frequently noted. Other organs that were less commonly affected were liver (35 percent), adrenal (26 percent), spleen (20 percent), and pancreas (1 percent). Up to 50 percent of patients had skin involvement manifested as superficial necrosis and gangrene, splinter hemorrhages, and purpura.

Diagnosis

The diagnosis of catastrophic APS can be difficult, and the differential diagnosis includes DIC, TTP, and SLE nephritis. Furthermore, Drenkard and colleagues reported a decrease in anticardiolipin antibody titer at the time of thrombosis in six patients with previously high antibody titers. The authors speculate that acute thrombosis may cause transient antibody consumption, which could complicate the diagnosis of APS at the time of the acute event. The laboratory diagnosis of catastrophic APS can be made by the presence of lupus anticoagulant and high titers of anticardiolipin IgG antibodies, both of which are detected in approximately 95 percent of patients. Patients may also demonstrate thrombocytopenia and anti-ds DNA if they also carry a diagnosis of SLE. There may also be evidence of hemolytic anemia and laboratory values consistent with DIC.

Treatment

There is no standard treatment for catastrophic APS. Patients often are critically ill and require admission to intensive care units. Supportive treatment depends on presenting symptoms, and may include aggressive antihypertensive therapy, assisted ventilation, dialysis, and vasopressors. Plasmapheresis has been recommended by some. However, others report improved outcome in patients who are treated with a combination of anticoagulation, steroids, and either intravenous immunoglobins or plasmapheresis in order to rapidly decrease the titer of antiphospholipid antibodies.

SUGGESTED READING

Arnett FC, Reveille JD, Wilson RW, et al.: Systemic lupus erythematosus: current state of the genetic hypothesis. *Semin Arthritis Rheum* 1984;14:24–35.

Asherson RA, Cervera R, Piette JC, et al.: Catastrophic antiphospholipid syndrome. Clinical and laboratory features of 50 patients. *Medicine (Baltimore)* 1998; 77:195–207.

Asherson RA, Piette JC: The catastrophic antiphospholipid syndrome 1996: acute multi-organ failure associated with antiphospholipid antibodies: a review of 31 patients. *Lupus* 1996;5:414–417.

Asherson RA: The catastrophic antiphospholipid syndrome. *J Rheumatol* 1992; 19:508–512.

Branch DW, Peaceman AM, Druzin M, et al.: A multicenter, placebo-controlled pilot study of intravenous immune globulin treatment of antiphospholipid syndrome during pregnancy. The Pregnancy Loss Study Group. *Am J Obstet Gynecol* 2000; 182:122–127.

Branch DW, Silver RM, Blackwell JL, et al.: Outcome of treated pregnancies in women with antiphospholipid syndrome: an update of the Utah experience. *Obstet Gynecol* 1992;80:614–620.

Bear RA: Pregnancy in patients with renal disease. A study of 44 cases. *Obstet Gynecol* 1976;48:13–18.

Burkett G: Lupus nephropathy and pregnancy. *Clin Obstet Gynecol* 1985;28:310–323.

Copel JA, Buyon JP, Kleinman CS: Successful in utero therapy of fetal heart block. *Am J Obstet Gynecol* 1995;173:1384–1390.

Cortes-Hernandez J, Ordi-Ros J, Paredes F, et al.: Clinical predictors of fetal and maternal outcome in systemic lupus erythematosus: a prospective study of 103 pregnancies. *Rheumatology (Oxford)* 2002;41:643–650.

Doria A, Cutolo M, Ghirardello A, et al.: Steroid hormones and disease activity during pregnancy in systemic lupus erythematosus. *Arthritis Rheum* 2002;47:202–209.

Englert HJ, Derue GM, Loizou S, et al.: Pregnancy and lupus: prognostic indicators and response to treatment. *Q J Med* 1988;66:125–136.

Fisher KA, Luger A, Spargo HB, et al.: Hypertension in pregnancy: clinical-pathological correlations and remote prognosis. *Medicine (Baltimore)* 1981;60:267–276.

Hayslett JP, Lynn RI: Effect of pregnancy in patients with lupus nephropathy. *Kidney Int* 1980;18:207–220.

Houser MT, Fish AJ, Tagatz GE, et al.: Pregnancy and systemic lupus erythematosus. *Am J Obstet Gynecol* 1980;138:409–413.

Houssiau FA, Vasconcelos C, D'Cruz D, et al.: Immunosuppressive therapy in lupus nephritis: the Euro-Lupus Nephritis Trial, a randomized trial of low-dose versus high-dose intravenous cyclophosphamide. *Arthritis Rheum* 2002;46:2121–2131.

Imbasciati E, Surian M, Bottino S, et al.: Lupus nephropathy and pregnancy. A study of 26 pregnancies in patients with systemic lupus erythematosus and nephritis. *Nephron* 1984;36:46–51.

Johnson MJ, Petri M, Witter FR, et al.: Evaluation of preterm delivery in a systemic lupus erythematosus pregnancy clinic. *Obstet Gynecol* 1995;86:396–339.

Julkunen H, Kaaja R, Palosuo T, et al.: Pregnancy in lupus nephropathy. *Acta Obstet Gynecol Scand* 1993;72:258–263.

Jungers P, Dougados M, Pelissier C, et al.: Lupus nephropathy and pregnancy. Report of 104 cases in 36 patients. *Arch Intern Med* 1982;142:771–776.

Kutteh WH: Antiphospholipid antibody-associated recurrent pregnancy loss: treatment with heparin and low-dose aspirin is superior to low-dose aspirin alone. *Am J Obstet Gynecol* 1996;174:1584–1589.

Lima F, Khamashta MA, Buchanan NM, et al.: A study of sixty pregnancies in patients with the antiphospholipid syndrome. *Clin Exp Rheumatol* 1996;14:131–136.

Lockshin MD, Bonfa E, Elkon K, et al.: Neonatal lupus risk to newborns of mothers with systemic lupus erythematosus. *Arthritis Rheum* 1988;31:697–701.

Lockshin MD: Lupus pregnancy. *Clin Rheum Dis* 1985;11:611–632.

Lockshin MD: Pregnancy does not cause systemic lupus erythematosus to worsen. *Arthritis Rheum* 1989;32:665–670.

Lockshin MD, Qamar T, Druzin ML: Hazards of lupus pregnancy. *J Rheumatol* 1987; 14(Suppl 13):214–217.

Lockshin MD, Reinitz E, Druzin ML, et al.: Lupus pregnancy. Case-control prospective study demonstrating absence of lupus exacerbation during or after pregnancy. *Am J Med* 1984;77:893–898.

Meehan RT, Dorsey JK: Pregnancy among patients with systemic lupus erythematosus receiving immunosuppressive therapy. *J Rheumatol* 1987;14:252–258.

Mintz G, Niz J, Gutierrez G, et al.: Prospective study of pregnancy in systemic lupus erythematosus. Results of a multidisciplinary approach. *J Rheumatol* 1986;13:732–739.

Packham DK, Lam SS, Nicholls K, et al.: Lupus nephritis and pregnancy. *Q J Med* 1992;83:315–324.

Petri M, Howard D, Repke J: Frequency of lupus flare in pregnancy. The Hopkins Lupus Pregnancy Center experience. *Arthritis Rheum* 1991;34:1538–1545.

Rider LG, Buyon JP, Rutledge, J, et al.: Treatment of neonatal lupus: case report and review of the literature. *J Rheumatol* 1993;20:1208–1211.

Tan EM, Cohen AS, Fries JF, et al.: The 1982 revised criteria for the classification of systemic lupus erythematosus. *Arthritis Rheum* 1982;25:1271–1277.

Varner MW, Meehan RT, Syrop CH, et al.: Pregnancy in patients with systemic lupus erythematosus. *Am J Obstet Gynecol* 1983;145:1025–1040.

Waltuck J, Buyon JP: Autoantibody-associated congenital heart block: outcome in mothers and children. *Ann Intern Med* 1994;120:544–551.

Zurier RB, Argyros TG, Urman JD, et al.: Systemic lupus erythematosus. Management during pregnancy. *Obstet Gynecol* 1978;51:178–180.

Index

Page numbers followed by italic *f* or *t* denote figures or tables, respectively.

Q

R

S

W

Z